Methods of Partial Deafness Treatment

Methods of Partial Deafness Treatment

Edited by
Henryk Skarżyński and
Piotr H. Skarżyński

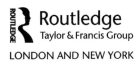

LONDON AND NEW YORK

Cover design - Monika Miaskiewicz
Images courtesy of Institute of Physiology and Pathology of Hearing, Warsaw, Poland

Thanks to the team collecting materials and working on translations: Kinga Wołujewicz, Olga Wanatowska, Aleksandra Mankiewicz-Malinowska.

Routledge is an imprint of the Taylor & Francis Group, an informa business

© 2022 Taylor & Francis Group, London, UK

British Library Cataloguing-in-Publication Data
A catalogue record for this book is available from the British Library

Library of Congress Cataloging-in-Publication Data
Names: Skarżyński, Henryk, editor. | Skarżyński, Piotr H., editor.
Title: Methods of partial deafness treatment / edited by Henryk Skarżyński and Piotr H. Skarżyński.
Description: Boca Raton : CRC Press, [2021] | Includes bibliographical references and index.
Identifiers: LCCN 2020056845 (print) | LCCN 2020056846 (ebook) |
Subjects: MESH: Cochlear Implantation—methods | Hearing Loss—surgery | Cochlear Implants | Hearing Loss—diagnosis
Classification: LCC RF305 (print) | LCC RF305 (ebook) | NLM WV 274 | DDC 617.8/9—dc23
LC record available at https://lccn.loc.gov/2020056845
LC ebook record available at https://lccn.loc.gov/2020056846

Published by: Routledge
          Schipholweg 107C, 2316 XC Leiden, The Netherlands
          e-mail: Pub.NL@taylorandfrancis.com
          www.routledge.com – www.taylorandfrancis.com

ISBN: 978-0-367-75960-5 (Hbk)
ISBN: 978-0-367-75961-2 (Pbk)
ISBN: 978-1-003-16487-6 (eBook)

DOI: 10.1201/9781003164876

Typeset in Times New Roman
by codeMantra

Contents

Preface

The newest developments in audiology, otology, and otosurgery, combined with the latest medical technologies, allow physicians to provide an effective treatment for practically all deaf and hard-of-hearing patients. The monograph *Methods of Partial Deafness Treatment* presents the overview of rationale and possibilities of preserving the ear's structures and functions in different hearing impairments from various perspectives: medical, surgical, audiological, educational, developmental, or diagnostic. The partial deafness treatment (PDT) method has been developed and perfected since 1997, when I had presented its first results at the 5th International Cochlear Implant Conference in New York, NY, USA. Since that time, the eponymous program that I have initiated and conducted in the World Hearing Center of the Institute of Physiology and Pathology of Hearing in Warsaw has encompassed more than seven thousand patients. It is the largest group of patients with partial deafness worldwide.

This monograph draws on the authors' experience amassed in the long-term follow-up of that enormous study material to present the reader with exhaustive information about the operative techniques and the current state of knowledge about the PDT method. The surgical method's essence is to preserve preoperative hearing regardless of its level and supplement it with electric stimulation through a cochlear implant. This innovation has the potential to improve the lives of millions of patients worldwide whose hearing in the low frequencies is normal but needs amplification in the medium- and high-frequency range. Before the PDT method, these patients were beyond the scope of feasible help.

The greatest challenge of the method is preserving the intact ear structures and function. Teaching the surgical technique perfected for achieving the optimal cochlear implantation results in partial deafness treatment is an integral part of the method. Over 13 years, in the World Hearing Center, our team in cooperation with hearing implant producers Med-El, Cochlear®, Advanced Bionics, and Oticon has been organizing specialized Window Approach Workshops (WAW) for otosurgeons from all continents looking to enrich their knowledge and raise qualifications in the use of implants for the treatment of total and partial deafness. So far, over 4.5 thousand people from around the world have participated in 57 workshops. In that time, I performed more than 1.2 thousand demonstration surgeries.

This monograph presents in greater detail topics taught during the workshops and adds several chapters presenting novel approaches to the partial deafness treatment. The issues discussed in the monograph include the following:

- Treatment of patients with various types of total and partial deafness and the results of multiple therapies applied in different groups of patients;
- Principles of diagnostics and patients' selection for different types of auditory implants (middle ear, cochlear, and bone conduction implants), including indications and contraindications;
- Strategies of hearing and structure preservation and minimally invasive surgical techniques, including original surgical procedure and appropriately selected implantable devices;
- Results of early and long-term observation of hearing preservation after cochlear implantation;
- Pharmacological treatment in patients undergoing cochlear implantation;
- Otoneurological aspects of cochlear implantation;
- Possible genetic markers predisposing children with prelingual congenital deafness to better respond to cochlear implantation;
- Electrophysiological and acoustic objective methods of hearing evaluation;
- Application of functional magnetic resonance and presentation of tonotopic organization of auditory cortex in patients with partial deafness;
- Auditory development, speech perception, and rehabilitation;
- Different psychological perspectives of partial deafness: subjective, auditory perception and communication, and social;
- Research on the plasticity of the auditory cortex and brain.

The clinical material presented in the monograph comprises almost 100 cases in which all available models of the cochlear, middle ear, and bone conduction implants were used in practice.

In the *Methods of Partial Deafness Treatment*, we present the clinical and scientific approach to partial deafness treatment supported by unique clinical cases. The reader will have the opportunity to learn firsthand from the pioneers of the method about the diagnostics, treatment, rehabilitation process, and related scientific implications of partial deafness treatment.

Prof. Henryk Skarżyński, M.D., Ph.D., dr. h.c. multi

Editors

Prof. Henryk Skarżyński, M.D., Ph.D., dr. h.c. multi, is a world-known otosurgeon, and an expert in otorhinolaryngology, audiology, and phoniatrics. He has been a National Specialist for Audiology and a National Consultant for Audiology and Phoniatrics, since 1994, and a National Consultant in Otorhinolaryngology since 2011. He was the first surgeon in Poland performing cochlear implantations (1992), and middle ear implantations (2003). Professor Skarżyński performed over 200 thousand hearing-improving surgeries. Within two decades of his activity, Poland has become one of the leading countries implementing and conducting hearing screening in children of various ages. He is an author and co-author of over 3,200 scientific publications. He runs an extensive educational activity for students, doctors, and specialists from Poland and abroad.

He was awarded the titles of Honorary Professor of Brigham Young University Provo, USA (1998), and the National Medical University "Nicolae Testemitanu" in Chisinau, Moldova (2013), and the Institute of Mother and Child in Bishkek, Kyrgyzstan (2016); he was honored with the title doctor honoris causa of Maria Grzegorzewska University (2011), Warsaw University (2012), and Maria Curie-Sklodowska University, Lublin (2014).

During the Polish Presidency of the European Union Council, Professor Henryk Skarżyński has initiated and coordinated several activities within the project of "Equal opportunities for children with communication disorders in European countries". The final achievement of the Polish Presidency was the preparation of the "EU Council Conclusions on early detection and treatment of communication disorders in children, including the use of e-Health tools and innovative solutions" and its endorsement by the Member States on December 2, 2011.

Professor Skarżyński is the organizer of domestic, international, and continental scientific meetings and conferences. He was the President of the high-level meetings, including 9th European Symposium on Paediatric Cochlear Implantation (ESPCI-2009), 10th European Federation of Audiology Societies Congress (EFAS-2011), XXV International Evoked Response Audiometry Study Group Biennial Symposium (2016), 1st World Tinnitus Congress (2018), 4th International Symposium on Otosclerosis and Stapes Surgery (2018), and 35th Politzer Society Meeting (2019).

In 2022, he will preside over the 35th World Congress of Audiology in Warsaw, Poland.

Professor Henryk Skarżyński is also the author of the libretto for the *Broken Silence* musical, which was premiered in September 2019 in the Warsaw Chamber Opera in Poland.

Prof. Piotr H. Skarżyński, M.D., Ph.D., M.Sc; his scientific career is tied to the World Hearing Center of the Institute of Physiology and Pathology of Hearing and the Institute of Sensory Organs. He is a member of numerous scientific societies. He participated in the third Stakeholders Consultation meeting during which the World Hearing Forum of the WHO was announced. He is a member of the Consultant Committee of International Experts of the CPAM-VBMS (for special invitation), an Honorary Member of the ORL Danube Society, and a member of the Roster of Experts on Digital Health of the WHO. He is also a Vice Chairman of the Junior ERS (2010–2014), Member of Board (2014–2016), Member of Congress and Meeting Department of the EAONO, Representative Board Member (till 2019) and Vice President and Institutional Representative (since 2019) of the IfSTeH, Regional Representative of Europe in the ISA, and Board Secretary of the Society of Otorhinolaryngologists, Phoniatrists, and Audiologists. He is also a Vice President of the Hearring Group, a Member of the Hearing Committee of the AAO-HNS, and an Auditor of the EFAS. He is an active participant of many conferences – over 1,838 presentations (116 as an Invited Speaker, 126 round tables, 128 courses as an Instructor) and 934 publications (IF – 192,225, IC – 47702,90, scientific points of the Ministry of Science and Higher Education – 10449). He also serves as a reviewer for 38 national and international scientific journals.

Contributors

Jillian N. Bushor
NeuroAudiology Lab
Department of Speech, Language and
  Hearing Sciences,
University of Arizona
Tucson, USA

Katarzyna Cieśla
Bioimaging Research Center
Institute of Physiology and Pathology of
  Hearing
Kajetany/Warsaw, Poland

Carrie M. Clancy
NeuroAudiology Lab
Department of Speech, Language and
  Hearing Sciences
University of Arizona
Tucson, USA

Joanna Ćwiklińska
World Hearing Center
Institute of Physiology and Pathology of
  Hearing
Kajetany/Warsaw, Poland

Beata Dziendziel
World Hearing Center
Institute of Physiology and Pathology of
  Hearing
Kajetany/Warsaw, Poland

W. Wictor Jedrzejczak
World Hearing Center
Institute of Physiology and Pathology of
  Hearing
Kajetany/Warsaw, Poland

Joanna Kobosko
World Hearing Center
Institute of Physiology and Pathology of
  Hearing
Kajetany/Warsaw, Poland

Krzysztof Kochanek
World Hearing Center
Institute of Physiology and Pathology of
  Hearing
Kajetany/Warsaw, Poland

Artur Lorens
World Hearing Center
Institute of Physiology and Pathology of
  Hearing
Kajetany/Warsaw, Poland

Monika Matusiak
World Hearing Center
Institute of Physiology and Pathology of
  Hearing
Kajetany/Warsaw, Poland

Frank E. Musiek
NeuroAudiology Lab
Department of Speech, Language and
  Hearing Sciences
University of Arizona
Tucson, USA

Anita Obrycka
World Hearing Center
Institute of Physiology and Pathology of
  Hearing
Kajetany/Warsaw, Poland

Agnieszka Pankowska
World Hearing Center
Institute of Physiology and Pathology of
  Hearing
Kajetany/Warsaw, Poland

Madelyn Schefer
NeuroAudiology Lab
Department of Speech, Language and
  Hearing Sciences
University of Arizona
Tucson, USA

Magdalena B. Skarżyńska
Institute of Sensory Organs
Kajetany, Poland

Henryk Skarżyński
World Hearing Center
Institute of Physiology and Pathology of
  Hearing
Kajetany/Warsaw, Poland

Piotr H. Skarżyński
World Hearing Center
Institute of Physiology and Pathology of
  Hearing
Kajetany/Warsaw, Poland

Lech Śliwa
World Hearing Center
Institute of Physiology and Pathology of
  Hearing
Kajetany/Warsaw, Poland

Magdalena Sosna-Duranowska
World Hearing Center
Institute of Physiology and Pathology of
  Hearing
Kajetany/Warsaw, Poland

Elżbieta Włodarczyk
World Hearing Center
Institute of Physiology and Pathology of
  Hearing
Kajetany/Warsaw, Poland

Tomasz Wolak
Bioimaging Research Center
Institute of Physiology and Pathology of
  Hearing
Kajetany/Warsaw, Poland

Małgorzata Zgoda
World Hearing Center
Institute of Physiology and Pathology of
  Hearing
Kajetany/Warsaw, Poland

Chapter 1

The strategy of preservation of preoperative hearing and inner ear structures in hearing implant surgery

Henryk Skarżyński
Institute of Physiology and Pathology of Hearing

CONTENTS

INTRODUCTION

For a long time, better and better results obtained in the treatment of profound hearing loss and deafness with cochlear implants, especially in younger and younger children, have been an incentive for scientists and clinicians to steadily expand cochlear implantation indications (Blamey et al. 2012). The research was conducted independently in Europe, the USA, and Australia. Initially, it was focused on electric stimulation of one ear with an implant, while the other ear, with slightly better hearing, was aided with a hearing aid. Less often, researchers studied the possibilities of ipsilaterally combined acoustic and electric stimulation (Skarżyński et al. 1997b, 2003, Ilberg Ch. et al. 1999, Gantz et al. 2004).

In 1997, the principles of the minimally invasive surgical technique developed for preserving the preoperative residual hearing in low frequencies were presented at a conference in New York, USA (5th International Cochlear Implant Conference) (Skarżyński et al. 1997b). In 2000, results of the first group of 67 children whose preoperatively nonfunctional residual hearing and inner ear structures have been preserved during implantation were presented at the European ESPCI congress in Antwerp, Belgium (Skarżyński et al. 2000). All these patients had in the same ear acoustic stimulation through a hearing aid in low frequencies and electric stimulation through a cochlear implant in the rest of the frequency range. In 2 to 3 years of follow-up, these children have shown improved and faster development of auditory skills, which confirmed this approach's utility. In 2000, results of the same application of cochlear implants with preservation of the residual hearing in the first group of adults were presented at the EUFOS congress in Berlin (Lorens et al. 2000).

Subsequently, several-year-long observations of implanted patients with a better and better residual hearing before implantation demonstrated the validity of broadening the accepted cochlear implantation indications to include the electric complementation of hearing entirely normal in frequencies up to 500 Hz (Skarżyński et al. 2002).

DOI: 10.1201/9781003164876-1

Electric complementation of normal low-frequency hearing was used for the first time by H. Skarżyński in an adult in 2002 and a child in 2004 (Skarżyński et al. 2003, 2004a).

Extension of cochlear implant indications was based on reported effects of hearing preservation and surgical procedure proposed by Skarżyński et al. (2006). It involves the approach to the tympanic duct through the round window as the most physiological way to insert an electrode into the inner ear and comprises six surgical steps (Skarżyński et al. 2010, 2012b). Longitudinal observation of the growing group of patients, which initially numbered hundreds and presently has overpassed six thousand, indicates the validity of extending indications for cochlear implantation in partial deafness. It has been corroborated by the numerous subsequent reports and presentations of the research material on all continental and global congresses and conferences dedicated to the hearing implants, audiology, and otology organized in recent years. It aimed to systematically present new target groups of patients and preservation of the preoperative hearing in a longer and longer time of follow-up. In recent years, it also involved presenting new technologies regarding the length and flexibility of cochlear implant electrodes and presenting the Polish school in that field of science and medicine.

During the 9th European Symposium on Pediatric Cochlear Implantation ESPCI in Warsaw in 2009, H. Skarżyński presented the new concept of partial deafness treatment that included the surgical procedure, length of electrodes, combination of acoustic and electric stimulation, and preservation of the preoperative hearing and inner ear structures (Skarżyński & Lorens 2010b) (Table 1.1 and Figure 1.1). In 2013, H. Skarżyński and 43 invited experts from all over the world had developed the first classification for the assessment of the results of preservation of preoperative hearing (Skarżyński et al. 2013).

The results of more than six thousand operated patients corroborate the strategy of preservation of preoperative hearing. All implantations with different cochlear implants were performed using the six-step procedure to preserve the existing structure

Table 1.1 The newest concept of applying the acoustic and electric stimulation in the treatment of different hearing impairments and partial deafness, according to Skarżyński et al. (2014b)

No.	Groups of patients with partial deafness
1.	Acoustic amplification of hearing with a hearing aid, bone conduction device, or middle ear implant [PDT – acoustic stimulation (PDT-AS)].
2.	Combined natural-electric stimulation: amplification of the preserved efficient hearing up to 1.5 kHz through electric stimulation [PDT – electro-natural stimulation (PDT-ENS)].
3.	Electric complementation of existing good hearing in low frequencies up to 0.5 kHz [PDT – electric complementation (PDT-EC)].
4.	Combined acoustic-electric stimulation with acoustic amplification of the preserved residual hearing in low and mid-frequencies with a hearing aid or a duet/hybrid system, and electric stimulation of the remaining part of the same ear [PDT – electric-acoustic stimulation (PDT-EAS)].
5.	Only electric stimulation in the case of an existing but nonfunctional residual hearing on different frequencies with preservation of inner ear structures [PDT – electric stimulation (PDT-ES)].

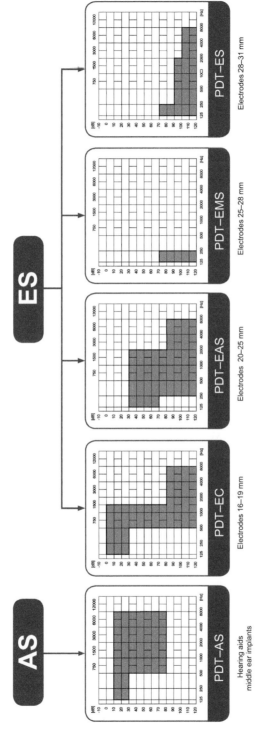

Figure 1.1 Comparison of stimulation ranges: acoustic (hearing aid or middle ear/bone conduction implant), electric (cochlear implant), and natural hearing, according to Skarżyński et al. (2010).

of the inner ear (Skarżyński et al. 2003, 2010, 2012b). Alongside the development of the surgical method and steady extension of indications for cochlear implantation in a larger and larger group of patients, the subsequent milestones were related to the impact of these actions on the development of new technologies, such as very flexible cochlear implant electrodes of different length (Skarżyński & Podskarbi-Fayette 2010, Skarżyński et al. 2012b, 2014a, Skarżyński P.H. et al. 2019). A new element of the development of that strategy was a modification of a limited electric stimulation with the electrodes of the length between 19–20 mm and 24, 25, and 28 mm as the complementation of a typical hearing preserved at 0.25, 0.5, 0.75, 1, and 1.5 kHz (Skarżyński et al. 2011, Skarżyński P.H. et al. 2019).

The crucially important step in developing the concept of partial deafness treatment was elaborating the previously mentioned, first in the world classification of partial deafness, according to Skarżyński et al. (2010). It is essential for continued study of the results of homogenous groups of patients with different levels of preserved preoperative hearing after cochlear implantation. The results obtained in various homogenous groups of patients presented by different authors and involving applying different technological solutions should be followed and form the basis for further extension of indications and popularization of the partial deafness treatment method. It has a significant effect on the development and application of new technologies in managing postoperative care, e.g., the creation of telemedical networks and the application of telefitting in everyday patient service. The satisfaction of patients and their families with the results of treatment of partial deafness in the World Hearing Center of the Institute of Physiology and Pathology of Hearing (WHC) and the subsequent growing interest in that method had the decided impact on the decision to expand the infrastructure of the WHC.

In recapitulation, it should be underlined that modern therapy can be developed to use acoustic stimulation with a middle ear implant or a bone conduction implant in many such situations. It is possible in some patients in the whole frequency range, but there are groups of patients where it is not because a small part of the ear, e.g., above 3 or 4 kHz, is deaf. For that reason, the PDT-AS (partial deafness treatment – acoustic stimulation) group has been included in the whole concept of treatment of different levels of partial deafness, but only with the application of acoustic stimulation. Indeed, continued longitudinal observation of good preservation of preoperative hearing up to 1.5 kHz should enable a further extension of cochlear implantation criteria, with hearing preserved in a broader range. It may be crucial to eliminate or reduce tinnitus's sensation caused by hearing loss over 2 and 3 kHz.

Twenty-three years has passed since the first surgeries of patients with preserved preoperative hearing in 1997. Since that time, the PDT strategy has been used in more than 5 thousand patients from 9 months to 84 years of age. In that group, children and youths up to 18 years constituted 37.2% and adults 62.8%. In children older than 5 years and adults, the preoperative hearing threshold was determined with audiometry. In younger children, the preoperative hearing threshold was tested with the ABR (auditory brainstem response) performed for 0.5, 1, 2, and 4 kHz. It should be underlined that the two most important groups were patients with normal or fully socially efficient hearing up to 500 Hz, 750 kHz, or 1,500 Hz – PDT-EC^{500}, PDT-EC^{750}, and PDT-ENS. These three groups of patients who need only electric complementation of the existing hearing are the most challenging for the surgeon. Still, at the same time, they are apt to obtain the best and fastest effects in postoperative rehabilitation. The fourth group, PDT-EAS (PDT – electric-acoustic stimulation), comprised patients with indications for the combined electric-acoustic stimulation, has been the most numerous. It was likely related to the fact that for these patients using the acoustic-only stimulation had little or negligible effects, so they were the most determined to undergo cochlear implantation. The PDT-ES (PDT – electric stimulation) group was not very numerous and comprised two subgroups. The first subgroup was adults with sudden deafness, including profound but not total hearing loss. The other, more numerous group was children in whom the ABR test showed residual reactions to acoustic stimuli in the capacity range of the measuring device at 0.5 or 1 kHz up to 100 dB.

OTOSURGICAL METHOD USED IN THE STRATEGY OF PRESERVING THE PREOPERATIVE HEARING AND INNER EAR STRUCTURES

The basis of this surgical method is the approach to the tympanic duct made through the round window. In 99.6% cases, the approach to the round window niche was possible through posterior tympanotomy, and in 0.4% cases, double access was needed – through posterior tympanotomy and the external ear canal (EAC). The latter group was patients in whom anatomical situation was such that even a wide tympanotomy did not enable visualizing the round window, which is essential for proper introduction of an electrode into a cochlea. In these cases, the round window niche was approached through the EAC access, and the electrode was inserted through the earlier made but insufficient posterior tympanotomy. In this way, it was possible in all ears to delicately introduce the electrode to the desired depth through the incision made in the round window membrane. The entire surgical procedure was conducted according to the standard proposed by H. Skarżyński, which comprises six principal steps (Table 1.2) (Skarżyński et al. 2003, 2010, 2012b).

The first step of the otosurgical procedure consists of performing a limited conservative antromastoidotomy. It means that the opening of the mastoid cavity should not be too wide but only sufficient to allow the electrode's unimpeded insertion. Before opening the mastoid, especially in children, it is recommended to remove a chip of the mastoid's cortical layer with a chisel. At the end of the procedure, that chip can be used

Table 1.2   The surgical procedure of the treatment of partial deafness with a cochlear implant according to Skarżyński

Step	Description
1.	Conservative limited antromastoidotomy.
2.	Posterior tympanotomy to visualize the round window niche and membrane.
3.	Puncture and incision of the round window membrane.
4.	Atraumatic insertion of the electrode into the tympanic duct through the round window.
5.	Sealing of the electrode in the round window niche.
6.	Fixation of the internal part of the implant in the niche under the skin-muscle-periosteum flap.

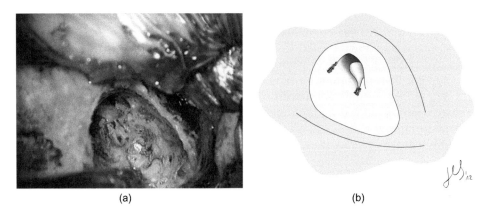

(a)   (b)

Figure 1.2 Limited antromastoidectomy – 'the first step': (a) intraoperative photo, (b) schematic drawing.

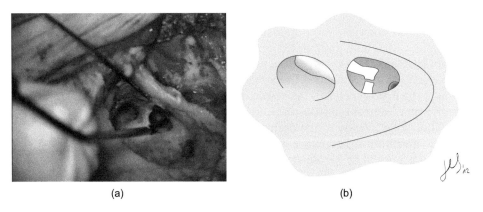

(a)   (b)

Figure 1.3 Posterior tympanotomy with access to the round window niche and membrane – 'the second step': (a) intraoperative photo, (b) schematic drawing.

to isolate the mastoid cavity from the pocket made under the skin-muscle-periosteal flap, in which the internal part of the implant is fixed (Figure 1.2).

The second step of the otosurgical procedure is the posterior tympanotomy (Figure 1.3). The primary goal of that action is to open the way into the tympani duct to allow visual control when introducing the electrode to the round window niche area. In some cases, it is necessary to remove the lateral bony lip at 0.2–0.5 mm from its free border, which obscures or limits the window membrane's visibility. It can help achieve the optimally safe conditions for the electrode's controlled insertion into the tympanic duct and its subsequent sealing. In the very few cases, as said before, when the round window niche cannot be well visualized, it is possible to make the secondary approach through the EAC that enables full control of the electrode during its insertion.

The third step of the procedure consists of performing a delicate puncture with the left- or right-curved hook and then a longitudinal incision of the round window membrane (Figure 1.4).

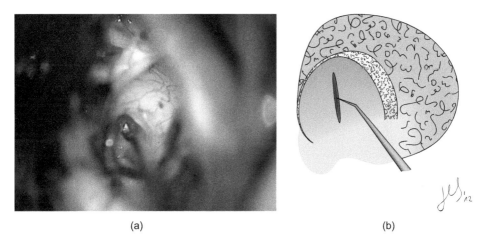

(a)   (b)

Figure 1.4 Incision of the exposed round window membrane – 'the third step': (a) intra-operative photo, (b) schematic drawing.

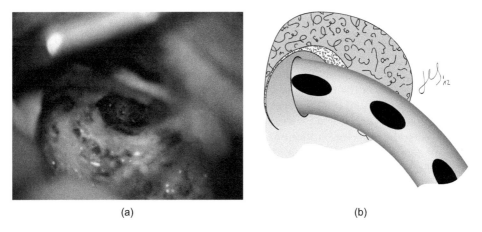

(a)   (b)

Figure 1.5 Insertion of the electrode into the tympanic duct – 'the fourth step': (a) intra-operative photo, (b) schematic drawing.

The fourth step of the procedure is the most critical because it consists of the electrode's delicate insertion into the tympanic duct. The electrode must be introduced at an angle possibly closest to perpendicular to the round window membrane (Figure 1.5). The author of this procedure believes that the electrode's position allows its least traumatic insertion into the inner ear, ensuring that it is not damaged in the process, and the preoperative hearing is preserved. In the first phase of the insertion, the electrode should be held in fingers to feel the possible resistance better. Notably, it is crucial with the most flexible electrodes that are preferred in the PDT strategy. Only the final stages of the electrode's insertion into the tympanic duct should be made with forceps or extra guiding pins. In electrodes equipped with an internal stylet for insertion, it is

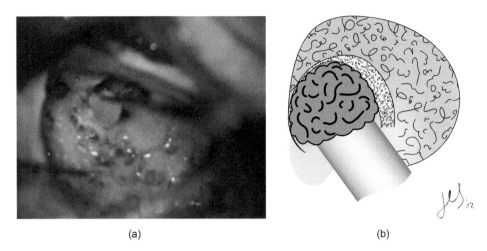

(a)   (b)

Figure 1.6 Sealing and fixing of the electrode – 'the fifth step': (a) intraoperative photo, (b) schematic drawing.

necessary to use forceps to introduce the electrode and another to slide out the stylet. That type of electrode is less preferred in the surgical treatment for partial deafness due to the higher risk of destroying good preoperative hearing or nonfunctional residual hearing and the unimpaired inner ear structures.

The fifth step of the procedure involves sealing the area where the electrode enters the tympanic duct and fixating the electrode in the posterior tympanotomy area using a fascia fragment and fibrin glue (Figure 1.6). The sealing must be delicate and cannot touch the stapes to avoid adhesions that would impair ossicles' mobility and lead to hearing deterioration. The remaining part of the electrode is coiled in the tympanic cavity. Entry to the cavity is closed with a fragment of compressed spongostan and a bony chip harvested at the start of the procedure, fixed with fibrin glue. In this way, the middle ear space is separated from the bony niche containing the implant's inner part.

The last, sixth step of the surgical procedure consists of placing the implant's inner part in the specially made bony niche or on the leveled surface of the temporal bone. Usually, a recess is hollowed out in the bone to contain the body of the inner part of the implant (implants made by Med-El Medical Electronics, Cochlear®, and Advanced Bionics); sometimes, the inner part of the implant is fastened with screws to the surface of the bone (Oticon implants). Sometimes, it is necessary to fix the implant with ionomeric cement or non-absorbable sutures (Figure 1.7). If there is a risk of bleeding from tiny vessels in bone or soft tissues, a suction drain can be placed for 1–2 days. Usually, if the periosteum layer with the whole flap was carefully detached from the surface of the temporal bone squama, there is no need to place the drain, and the compression dressing is enough. Before applying the dressing, the wound should be closed with two layers of sutures (Figure 1.8).

During the last 25 years, the approach at that final stage of surgery evolved. At the beginning of our program, the recommended method had been to strip a relatively wide area of the temporal bone surface to prepare a full bony niche for an implant's

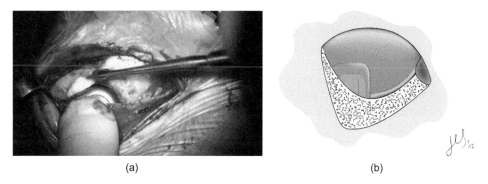

(a)   (b)

Figure 1.7 **Fixation of different kinds of the internal part of the implant in the skull bone: (a) intraoperative photo, (b) schematic drawing.**

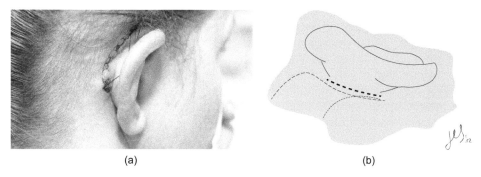

(a)   (b)

Figure 1.8 **The line of the incision after the placement of sutures behind the ear: (a) intra-operative photo, (b) schematic drawing.**

internal part. An additional precaution against the implant's displacement was glass-ionomer cement or non-absorbable sutures. Later, with the advances in cochlear implants' construction, a shallow bony niche suffices to prevent the device's internal part from moving. Subsequent improvements of the implant's structure were aimed at making the procedure more secure and straightforward. These solutions include fixing the implant's internal part to the skull with special screws or pins. Continued miniaturization of implants involved flattening and thinning of the internal part of the device. In many cases, it is now possible to resign from carving out the bony niche. It is particularly advantageous in small children whose skull bone is thin. In these cases, the surgeon may limit the drilling to flatten the bone surface or even forgo that stage and slide the device's internal part into a tight pocket under the skin-muscle-periosteal flap. That solution also eliminates the necessity of the suction drain that typically would be placed for 1–3 days. Intact periosteum makes it possible that the implanted device fits closely into a bone imprint that forms naturally over time. An additional necessary condition is that the skin incision is short, about 2.5 cm long, and made in the shape of an elongated 'S.'

In the treatment of partial deafness, different systems of cochlear implants are used. Med-El implants were used with electrodes from 19 to 28 mm long, including Flex20, Flex24™, Medium, and Flex28™ placed in the tympanic duct. In the first stage of the partial deafness treatment program, only one electrode was available – the standard electrode, which was then used with partial insertion. In PDT cases, insertion exceeding 25 mm is a deep insertion. Different lengths of electrodes were used in cases of PDT-ENS, PDT-EC, PDT-EAS, and PDT-ES. The second type of implant was Cochlear with electrodes CI522 and CI422/SRA developed according to Skarżyński's concept (Skarżyński & Podskarbi-Fayette 2010, Skarżyński et al. 2012a, 2014a). The latter electrode is 20 mm long with a possibility of deeper, up to 25 mm insertion. They were used in the PDT-EC and PDT-EAS types of hearing loss. Advanced Bionics (AB) implants with the HiFocus™ SlimJ electrode were used in partial deafness types PDT-EAS and PDT-ES. Oticon implants with the Neuro Zti EVO electrode were used only in cases of residual hearing in PDT-EAS and PDT-ES. In cases of combined electric-acoustic stimulation, initially, hearing aids were used regardless of the implant type. Later, Duet or Hybrid™ systems became commercially available. The process of postoperative fitting and further rehabilitation is described elsewhere.

The strategy of partial deafness treatment using cochlear implants in patients who before surgery had preserved good hearing in the low- and medium-frequency range or a significant but nonfunctional residual hearing had been the milestone in otosurgery. The introduction of this new method has presented the full picture of possibilities of acoustic and electric stimulation of the inner ear, and significantly widened the earlier indications for surgical treatment of different, acquired, and congenital hearing impairments with cochlear implants with different-length electrodes. The most critical and most challenging task was the introduction, for the first time in the world in 2002, of the program of the electric complementation of the extant good hearing in low frequencies up to 0.5 kHz (PDT-EC). It had been a breakthrough showing that it is possible to preserve small residual hearing and inner ear structures while providing electric complementation of normal hearing up to 0.5 kHz both in adults and in children. It has been preceded with a 5-year-long experience (since 1997) of performing cochlear implantation according to the original '6-step procedure' developed to preserve residual hearing and intact anatomical structures of the inner ear. After 10 years of follow-up of good and excellent results in PDT-EC, another breakthrough became possible – combining the preserved natural hearing up to 1.5 kHz with electric hearing. It opened the possibility of using cochlear implants in millions of patients, including the eldest and those after various traumas with extant normal hearing up to 750, 1,000, or 1,500 Hz. Implantation of a cochlear implant with an appropriate electrode had given them natural-electric hearing (PDT-ENS).

In hearing tests performed before implantation, speech comprehension in silence was on average at the level of 40%–50%, but it would drop to 25%–35% in noise. After cochlear implantation, speech understanding in noise may be as high as 100% or, in particularly unfavorable conditions, 70%–80%. Particularly noteworthy is the excellent preservation of preoperative hearing in the long term, especially in the crucial range of low frequencies in the middle range. The most significant deterioration, usually temporary, was observed at 1,000 Hz in the first 6 months. For the period up to 2 months, hearing thresholds could be, on average, lower by about 10–15 dB at all frequencies at the time of the first postoperative evaluation at about one month. The changes between the 3rd and 6th months were minimal, so the results at 6 months after cochlear implantation formed the long-term assessment base. From 12 months to 9–10 years, there was no longer any significant hearing deterioration observed in the critical low frequencies in the first group of implanted patients with PDT-EC who had electric complementation of hearing.

For the first 2 years (2002–2004), the only patients qualified for surgery in the PDT-EC group were adults whose hearing levels had been stable for about ten years before surgery. So it may be said that the treatment method had been evaluated based on the preservation of hearing directly before the surgery and then verified in the period from 6 months to 10 years post-implantation. In 2004, the PDT-EC program had been expanded to include children. The follow-up results in both groups of patients have led to another breakthrough and identification of a new, huge target group – the PDT-ENS group (Skarżyński et al. 2015, 2019a, 2019b). The PDT-ENS group (that is, the electro-natural hearing in partial deafness treatment) included adults and children.

A crucial observation made by Lorens et al. (2008) had been the possibility of adjusting the sound processor's fitting when hearing deteriorates further because of the progression of the primary pathology in both ears. Bilateral drop in auditory thresholds excludes the cochlear implantation surgery as the cause of hearing loss progression. The reprogramming of the sound processor in conjunction with auditory training means that there is no need to remove, e.g., 20 mm electrode to replace it with the 24 or 28 mm electrode. The speech processor settings' adjustment allows compensating lost acoustic hearing with the electric hearing (Lorens et al. 2008, 2012). These observations of the engineering and rehabilitation team have allowed separating from the PDT-ENS and PDT-EC group another subgroup: PDT – modified electric stimulation (PDT-MES). It includes patients with deteriorating hearing thresholds, whose electric stimulation parameters were modified according to the new hearing status (Skarżyński & Lorens 2010b).

At each stage of extending indications for cochlear implantation in partial deafness treatment, the primary group was adult patients. Excellent results obtained in the group of adults allowed implanting, for the first time in the world, a child with good low-frequency hearing up to 0.5 kHz (PDT-EC). The implantation was performed by Skarżyński in 2004 (Skarżyński et al. 2007a, Skarżyński & Lorens 2010a).

Observation of the post-cochlear implantation results in a growing group of small (younger than one year) and a little older children allowed developing a new standard surgical approach. It aims to preserve any preoperative hearing and inner ear structures (Skarżyński et al. 2016). Thus, children implanted today would have no limitations in taking advantage of future technologies for restoring hearing that may appear in 10 or 20 years. Application of the most flexible of the available electrodes will enable, if such need arises, their most minimally invasive surgical replacement.

Ten-year and longer observation time of children and adults in the treatment for partial deafness showed that results obtained in this method are stable. It leads to an optimistic conclusion that this approach to the treatment of partial deafness is an optimum solution for treating these impairments in the elderly patients, in whom classic hearing aids are not useful, because their speech understanding is affected by increased audiometry thresholds in the high-frequency range. As this type of hearing loss affects about 65% of people over 75, this extension of indications has an enormous social impact.

Simultaneously, the data on patients operated in the WHC shows that 53.4% of them had a slight, gradual progression of hearing loss in both ears in about 10 years before cochlear implantation. It may mean that a small progression of hearing loss would continue in these ears after implantation in the operated and contralateral ear. Significant benefits related to cochlear implantation performed in the way described here mean that the strategy, gradually introduced into the clinical practice, is justified as the procedure of choice. Further explanation of this phenomenon will probably be possible after collecting and analyzing the longitudinal results – in 10 to 15 years of follow-up – in a larger group of implanted patients. It will be the subject of a separate, multifaceted analysis of preservation of preoperative hearing and long-term patient satisfaction.

In this context, the most critical aspect of operated patients' results becomes speech understanding tests. Results obtained by the presently implanted patients are very stable in long observation, providing they receive regular rehabilitation. The level of speech understanding both in silence and in noise is much higher in a group of patients with the electro-natural hearing (PDT-ENS) and electric complementation of hearing (PDT-EC) than in patients with combined electric and acoustic stimulation (PDT-EAS) (Skarżyński et al. 2019a, 2019b).

Summarizing the subsequent stages of introducing the strategy, and gradual widening of indications for cochlear implantation in different hearing loss configurations have made it possible to present a coherent conception of partial deafness treatment. In the subsequent stages of development, this method has encompassed both adult and pediatric patients. This publication presents the development of hearing preservation possibilities in the years 1997–2000, in the first and the largest group of partially deaf patients globally – patients of the WHC. Stable results obtained with this approach confirm that the developed classification system and surgical strategy are valid (Gifford et al. 2013). In the literature of the subject, there are reports from other centers that have introduced a similar surgical strategy and patient selection criteria as described above, following the WHC example (Dorman & Gifford 2010, Van de Heyning et al. 2013, Rajan et al. 2018).

The above facts confirm that the Polish school of partial deafness treatment in children and adults in modern science and medicine is steadily becoming more popular.

It is illustrated in the original international series of 56 surgical training workshops – Window Approach Workshop (WAW) conducted in 2007–2020. The series has included more than 1,200 'live' demonstration surgeries of different cases of partial deafness in children and adults for about 4.5 thousand ear surgeons from all continents. It provides an excellent way to disseminate information about the partial deafness treatment results and the impact of that strategy on the development of new technologies, including the creation of a series of novel flexible electrodes of different lengths – from 19 to 34 mm. The workshops' organization involved cooperation with leading global producers of cochlear implants: Med-El, Cochlear, AB, and Oticon. For the organizers, scientific collaboration with these companies, with their extensive research and implementation facilities, has been a vital impulse in developing the partial deafness treatment strategy.

CONCLUSIONS

Twenty years of observations collected in a very large and diverse group of patients allows formulating the four principal conclusions.

A. A very long follow-up time of the growing group of patients of different ages has shown the need for expanding the indications for cochlear implantation to ever-larger residual hearing and normal preoperative hearing in the low and widening frequency range, which significantly improves speech understanding in silence and noise and increases the ability to communicate.
B. Stability of the results, documented in long observation, as well as good and excellent effects of preservation of preoperative hearing, has confirmed that choice of the surgical strategy with the most physiological approach to the tympanic duct through the round window is optimal in terms of electrode insertion as well as its secure fixation.
C. Clinical results presented in further chapters of this monograph have considerably speeded up the progress of new technologies, including new, flexible cochlear implant electrodes and different systems for the combined electric and acoustic stimulation. That approach is crucial to preserving and taking advantage of the preoperative hearing and protecting the inner ear structures.
D. Implementation of the strategy described in this chapter has allowed demonstrating the very high effectiveness of preserving the preoperative hearing. It significantly affected elaborating new strategies of early detection of different partial hearing impairments based on the universal, population-wide screening tests in school-age children that have encompassed over 1.5 million people in Poland and large groups on four continents. It has shown several new directions for developing the infrastructure and application of the information and communication technologies to extend eHealth in regular postoperative care and improve the effects of rehabilitation.

Chapter 2

Audiological aspects of the partial deafness cochlear implantation with hearing preservation

Artur Lorens
Institute of Physiology and Pathology of Hearing

CONTENTS

INTRODUCTION

Prosthetic correction for sensorineural hearing loss most often involves fitting the appropriate hearing aids and, when that method fails, a cochlear implant. Hearing aids are used primarily in mild to severe hearing impairment cases, while profound or total hearing loss remediation requires a cochlear implant (Skarżyński et al. 2005). A cochlear implant operates by bypassing the damaged fragment of the auditory pathway and providing electric stimulation to the extant nerve fibers to enable the reception of the surrounding sounds. The electric stimulation of the auditory nerve gives patients a new kind of hearing. This so-called electric hearing replaces the natural hearing mechanism (Zeng 2004). There was an expectation that the new electric hearing would enable deaf patients to hear the environmental sounds and improve their phonic communication by supplementing lip-reading. However, research shows that most adult cochlear implant users can understand a considerable part of phonic communication using only the auditory pathway without lip-reading (Skarżyński et al. 1997a).

Although modern hearing aids are becoming more and more effective, many patients find them unsatisfactory. Those patients have a hearing loss characterized by normal hearing or slight hearing loss in the low-frequency range and nearly total deafness in high frequencies (Ching et al. 1998). That configuration of hearing loss is now called the 'partial deafness' to differentiate it from the 'residual hearing,' which is commonly used in the literature to describe a hearing loss characterized by thresholds measured typically at 80–120 dB (Skarżyński et al. 2003). Correction with hearing aids

DOI: 10.1201/9781003164876-2

in patients with partial deafness does not bring any satisfactory effects because the absence of hearing in high frequencies makes it impossible to adequately compensate for the impairment by acoustically amplifying the sounds with hearing aids. Patients with partial deafness find it very difficult to understand speech, especially when there are many competing sound sources. It causes many communication problems, often complicating, and sometimes even preventing social and professional activities (Halpin & Rauch 2009). According to the criteria and guidelines developed during the ten years of the cochlear implant program in Poland, failure to improve speech discrimination after receiving a hearing aid was an indication to consider the decision of cochlear implantation (Skarżyński et al. 2005). However, for a long time, these patients had not been qualified for cochlear implantation because of the fear that surgical intervention would damage the cochlea's still-functioning fragment (Boggess et al. 1989, Adunka et al. 2005).

In 2002, H. Skarżyński had performed the first in the world cochlear implantation in a patient with partial deafness, successfully complementing her normal hearing in frequencies below 500 Hz. Thus, he and his team had started the program of partial deafness treatment (PDT) (Skarżyński et al. 2003, 2006, 2007a, 2007b, 2010, Lorens et al. 2008, Skarżyński & Lorens 2010a, 2010b). Preservation of low-frequency hearing obtained by Skarżyński has enabled to introduce a novel concept of combining partially functional acoustic hearing and new electric hearing in the same ear. The concept involves electric stimulation of the auditory nerve with the cochlear implant system and simultaneous acoustic stimulation of the auditory receptor functioning normally in the low-frequency range. The concept is based on the assumption that electric stimulation with a cochlear implant that restores hearing in high frequencies, combined with the preserved natural low-frequency hearing, would significantly improve speech discrimination in patients with partial deafness (Skarżyński et al. 2003).

The initiation of this new method of treatment of hearing loss was a remarkable scientific and medical achievement. It made it possible to improve the facility of phonic communication in patients with hearing loss. Moreover, it broke down into two limitations of medical intervention that were restricting the possibilities of efficient treatment. The prevailing opinion in the literature of the subject at that time was that cochlear implantation must unavoidably damage the cochlea (Boggess et al. 1989) and that any residual hearing must be irreversibly destroyed. Surgical access to the inner ear through the round window, proposed and implemented by H. Skarżyński, proved to be the effective method enabling the preservation of low-frequency hearing during cochlear implantation (Skarżyński et al. 2003, 2007b, 2009, 2010). The second conjectured limitation involved the possibility of integration of two modes of information, obtained through electric and acoustic stimulation of the hearing receptor, in the auditory centers of the central nervous system. Later studies have shown that using a procedure of fitting of the cochlear implant system specially developed for patients with partial deafness, such integration of information can be supported (Lorens et al. 2008).

In the course of development of the program of PDT, the range of application of that strategy was extended to include other groups of patients, described in detail in the article *Expanding pediatric cochlear implant candidacy: A case study of electro-natural stimulation (ENS) in partial deafness treatment* by Skarżyński et al. (2015).

ASSESSMENT OF THE PRESERVATION OF HEARING AFTER COCHLEAR IMPLANTATION

In the literature, there are many definitions of preservation of hearing sensitivity after cochlear implantation. Depending on a study, it was defined as:

A. Preservation of the hearing threshold value in the free field within the audiometer capacity range in hearing aids (Rizer et al. 1988).
B. Postoperative increase of hearing thresholds not higher than 5 dB registered for frequencies 250, 500, 1000, 2000, and 4000 Hz (Boggess et al. 1989).
C. Obtaining in the postoperative test the responses within the audiometer capacity range for at least one of the three tested frequencies 500, 1000, and 2000 Hz, regardless of the size of the loss (Barbara et al. 2000).
D. Postoperative mean threshold calculated for frequencies 125, 250, and 500 Hz within the range of ±5 dB of the preoperative value (Skarżyński et al. 2002).
E. Postoperative increase of the hearing threshold not higher than 10 dB registered for 125, 250, 500, and 1,000 Hz (Kiefer et al. 2004).
F. Postoperative increase of hearing threshold value not higher than 15 dB registered for all frequencies (125, 250, 500, 750, 1,000 Hz) in audiometry (Gantz & Turner 2004).
G. Postoperative increase of the hearing threshold value not higher than 10 dB registered for frequencies 125, 250, 500, 1000, 2000, and 4000 Hz (Skarżyński et al. 2007b).

  Some authors had been using the concept of the partial preservation of hearing sensitivity that was defined as:

a. Postoperative increase of hearing threshold higher than 10 dB but not exceeding the audiometer range for at least one of the three frequencies 125, 250, and 500 Hz (Skarżyński et al. 2002).
b. Increase in hearing threshold higher than 10 dB but not higher than 20 dB registered for 125, 250, 500, and 1,000 Hz (Kiefer et al. 2004).
c. Increase of hearing threshold not higher than 40 dB registered for 125, 250, 500, and 1,000 Hz (Gstoettner et al. 2004).
d. Increase of hearing threshold higher than 10 dB registered for 125, 250, 500, 1000, 2000, and 4000 Hz, but not exceeding the audiometer range (Skarżyński et al. 2007b).

  Besides quoting the percentage value of hearing sensitivity preservation, many authors also specify the mean value of the pre- and postoperative thresholds for the group at the individual frequencies. In many studies, the postoperative thresholds' values at some frequencies exceeded the audiometer range (nonmeasurable values, NM). There were several different methods used in various studies for calculating the mean:

a. Elimination of the NM,
b. Assigning of a specific maximum value (mostly the maximum output level of the audiometer for individual frequencies),
c. Using the median value instead of the mean.

It is common knowledge that the arithmetical mean is the parameter sensitive to the outlying values in the analyzed data set. Median, on the other hand, is more robust against the outliers. The mean and median are consistent and unbiased estimators of the population's expected value for the specific distribution type. Depending on the adopted methodology, the final result shows different values of pre- and post-intervention change; this lack of a unified approach makes it impossible to compare the results (James et al. 2005).

The analysis of different definitions and calculation methods cited here allows concluding that the obtained level of preservation of hearing sensitivity is highly dependent on the adopted definition and methodology. The literature review shows significant divergences in preserving hearing sensitivity after cochlear implantation in different studies, ranging from different dimension of spaces. For this reason, there was an attempt undertaken to develop a uniform classification of hearing preservation – the HP classification system. This classification was presented in the article published by Skarżyński et al. (2013), *Towards a consensus on a hearing preservation classification system.*

THE POSSIBILITIES OF HEARING PRESERVATION OBTAINED IN THE PARTIAL DEAFNESS TREATMENT PROGRAM

To increase the effectiveness of the hearing sensitivity preservation, Skarżyński had proposed the surgical technique of introducing the implant's electrode to the inner ear through the round window (Skarżyński et al. 2003). Audiometric and electrophysiological measurements in the implanted ear were made before and after implantation to assess the preservation of the level of hearing after cochlear implantation through the round window. It was the first reported study of the preservation of hearing in a patient with the slightly increased hearing threshold in low frequencies and almost total deafness in the high-frequency range in preoperative tests (Skarżyński et al. 2003). Audiometric tests were conducted according to the above-described method. The auditory brainstem response (ABR) test was performed using click stimuli of ranged intensity and short tone bursts of 500 and 1,000 Hz, on the Eptest system with electrodes placed on the forehead and mastoids, through air conduction in-ear headphones Madsen. The amplifier band was 200–2,000 Hz (drop 6 dB/octave). The repetition rate of the stimuli was 37/s, with alternating polarity. The response analysis time was 20 ms. The audiometric thresholds measured preoperatively for 125, 250, 500, and 1,000 Hz were 10, 20, 40, and 100 dBHL, respectively. Postoperative hearing thresholds for 125 and 250 Hz were unchanged. For 500 and 1,000 Hz, a decrease in a hearing level was observed, 30 and 10 dB, respectively. The mean value of the hearing threshold has increased by 15 dB. The difference in hearing thresholds for 500 Hz in the electrophysiological measurement was 30 dB. The level of hearing in the low-frequency range had been in the large degree preserved, as confirmed by audiometric and electrophysiological tests (Skarżyński et al. 2003).

This case report has started a series of studies on hearing preservation in patients with partial deafness. The study performed in ten adult patients with partial deafness using the research method described above has shown preservation of hearing in 90% of patients (Lorens et al. 2005, Skarżyński et al. 2007b). These studies were different from the other, previously published reports because patients had lower hearing threshold values. The recorded hearing preservation rate was higher than that reported by other study groups – 86% reported by Kiefer et al. (2004) and 75% by Gstoettner et al. (2008).

In the next series of tests, the preservation of hearing was assessed in the group of 18 adults and 10 children using the cochlear implant systems produced by one company, with different types of electrodes (Skarżyński et al. 2009). The hearing was preserved in 88% of cases. This result was comparable to the previous studies (Skarżyński et al. 2007b), and thus, the feasibility of hearing preservation was confirmed on more extensive study material. Moreover, this study has demonstrated that the type of electrode has no impact on hearing preservation.

Two separate studies have been conducted in the pediatric population (Skarżyński et al. 2007a, Skarżyński & Lorens 2010a).

In the first study, performed on nine children, preservation of hearing had been observed in 100% cases. Looking to better describe the possibilities of electric-acoustic stimulation after implantation, the authors have proposed three categories of the level of hearing preservation:

1. Full hearing preservation – when postoperative hearing thresholds are within the range of ±10 dB from the preoperative values;
2. Partial hearing preservation – when postoperative hearing thresholds do not exceed the audiometer's capacity range, but the threshold change is more than 10 dB;
3. Functional hearing preservation – when postoperative hearing thresholds are lower than 80 dB HL, enabling application of the electric-acoustic stimulation.

In this study group, functional hearing preservation had been obtained in 89% of cases. For the first time, preservation of hearing after cochlear implantation in children with partial deafness was reported and published.

The second study compared the preservation of hearing between two groups of children: with lesser hearing loss before implantation implanted with a shorter 20 mm electrode, and greater hearing loss and longer 30 mm electrode. No statistically significant differences in hearing preservations between these groups were observed. According to the adopted criteria, in the whole study material (25 children), preservation of hearing was obtained in 100% cases, and the functional preservation of hearing in 88% cases. The results of hearing preservation in this study were similar to the former, indicating that the applied surgical technique was effective and reproducible. Therefore, it is possible to use the electric-acoustic stimulation in children with partial deafness who received cochlear implants.

Hearing preservation rate was also assessed using the masking with a composite sound – Schroeder's harmonics compound. It has shown that after cochlear implantation, it is possible to preserve hearing thresholds and such perception features as temporal resolution, related to the nonlinear processes in the inner ear (Lorens et al. 2001, Gifford et al. 2008).

FITTING OF A COCHLEAR IMPLANT SYSTEM AIMED AT OBTAINING THE OPTIMAL ELECTRIC-ACOUSTIC STIMULATION OF THE AUDITORY RECEPTOR

To ensure the electric-acoustic stimulation of the auditory receptor in patients with partial deafness (who have close to normal hearing in the low-frequency range and no hearing in high frequencies), the surgeon must insert the electrode into the cochlea in such a way that the low-frequency hearing is preserved (Skarżyński et al. 2003). The implant electrode transmits electric impulses that stimulate the auditory nerve. In partial deafness, only the fragment of the auditory nerve responsible for hearing in high frequencies should be stimulated (Lorens et al. 2005). To this end, the electrode length is adjusted according to Greenwood's equation (Greenwood 1997), determining the location of stimulation in a cochlea relative to sound frequency. Assuming that the preserved level of hearing is up to about 1,000 Hz, we can calculate from Greenwood's equation that a 1,000 Hz tone causes the maximum displacement of the basilar membrane at the distance of about 20 mm from the cochlea's windows (Skarżyński et al. 2003). Due to the spatial dispersal of the electric charge in the cochlea, it is impossible to define a precise stimulation location caused by an electrode placed 20 mm from the cochlear case (Walkowiak et al. 2004).

A speech processor used for the electric-acoustic stimulation combines in one casing an acoustic part (a hearing aid) and an electric part (a speech processor) (Lorens et al. 2008). The acoustic part had been optimized for amplifying the low-frequency sounds. The electric part (the speech processor) can be fitted to transform sounds for the electric stimulation starting from the selected border frequency (Lorens et al. 1999). Depending on the selection of parameters of electric stimulation (setting of the bottom border frequency of the acoustic signal processed into the electric stimulation), it is possible to obtain (Lorens et al. 2004):

1. Overlap of the electric and the acoustic hearing, i.e., a situation when sounds from a specific frequency range simultaneously cause the electric and acoustic stimulation in a section of the auditory nerve.
2. Separation of the electric and the acoustic hearing so that the area stimulated acoustically is discrete from the site stimulated electrically.
3. Separation of the regions stimulated acoustically and electrically with an additionally created gap between these regions.

    A choice of one of the three above conditions may impact the subjective assessment of the quality of sound that the patient hears and the rate of speech discrimination (Gantz and Turner 2003, 2004, Vermeire et al. 2008).

A study was conducted (Lorens et al. 2008) to determine which setting of the lower-frequency border of the electric stimulation enables patients with partial deafness a maximum level of speech discrimination. The best speech discrimination results were obtained when regions stimulated acoustically and electrically were separated without a gap.

ASSESSMENT OF SPEECH DISCRIMINATION IMPROVEMENT AFTER APPLYING THE NEW METHOD OF PARTIAL DEAFNESS TREATMENT

A combination of information obtained through the acoustic pathway and the electric stimulation can be for patients with partial deafness, an effective method of increasing the degree of speech understanding in noise (Skarżyński et al. 2003). It can be assumed that if hearing thresholds in the low-frequency range are preserved, the perception of high-frequency sounds will be restored through a cochlear implant system. Thus, the obtained electric-acoustic stimulation of the auditory receptor could create better conditions for transmitting more information about the speech signal than the electric or the acoustic stimulation used separately.

In order to test that hypothesis, a study was conducted to assess speech discrimination after electric-acoustic stimulation in a patient with partial deafness (Skarżyński et al. 2003). After three months of using a cochlear implant, the patient's rate of identification of monosyllable words in silence increased by 67% and in noise by 65%. Improvement in silence was higher by 23% than the typically observed change of the monosyllable words' identification rate in cochlear implant users relying only on the electric stimulation. Improvement of speech discrimination in noise was 55% higher than the typically obtained through the electric stimulation only (Hamzawi et al. 2003). This significant increase of speech understanding in the monosyllable words' test was the effect of combined electric and acoustic stimulation of the auditory receptor. The patient's word identification test results in our study in electric stimulation conditions only, and the acoustic stimulation only, 23% and 40%, respectively, were a confirmation of the hypothesis. We observe the effect of synergy, where a combination of two different factors (electric stimulation and acoustic stimulation) produces an effect more massive than the sum of separate effects (90% > 23% + 40%). Considering that the monosyllable words' test is one of the most difficult audiometric tests, these good results confirm the effectiveness of the auditory receptor's electric-acoustic stimulation in patients with partial deafness. The patient has achieved a speech discrimination level allowing her almost free verbal communication, even in noisy conditions. These results have confirmed the validity of the application of cochlear implants in patients with partial deafness. The electric-acoustic stimulation has, to a significant degree, eliminated the problems with the speech-in-noise understanding related to the technological constraints of cochlear implant systems.

Another study of speech discrimination in patients with partial deafness using cochlear implants was conducted on a group of ten persons (Skarżyński et al. 2006). The tests of identification of monosyllable words in the conditions of electric-acoustic stimulation of auditory receptor in silence and noise were conducted at the following intervals: one month before surgery, and one, 3, 6, and 12 months after the activation of a cochlear implant. The results show a statistically significant change of word identification rate in time, both when listening in silence and listening in noise. The statistically significant improvements have been observed in tests performed three months after activation compared to tests 1 month after activation, and 6 months after activation compared to 3 months after activation. There was no statistically significant difference in speech discrimination rate between the tests performed 12 months and 6 months after cochlear implant activation. The largest change of the monosyllable words' identification was observed in the test conducted 1 month after activation compared to the preoperative result, showing a significant improvement in the short time from implant activation. After 12 months from the cochlear implant system's activation, the rate of monosyllable words' identification has grown on average to 90% in silence and 65% in noise.

These results can be compared with the results obtained with the application of an implant and a hearing aid in one ear reported by Kiefer et al. (2004). In the latter study, patients with partial deafness using a hearing aid in the implanted ear achieved, on average, 56% of monosyllable words identification in silence. That result, markedly worse than in the Program of PDT, demonstrates that in patients with partial deafness, the electric-acoustic stimulation promotes speech understanding better than a hearing aid and cochlear implant in patients with residual hearing.

Speech discrimination results have also been evaluated in the pediatric population (Skarżyński et al. 2007a, Skarżyński & Lorens 2010a). In a short time after implant activation, all children have shown a significant improvement of monosyllable words' discrimination.

DISCUSSION AND CONCLUSIONS

Ensuring the auditory receptor's adequate electric-acoustic stimulation is a crucial part of the clinical management in the novel PDT method (Skarżyński et al. 2003).

The necessary condition enabling such stimulation is the adequate level of low-frequency hearing before implantation and preservation of that hearing after the electrode's insertion into the inner ear (Skarżyński et al. 2002). Preservation of hearing has been demonstrated in 90%–100% cases depending on the study group. Therefore, it is possible to conclude that most patients implanted with the new PDT method can benefit from the electric-acoustic stimulation of the auditory receptor (Skarżyński et al. 2007a, 2007b, 2010, 2011, Gifford et al. 2008).

Another audiological challenge was optimizing the electric-acoustic stimulation of the auditory receptor for the maximum benefit from the proposed clinical management. In particular, the research focused on the effect of the lower-frequency border of the electric stimulation on maximizing speech discrimination of patients with partial deafness after applying the electric-acoustic stimulation of the auditory receptor. The results enabled developing the cochlear implant fitting procedure guidelines for the auditory receptor's electric-acoustic stimulation (Lorens et al. 2008).

In all cases, improved speech understanding was observed; in most cases, the improvement was significant (Lorens et al. 2008, Skarżyński et al., 2006, 2007b, 2010). The gain obtained in the proposed intervention was much higher than the risk of adverse effects. Moreover, the comparison of the alternative management strategies using the quantitative methods of investigating management outcomes shows that the benefits of the electric-acoustic stimulation of the auditory receptor outweigh the benefits of using only the electric stimulation with cochlear implants or only the acoustic stimulation with a hearing aid (Lorens et al. 2008).

Chapter 3

Intraoperative monitoring of hearing preservation with ECochG in treatment of partial deafness

Piotr H. Skarżyński
Institute of Physiology and Pathology of Hearing

CONTENTS

INTRODUCTION

As auditory benefits of deaf and hard-of-hearing patients provided with cochlear implants (CIs) become better and better, the inclusion criteria for CIs with electrodes of various lengths expand. It has been happening for over 20 years, particularly concerning preserved functional postoperative hearing and combined acoustic and electric stimulation. We know that many CI users have useful residual hearing or good low-frequency hearing in the ear intended for cochlear implantation from the currently applied diagnostic measures. While residual hearing alone is usually not sufficient to understand speech and support communication, appropriate surgical techniques allow the surgeons to preserve it during the electrode array insertion (Kennedy 1987, Giordano et al. 2014, Skarżyński et al. 2019). In these situations, as described in Skarzynski's partial deafness treatment concept (Skarżyński et al. 2010), it is possible to apply combined electric-acoustic stimulation (EAS) or electric complementation in the deaf part of the ear. This approach is called the partial deafness treatment – electric complementation (PDT-EC) or the partial deafness treatment – electro-natural stimulation (PDT-ENS). This approach requires electric stimulation for high-frequency sounds and existing acoustic hearing on lower frequencies (Friedmann et al. 2015). EAS has been shown to enable better pitch perception, sound quality, and speech intelligibility in noise than electric stimulation alone (Incerti et al. 2013). Significantly, users prefer combined stimulation to electric-only stimulation with an implant, if available (Skarżyński et al. 2014b). Even if a patient does not have residual hearing that could be preserved during the surgery, the preservation of the inner ear structures and the gain obtained from the CI are better in situations where the

DOI: 10.1201/9781003164876-3

damage to the inner ear was minimized during the surgery (Aschendorff et al. 2007, Finley et al. 2008).

INSERTION OF THE ELECTRODE USING ECOCHG

The correlation between the preservation of the delicate anatomy of the cochlea and the results of hearing and speech understanding after cochlear implantation is well known. During the electrode insertion to the cochlea, the surgeon can gently operate insertion parameters such as angle and speed. Their modifications are often a part of the standard cochlear implantation procedure. However, hearing and cochlear structure preservation depend on atraumatic electrode insertion. The conventional insertion mechanism's actual status does not provide the surgeon with feedback on location, time, or kind of structures' damage. Therefore, it is essential to have a tool that provides the surgeon with real-time information regarding trauma inside the cochlea and its potential impact on hearing. The application of electrocochleography (ECochG) is one of the possible ways to obtain such information.

The ECochG measurement signal is an objective electrophysiological reflection of the peripheral electric-acoustic interactions within the cochlea. During the ECochG measurement, a short sound stimulus of a particular frequency and level is delivered to the external ear canal and induces the natural physiological movement of the cochlea's external and internal hair cells. These movements generate small electrical potentials that can be detected through a recording electrode placed near the cochlea (e.g., formerly located on the promontory or in the area of the round window) (Finley et al. 2008, Mandalá et al. 2012). Averaging these potentials' records, synchronized with the acoustic stimulus, allows amplifying the weak ECochG signal while eliminating physiological and electrical noise. ECochG measurement enables the verification of the functional integrity of various elements of the peripheral auditory system. The ECochG measures, particularly crucial for cochlear implantation, include CM – cochlear microphonic, generated by external auditory cells of the cochlear, AP – action potential (nerve impulse), and ANN – auditory nerve neurophonic. Comparing the recorded signal's energy for the measured frequency with the signal stimulus level, one can estimate the audiometric pure-tone hearing thresholds with an accuracy of ±10 dB (Koka et al. 2017).

INTEGRATED SYSTEM ECOCHG ADVANCED BIONICS AIM™

Advanced Bionics' (AB) CI system has a built-in back-telemetry capability. Initially, it served to conduct impedance measurements confirming the system's proper functioning. Later, the back-telemetry system was also adopted by other CI producers and improved to register electrically evoked compound action potential (ECAP), which is a physiological signal resulting from electric stimulation of the auditory nerve. ECochG registration applying back-telemetry is a new type of measurement that may become an essential clinical tool, as the number of CI users with preserved hearing is growing. The latest version of the integrated ECochG measurement system is the AB's Active Insertion Monitoring AIM™ platform (Figure 3.1). It is the first device commercially available introduced to clinical practice. The system includes a tablet computer with

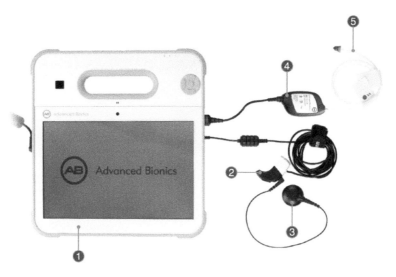

Figure 3.1 Active Insertion Monitoring AIM™ system: (1) a central unit of the system AIM, (2) processor Naida CI Q, (3) transmitter UHP, (4) insert earphone, (5) sterile sound tube with a dome. (Source: Advanced Bionics with permission.)

a sound processor, a programming interface, a transmitter, and measurement equipment. An integrated sound card and an earphone are used for acoustic stimulation. A dedicated software package controls and synchronizes the operation of the integrated system. The original version of the AB ECochG system has been described and successfully used in several clinical trials (Koka et al. 2017). AB's system enables data acquisition with sufficient precision and speed to identify significant markers associated with potential cochlear damage, providing the surgeon with the real-time visual and audible feedback during electrode insertion.

In comparison with previous significant solutions, where ECochG was registered near the cochlea before and after the electrode insertion, ECochG recording from distal electrode contact in the cochlea during insertion has an advantage – the part of the electrode is closer to the ECochG signal generators (meaning cochlear auditory cells and auditory nerve). This solution results in a greater amplitude of the signal being registered. Thus, a surgeon gets faster feedback and information in the event of a change of these potentials (Figure 3.2).

For example, if the CI electrode touches delicate structures (such as a basilar membrane or spiral ligament) of the cochlea during insertion, the ECochG potential's amplitude decreases. With the real-time measurement system used during the electrode insertion, it is possible to observe decreasing ECochG potentials. The surgeon may intentionally apply a chosen modification of the electrode insertion technique, for example, changing the insertion angle to avoid translocation. The expected functional benefits of cochlear structure preservation using this novel method of real-time insertion monitoring include improved indicators of hearing preservation (HP) and enhanced speech perception after cochlear implantation.

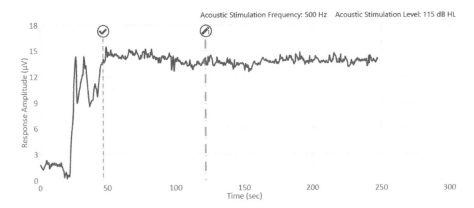

Figure 3.2 An example registration of ECochG measurement performed intraoperatively during electrode insertion. (Source: Advanced Bionics with permission.)

IMPLEMENTATION OF ECOCHG IN THE ASSESSMENT OF HEARING PRESERVATION AFTER COCHLEAR IMPLANTATION

Additionally, the intracochlear electrodes' application in the ECochG test allows the monitoring of potentials after surgery. In some cases, residual hearing presence is confirmed by pure-tone audiometry (PTA) performed several days after implantation. Still, it has also been observed that it may disappear shortly or long after the implantation. The ECochG test is an objective hearing monitoring method at regular intervals in the early and late postoperative periods. The ECochG measurement recording can reveal the moment of hearing loss and help identify factors contributing to hearing loss. The below figures present examples of the results of two patients. The results were obtained by applying the above-discussed method and Skarzynski's Hearing Preservation Classification.

Patient #1

Patient's #1 PTA thresholds before implantation and at 1 and 3 months after the implantation are shown in Figure 3.3. Figure 3.4 shows the estimated ECochG hearing thresholds registered intraoperatively and at 1 and 3 months after the implantation. Figure 3.5 shows Patient's #1 rate of preservation of hearing after cochlear implantation calculated using Skarzynski's Hearing Preservation Classification method for measurements performed 1 month after surgery and 3 months after surgery. When the calculated HP numerical rate is converted to a categorical scale, we can see that Patient #1 has obtained complete HP in both follow-up examinations. The HP rate in the longer follow-up was better.

Patient #2

Patient's #2 PTA thresholds before implantation and at 1 and 3 months after implantation are shown in Figure 3.6. Figure 3.7 shows the estimated ECochG hearing thresholds registered intraoperatively and at 1 and 3 months after the implantation.

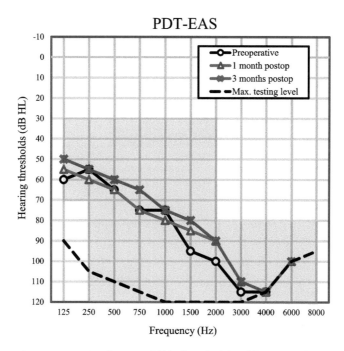

Figure 3.3 Pre- and postoperative hearing PTA thresholds of Patient #1.

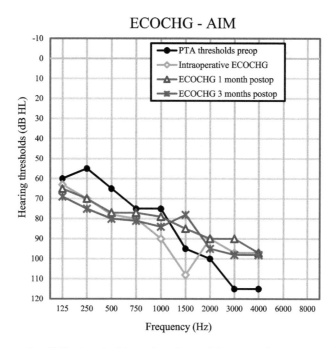

Figure 3.4 Preoperative PTA thresholds and estimated intra- and postoperative ECochG hearing thresholds of Patient #1.

Hearing Preservation, Calculation in [%]			
Legend:		Follow-up	
S	Hearing Preservation	1 month	3 months
75-100%	Complete HP		
26-74%	Partial HP	S=107.7%	S=121.2%
1-25%	Minimal HP		
No detectable hearing	Loss of hearing		

Figure 3.5 Postoperative percentage of hearing preservation of Patient #1 according to Skarzynski's Hearing Preservation Classification.

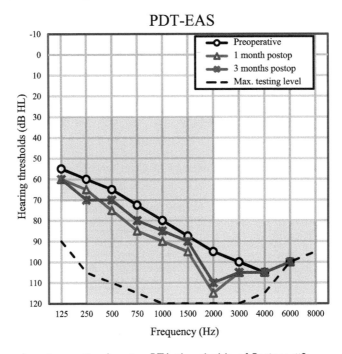

Figure 3.6 Pre- and postoperative hearing PTA thresholds of Patient #2.

Figure 3.8 shows Patient's #2 rate of preservation of hearing after cochlear implantation calculated using Skarzynski's Hearing Preservation Classification method for measurements performed 1 month after surgery and 3 months after surgery. When the HP rate of Patient's #2 is converted to a categorical scale, we see that he had partial HP 1 month after implantation, and it improved to complete HP 3 months after surgery.

SUMMARY

The monitoring of auditory functions with electrocochleography has gained a new meaning thanks to the possibility of using the CI electrode to take the measures.

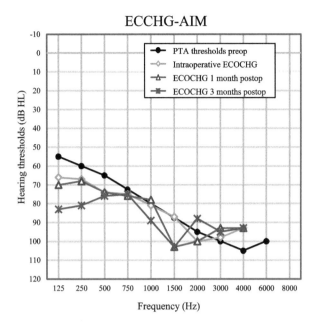

Figure 3.7 Preoperative PTA thresholds and estimated intra- and postoperative ECochG hearing thresholds of Patient #2.

Hearing Preservation, Calculation in [%]			
Legend:		Follow-up	
S	Hearing Preservation	1 month	3 months
75-100%	Complete HP		
26-74%	Partial HP	S=74.6%	S=81.4%
1-25%	Minimal HP		
No detectable hearing	Loss of hearing		

Figure 3.8 Postoperative percentage of hearing preservation of Patient #2 according to the Skarzynski's Hearing Preservation Classification.

ECochG, which used to be a limited examination applied to measure the functional integrity of selected elements of the peripheral auditory system, has now become a tool supporting a surgeon during cochlear implantation and allowing for objective monitoring of hearing after implantation.

The real-time feedback on the condition of the cochlea function during implantation obtained by the surgeon during the measurement may, in the future, allow scientists to modify their surgical methods and the design of the electrode bundles themselves. Hearing threshold estimation based on ECochG measurement, apart from the objective insight into the quantitative assessment of hearing loss, provides essential information on the physiology of hearing and processes taking place in the cochlea after implantation. It has the potential to predict HP in individual clinical cases, which in turn markedly increases the safety of the procedure and provides the opportunity to expand indications for implantation in partial deafness cases.

It should be emphasized that the ECochG measurement method using the Advanced Bionics AIM system is in the initial phase, assessing its new clinical applications. For now, we may state the tremendous clinical value it brings as a tool used in surgical and audiological practice.

Chapter 4

Genetic biomarkers of neuroplasticity in the treatment of children with prelingual deafness with cochlear implantation

Monika Matusiak and Henryk Skarżyński
Institute of Physiology and Pathology of Hearing

CONTENTS

INTRODUCTION

Lack of auditory sensory stimulation in prelingually deaf children, such as children born with congenital deafness, results in the auditory system's deprivation, so a child cannot develop verbal communication. Cochlear implantation assures that the sensory cortex receives acoustic stimulation, which starts the cascade of molecular processes in neurons and promotes cortical synapses' formation. Neural tissue of a juvenile brain possesses a vast capacity to change neuronal connections' strength in response to environmental stimuli. On average, the functional results of cochlear implantation in small children are good. However, there is still a large variability of the outcomes. Identification of genetic biomarkers of neuroplasticity after cochlear implantation might facilitate clinical management of implanted children, giving them better chances of developing proficient spoken language.

This chapter discusses the findings of the research grant funded by the National Science Centre (SONATA UMO 2013/14/D/NZ5/03337). The study investigated the hypothesis that a specific set of matrix metalloproteinase-9 (MMP-9) and brain-derived neurotrophic factor (BDNF) gene variants predisposes children diagnosed with prelingual congenital deafness implanted before 2 years of age to better respond to cochlear implantation. The other hypothesis tested in that study was the relationship between plasma levels of MMP-9 and BDNF before cochlear implantation and hearing and speech rehabilitation results.

DOI: 10.1201/9781003164876-4

CONGENITAL DEAFNESS AND ITS TREATMENT IN CHILDREN YOUNGER THAN 2 YEARS

The incidence of prelingual congenital deafness is 1.3–4:1,000 births. For about 28 years in Poland and nearly 30 years worldwide, its typical treatment has been cochlear implantation (Kral & O'Donoghue 2010, Korver et al. 2017).

Neural tissue has the unique capability to encode information contained in the acoustic stimuli reaching the ear, transmit it to higher levels of the auditory pathway, and then transduce it for the cognitive processes. This process requires an intact sensorineural system from the receptor to the auditory cortex and stable delivery of the acoustic stimuli (Kral & O'Donoghue 2010, Kral et al. 2016). A cochlea malfunction results in a lack of sensory stimulation of the auditory pathway neurons and their progressive deprivation. Cochlear implantation, popularly used as a method of choice in treating profound prelingual sensorineural hearing loss, allows restoring cochlea function.

About 60% of cases of congenital deafness are caused by a genetic defect of the receptor. In about half of these cases, two pathogenic variants are detected in *GJB2*/*GJB6* genes (locus DFNB1), coding connexin 26 and 30, respectively. These proteins are critical for the physiology of the organ of Corti at the cellular level (Oziębło et al. 2020). It means that hearing impairment in this group of patients results from the blocked synthesis of one of the receptor cells' proteins, while the morphology of the labyrinth stays intact. Carriers of the pathogenic variants in DFNB1 fail newborn screening tests, and usually, no response is registered in the auditory brainstem evoked potentials test (500 Hz and 2–4 kHz). However, in some of these children, as they grow up and become able to perform pure-tone audiometry tests, some hearing thresholds can be registered at the level of 80 dB and lower, particularly in low frequencies such as 250 or 500 Hz. It shows that the diagnostics and cochlear implantation in children with DFNB1-conditioned deafness should be handled as partial deafness patients. This means application of the same very conservative surgical technique aimed at preservation of the labyrinth structures, especially the intracochlear elements. This approach may become crucial for possible future treatment methods, such as gene therapy or stem cell therapy.

The optimized of the surgical technique introduced to the clinical practice by H. Skarżyński is based on the maximally atraumatic insertion of the electrode array into the scala tympani. This approach aims to preserve inner ear structures and residual low-frequency hearing, or normal low- and mid-frequency hearing (Skarżyński et al. 2016). In congenitally deaf children, this technique also assures optimal stimulation of spiral ganglion neuron fibers. It thus provides maximum transmission of stimulation to the auditory pathway's upper levels (van der Marel et al. 2015). An implanted child is given access to acoustic information to acquire several developmental competencies, among which verbal communication is the most important one. Although this method of treatment is undoubtedly successful, its disadvantage is a large variability of the results. This is mostly seen in the youngest group of cochlear implant users, even in children without any comorbidities implanted at the same age with the same minimally invasive technique (Skarżyński et al. 2011, 2016). Some implanted children develop auditory skills with a learning curve similar to their normal-hearing peers. However, despite enormous effort, some patients never achieve age-appropriate norm in hearing (Kral & O'Donoghue 2010, Kral et al. 2016, Niparko et al. 2010, Rijke et al. 2019).

The indirect cognitive consequences of auditory deprivation at a young age, such as impaired development of working memory, attention, and executive functions, have been hitherto seldom reported but cannot be ignored (Rijke et al. 2019, Kronenberger et al. 2014, Kral et al. 2016). So far, identified factors influencing rehabilitation of hearing and speech after cochlear implantation include patient's age at diagnosis, age at implantation, comorbidities, environmental factors such as parents' education level, and others (Niparko et al. 2010, Kral et al. 2016). However, the aforementioned clinical conditions resulting from the vast variability of hearing and speech rehabilitation outcomes indicate a pressing need to search for and identify other contributing factors. Their identification would improve our understanding of the verbal communication skills' development process. It would also allow predicting the trajectory of language development in an individual child. That, in turn, would help to identify children who are at risk of rehabilitation failure and develop a therapeutical approach tailored to a child's individual needs.

NEUROPLASTICITY IN THE AUDITORY SYSTEM

Brain, a system in a dynamic balance, has the unique and fundamental capacity to change plastically in response to the environment's changes. In the auditory system, acoustic stimuli transduced to the auditory cortex just after birth, or even earlier, stimulate neuronal connectivity and increase the potential for synaptogenesis (Kral et al. 2016, Holtmaat & Caroni 2016). Modern scientific technology allows for a successful diagnosis of complex pathologies in an impairment of a singular molecular mechanism, so a synapse is treated as a functional unit of a brain (Beroun et al. 2019). In the brain cortex exposed continuously to sensory stimulation, synapses' formation is counterbalanced by eliminating existing connections (the so-called synaptic turnover). This balance forms the neuronal basis of the brain's computational power. That, in turn, is the ground for creating a memory trace (engram), which is recognized as a functional unit of memory and learning (Kral et al. 2016, Holtmaat & Caroni 2016, Reinhard et al. 2015). Electron microscopic studies of the human auditory cortex show that under stable sensory stimulation, the number of synapses increases from birth until adolescence, peaking between 1 and 4 years of life, and then decreases (the so-called synaptic pruning) (Huttenlocher et al. 1997, Kral & Sharma 2012). Studies of animal models and clinical observations allow concluding that there is a critical period in the early ontogenesis when the capability to form neuronal assemblies under sensory stimulation is the greatest. In these conditions, axons and dendrites of cortical neurons compete for their synaptic partner and form numerous dendritic spines capable of building a robust and stable synapse. Thus, the sensory cortex can easily develop a required number of stable synaptic connections, thus acquiring modality-specific competencies (Sharma et al. 2002, Kral & O'Donoghue 2010, Kral et al. 2016, Holtmaat & Caroni 2016, Reinhard et al. 2015). Cochlear implantation performed during the critical period enables the delivery of electric stimuli to spiral ganglion nerves and starts the cascade of synaptic changes in neurons of the auditory pathway, promoting its maturation. Otherwise, these neurons would undergo irreversible degeneration processes (Kral & Sharma 2012, Kral et al. 2016).

SYNAPTIC PLASTICITY – MOLECULAR GROUNDS

At the base of the nervous system's capacity to respond to stimuli coming from the continually altering environment, there is the capacity to modify synapse strength. The term 'synaptic plasticity' describing this phenomenon was coined by a Polish neurobiologist Jerzy Konorski – a pioneer of neuronal plasticity research working in the Institute of Experimental Biology in Warsaw in the years 1933–1973 (Konorski 1948). Changes in the strength of intrasynaptic interactions are based on a mechanism of complex genetic and molecular regulations between the pre- and postsynaptic membrane, between neurons and glial cells, and between neurons and extracellular matrix. The recent research results on the extracellular matrix's role suggest that it may play a significant role in synaptogenesis (Kral et al. 2016, Holtmaat et al. 2016, Rivera et al. 2010, Vafadari et al. 2016). It has recently been postulated that the extracellular matrix is the fourth regular part of a synapse. The other three are the presynaptic and postsynaptic membranes and glial invaginations (Rivera et al. 2010, Vafadari et al. 2016, Ferrer-Ferrer & Ditaytev 2018). The extracellular matrix undergoes proteolysis in the process of enzymatic cleaving; this attribute is thought to be a critical factor for communication between neurons and consequently for promoting *de novo* synaptogenesis (Reinhard et al. 2015, Rivera et al. 2010, Vafadari et al. 2016).

Matrix metalloproteinases (MMPs) are a group of 20 proteolytic enzymes, whose primary function is the cleavage of extracellular matrix proteins, promoting changes in the strength of synaptic connections and cleavage of membrane proteins, which results in synaptic reorganization (Beroun et al. 2019, Vafadari et al. 2016). One of the best-described MMPs involved in synaptic plasticity is MMP-9 – synthesized and released into the extracellular space as an inactive zymogen pro-MMP-9. In the brain, MMP-9 is expressed at a low level and released at a synapse due to neuronal stimulation. In the form of inactive proenzyme, MMP-9 is released into the extracellular matrix, where it is activated through proteolytic cleavage (removal of a propeptide), uncovering its active site (Szklarczyk et al. 2002, Bozdagi et al. 2007, Dziembowska et al. 2012). Animal studies have shown that MMP-9 participates in the synaptic plasticity processes on different levels of synaptic functions (Wang et al. 2007, Dziembowska et al. 2012, Rivera et al. 2010, Vafadari et al. 2016).

The ability to form synapses relies on two neuronal phenomena: long-term potentiation (LTP) and long-term depression (LTD) (Holtmaat & Caroni 2016, Nagy et al. 2006, Minichiello 2009). Numerous research studies have proven that MMP-9 plays a critical role in inducing the late phase of LTP (Nagy et al. 2006, Ethel & Ethel 2007, Okulski et al. 2007). Another protein engaged in the induction of early and late phases of LTP is the brain-derived neurotrophic factor (BDNF). Genes coding these molecules are characterized by single nucleotide polymorphism (SNP) (Rybakowski et al. 2009, Hariri et al. 2003, Cheeran et al. 2008, Ethel & Ethel 2007). The substitution of one nucleotide in a gene sequence leads to significant changes in the synthesized protein activity, in this case, in its synaptic influence.

The *MMP9* gene is localized in the chromosomal region 20q11.2-q13.1. It is known to have at least several polymorphisms (St Jean et al. 1995). Substitution of cytosine (C) by thymine (T) at position 1562 in the promoter region (rs 3918242, -1562C/T) influences the transcriptional activity of the gene (Rybakowski et al. 2009, Vafadari et al. 2016). A significant difference in the distribution of the C/C and C/T rs 3918242 genotype carriers has been observed in schizophrenia patients who statistically more frequently have the C/C genotype, which is connected with the gene's lower transcriptional activity (Rybakowski et al. 2009). Also, among patients treated for bipolar disorder, carriers of the C/C genotype had significantly higher cognitive test scores than the C/T genotype carriers. BDNF is a neurotrophin known for its modulatory role in neuroplasticity (Cheeran et al. 2008, Minichiello 2009, Bekinschtein et al. 2011, Wiłkość et al. 2016). It has been demonstrated that it plays a critical role in plasticity essential for learning and memory (Hariri et al. 2003).

The best-studied functional polymorphism is Val/Met substitution at codon 66 in rs 6265 gene (Hariri et al. 2003, Cheeran et al. 2008, Lamblin et al. 2002). It is located in the region coding pro-BDNF, so it does not affect the mature protein's function. However, it affects the intracellular transport and release of the mature form of BDNF (Hariri et al. 2003). It has been demonstrated that carriers of the Val/Val BDNF variant show higher potential for plastic changes in the motor cortex than those of Val/Met variant (Cheeran et al. 2008). It has also been demonstrated that Val/Val genotype carriers show increased hippocampus activity in fMRI tests performed during cognitive tasks (Hariri et al. 2003).

GENETIC BIOMARKERS OF THE RESULTS OF TREATMENT OF PARTIAL DEAFNESS WITH A COCHLEAR IMPLANT

Since 2016, the Institute of Physiology and Pathology of Hearing in Warsaw, in cooperation with the Nencki Institute of Experimental Biology, carried out the research grant funded by the National Science Centre (SONATA UMO 2013/14/D/NZ5/03337). The project aims to verify the hypothesis that carrying a specific set of MMP-9 and BDNF gene variants predisposes children diagnosed with prelingual congenital deafness implanted before 2 years of age to better cochlear implantation results. The second tested hypothesis assumes the relationship between plasma levels of MMP-9 and BDNF before cochlear implantation and results of hearing and speech rehabilitation. Seventy children participated in the project. They all had prelingual deafness, no comorbidities, and negative anamnesis; all had been implanted before 2 years old. A follow-up period in all children was over 18 months. During this period, their speech and hearing development were evaluated at three particular intervals. Genomic and proteomic tests were performed in all patients enrolled in the project to identify markers that could be used, particularly at the preimplant level, to single out children who may need individually targeted auditory development support after cochlear implantation.

These markers would be a handy clinical tool for early detection of children at risk of delayed language development and, according to the newest publications, delayed cognitive development. It would allow designing specially tailored intervention encompassing early implantation and extensive, multifaceted rehabilitation program (Kral et al. 2016).

The project has received funding from the National Centre of Science – Grant #UMO 2014/13/D/NZ5/03337.

Chapter 5

Otosurgical techniques in the application of various auditory implants

Henryk Skarżyński and Piotr H. Skarżyński
Institute of Physiology and Pathology of Hearing

CONTENTS

INTRODUCTION

Medical technologies and surgical techniques have reached such a level of development that practically all hearing impairments can be remediated by applying various hearing prostheses. The optimal management approach decision depends on which part of the hearing pathway is damaged, and the degree and configuration of hearing impairment. A comprehensive concept published by Skarżyński and Lorens (2010b) (presented earlier during the 9th ESPCI in 2009) is a decision support tool allowing for different configurations of a preoperative audiogram. The details of this concept are presented in Chapter 1. It divides patients into five groups according to the configuration of their hearing loss and recommended intervention. For patients with a mostly flat audiogram and mild to severe hearing loss (PDT-AS group), recommended options include hearing aids (HAs), bone conduction implants, or middle ear implants (MEIs).

    The conventional HAs have limitations such as an occlusion effect, auditory feedback, auricle irritation, or excessive secretion of ear wax. There may also be problems related to anatomical conditions such as congenital or acquired malformations of the

DOI: 10.1201/9781003164876-5

auricle or ear canal. Many patients refuse to wear HAs because they find them cumbersome, unsightly, or because they are afraid to be stigmatized as disabled or old. The implantable acoustic hearing devices allow bypassing the drawbacks of HAs.

There are two kinds of these devices presently commercially available for clinical use, based on different operating principles: conduction of sounds through the bone or delivery of mechanical vibrations directly to the middle ear (bone conduction implants and MEIs).

In Poland, the program of hearing implants, initiated by H. Skarżyński, dates back to the first cochlear implantations in adults and children with total deafness in 1992. In 1993, B. Rydzewski implanted the first bone conduction device (Baha®) in an adult patient. In 1997, H. Skarżyński performed the first such surgery on a child. The first MEI surgery in Poland took place in 2003, conducted by H. Skarżyński. Until 2020, more than a thousand patients received MEI and bone conduction implants in the Institute of Physiology and Pathology Hearing. Our program of hearing implants has collected a group of more than 10 thousand ears, and the whole ear surgery program has grown to over 15 thousand otosurgical procedures per year, comprising various hearing improving surgeries (Skarżyński 2018).

This chapter describes the surgical techniques of implantation of the middle ear and bone conduction devices most often used in our clinical practice. Bone conduction implants are Baha® Connect, Baha® Attract, Osia® (Cochlear Ltd., Sydney, Australia), and Bonebridge (Med-El Medical Electronics GmbH, Innsbruck, Austria). MEIs presented in this chapter are Vibrant Soundbridge (Med-El Medical Electronics GmbH, Innsbruck, Austria), Codacs™, and MET® (Cochlear Ltd., Sydney, Australia).

BONE CONDUCTION IMPLANTS – INDICATIONS AND INCLUSION CRITERIA

Bone conduction hearing implants are working on a principle of transferring sound to the inner ear by skull vibrations bypassing the outer and middle ear's conducting structures. For this reason, they are a perfect treatment solution if there is a conductive element of the hearing loss present.

They are recommended for the treatment of conductive and mixed hearing loss and single-sided deafness (SSD). In the latter case, rehabilitation of the deaf ear is not through direct acoustic stimulation; it is a CROS hearing that diverts the signal from the deaf side to the contralateral normal hearing ear.

Bone conduction implants are divided into percutaneous types such as Baha Connect System, where the element implanted in the skull bone penetrates the skin, and transcutaneous, fully implanted types such as Baha Attract, Osia, and Bonebridge systems.

Common indications for all the above bone conduction implants' models include unilateral or bilateral hearing loss of conductive or mixed type with an air-bone gap larger than 25–35 dB HL. The sensorineural component of mixed hearing loss will determine the sound processor's selection and varies from ≤45 dB HL at 0.5–3 kHz for Bonebridge, ≤55 dB HL for Osia, and ≤65 dB HL for Baha with the strongest processor.

In SSD cases, the air conduction threshold in the better hearing ear cannot exceed 20 dB HL for frequencies from 0.5 to 3 kHz. Moreover, the pre-implantation trial must show that patient will benefit better from this system than from a classic HA in CROS configuration.

Typical candidates for the bone conduction hearing implants are patients with outer and middle ear malformations, either congenital or acquired due to injury, obliterative otitis, and sclerotic lesions tympanoplasty, radical ear surgery, or other causes if the patient does not achieve a satisfactory improvement with a classic HA.

All bone conduction implants presented in this chapter have common inclusion criteria of stable bone conduction threshold, no central auditory processing disorders, and CT-confirmed anatomy of the temporal bone sufficient to accommodate the implantable bone conduction actuator. Moreover, all candidates for implantation must undergo a preoperative simulation test and prove that they are capable of benefiting from the bone conduction device. That simulation test should involve free-field audiometry in classic or bone conduction HA. Also, before the decision about implantation, all patients should undergo counseling to ensure strong motivation and realistic expectations.

The minimum age requirement varies for different implants. For Baha Connect and Baha Attract, the minimum age is ≥5 years in the USA (FDA approval); in Europe, there is no age restriction for these two systems, although they are not recommended in children younger than three months for practical reasons such as the minimum required thickness of temporal bone. The Osia system can be implanted in children ≥12 years old. Bonebridge is allowed for children ≥5 years in Europe (CE) and ≥12 years in the USA (FDA).

Contraindications for bone conduction implants are central auditory processing disorders, unstable hearing loss, and unfavorable anatomy seen in a CT image. For Baha Connect, an additional contraindication is an allergic reaction to the implant's materials.

MIDDLE EAR IMPLANTS – INDICATIONS AND INCLUSION CRITERIA

Generally speaking, (active) MEIs operate by mechanically amplifying the conductive apparatus's vibrations in the middle ear by vibrating the ossicles or the membrane window of the cochlea, depending on where they attach.

They have been developed to give an additional treatment option for patients who have limited success or are unable to wear traditional HAs because of ear malformations such as atresia, microtia, otosclerotic lesions, chronic or recurrent otitis with effusion, or the occlusion effect and sound quality issues when wearing a HA.

Two MEI systems presented in this chapter, Vibrant Soundbridge VSB and MET, are recommended for cases of moderate to severe conductive, mixed or sensorineural hearing loss, as well as SSD. Indications for these implants are middle and sometimes outer ear defects, congenital or acquired due to injury, inflammatory or sclerotic lesions, earlier reconstructive or radical ear surgeries. Also, other hearing disorders, in which simulation tests have shown a chance of better hearing benefit than the application of a HA, can be the indication for a VSB or MET.

Codacs system is indicated for bilateral and unilateral severe to profound mixed hearing loss in cases of advanced otosclerosis or tympanosclerosis with significantly diminished inner ear function. This MEI has been introduced to clinical practice fairly recently. There is a possibility that these basic indications will be expanded to include also congenital and acquired malformations in patients in whom other implantable solutions do not provide a good hearing effect.

All types of MEI described in this chapter are allowed for application in adult patients, while the VSB is also allowed in Europe (CE mark) for use in children aged 3 years and older. Inclusion criteria are stable bone conduction thresholds (also, in sensorineural hearing loss stable air conduction threshold), middle ear anatomy allowing for the placement of the transducer on a chosen structure, realistic expectations, and strong motivation on the patient's side. Moreover, all candidates must undergo audiometric tests in the free field with conventional HA to confirm that they can benefit from amplification. Contraindications for MEI are central or retrocochlear auditory disorders and chronic and active otitis media.

Patients with sensorineural hearing loss considered for VSB or MET should have mild to severe hearing impairment with stable air conduction thresholds and normal middle ear function confirmed by impedance measurements. Free-field audiometric tests in conventional HAs must prove that the patient is capable of benefiting from amplification. They must have speech understanding at least 50% in an open monosyllabic word test at the most comfortable level in headphones.

BONE CONDUCTION IMPLANTS – SURGICAL TECHNIQUE

Baha® Connect

The surgical procedure for Baha® Connect implantation has developed over the years since its introduction to clinical use in Poland in 2003. The approach presented below has been perfected based on a long time of observation of results obtained using different surgical techniques.

Presently, the surgery of Baha® Connect implantation comprises five steps, presented in Figure 5.1. First, the surgeon must measure the subcutaneous tissue thickness, select the optimum location for the titanium screw, and mark the incision. The incision should be located posterior to the pinna, in a straight line about 2–2.5 cm long. The next step is the incision and exposure of the surface of the temporal bone squama. Then, the surgeon drills a hole in the bone with a guide drill and widens it with a widening drill. The implant screw and the abutment are then placed in the temporal bone. Next, a hole is punched in the skin located over the abutment, and the skin flap eased over the abutment to close the wound. Finally, the wound is sutured and dressed, and a healing cap is applied to hold the abutment in place and protect it.

After surgery, the patient remains in the hospital for 2–3 days before discharge. The dressing and stitches can be removed 7–8 days after surgery as an outpatient procedure. The patient may experience pain in the area behind the ear for a few days after the surgery. It is a normal occurrence, and the pain will pass naturally. If needed, pain medicine may be administered.

The sound processor is fitted usually 4–5 weeks after the removal of stitches when the wound is sufficiently healed. The fitting is done in a clinic.

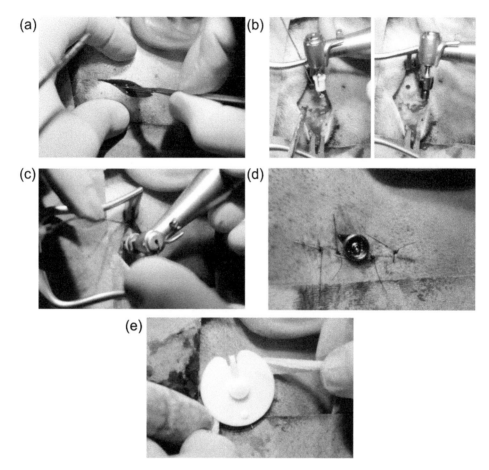

Figure 5.1 Surgical steps for the implantation of a titanium abutment for the Baha® Connect system: (a) incision of skin behind the pinna, about 2–2.5 cm long, to expose the surface of the temporal bone, (b) drilling a hole in the bone with guide drills, (c) screwing of the titanium implant into the temporal bone squama, (d) the abutment is eased through the skin flap and sutures applied, (e) placement of the healing cap.

In patients who have been correctly qualified for intervention according to the indications, complications are rare. As Baha Connect penetrates the skin, there is a possibility of dermatologic complications related to poor healing of a postoperative wound, although these are also infrequent.

Baha® Attract

Baha Attract is a relatively new solution increasingly popular among patients. It is a transcutaneous system, so it has cosmetic appeal and does not require daily cleaning

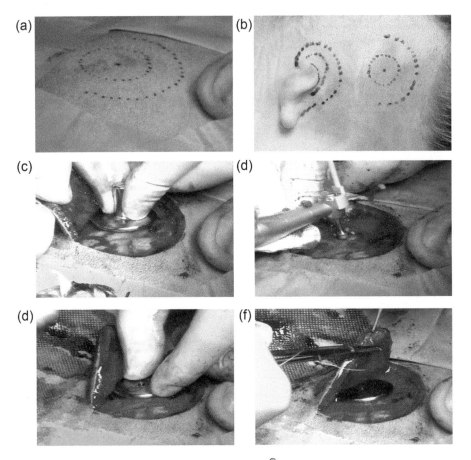

Figure 5.2 Surgical steps for implantation of the Baha® Attract system: (a) marking of the
location of skin incision and planned implant site behind the pinna, (b) if auricle
reconstruction is planned or in progress, the skin incision should be reversed
relative to the planned auricle, (c) exposing of the bone surface and locating
the optimum, possibly flat place for the implant magnet with the template,
(d) fixing of the titanium screw in the bone, (e) attaching the magnet plate
to the titanium screw, (f) closing of the periosteal flap over the implant and
suturing.

like Baha Connect. The surgical procedure is performed in six steps, which are presented in Figure 5.2.

The first step is to mark the site of skin incision and the area for placing the internal, implanted part of the device behind the auricle. The surgeon must also verify the
thickness of subcutaneous tissue, which for Baha Attract should not exceed 7 mm. If
auricle reconstruction is made or planned, the incision should be reversed in relation
to the future auricle.

Then, the surgeon makes the incision, exposes the surface of the temporal bone,
and identifies where the internal part of the implant is to be fixed. Next, the hole is
drilled using the guide and widening drills, and the titanium implant is screwed to the

bone. Then, the magnet plate is attached to the implant. Finally, the skin flap is placed back, and the wound is sutured and dressed.

The system can be activated about 4 weeks after surgery when the wound is sufficiently healed.

Osia® System

Osia System is a relatively new solution. In Poland, it has been for the first time implanted in the Institute of Physiology and Pathology of Hearing in 2018, and it had been one of the first countries that have introduced this system to clinical practice.

Osia is a transcutaneous implant using piezoelectric stimulation, unlike other bone conduction devices presented here that use electromagnetic stimulation.

The surgical procedure is shown in Figure 5.3. It is conducted in four basic steps. At the start, the surgeon must plan how to place the system's elements within the temporal bone. Next, the temporal bone surface is exposed, and a niche for the implant's inner part and the hole for the screw are drilled. Then, the implant elements are placed in the bone, the wound is sutured in layers, a drain is placed, and the wound is dressed.

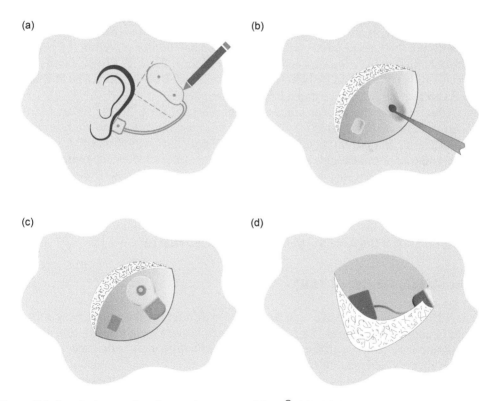

(a)

(b)

(c)

(d)

Figure 5.3 Surgical steps for the implantation of Osia® OSI100 System: (a) marking of the placement of all elements of the system in the temporal bone, (b) preparing of the implant niche and hole for the implant screw in the temporal bone, (c) fixing of the implant elements on the mastoid, (d) implants elements are placed, followed by suturing of the wound in layers and drain placement.

A drain should remain in place for at least 2–3 days. Sutures can be removed when the wound is sufficiently healed, usually 7–8 days later, in an outpatient procedure. About 6–8 weeks after surgery, the sound processor is fitted and activated.

Bonebridge System

The Bonebridge system comprises the implanted part and the external sound processor. The implanted part is the BCI that consists of the BC-FMT (bone conduction floating mass transducer) fixed in the hole in the temporal bone. There are two generations of BCI; the newer BCI 602 is thinner, requiring less drilling depth: 4.5 mm versus 8.7 mm in BCI 601. This bone bed can be even shallower, even as little as 3.5 mm, if using the specially designed BCI lifts.

The surgical procedure for implanting both models of BCI is similar. Succeeding steps are shown in Figure 5.4 and comprise the following actions. The first step involves marking the internal part's placement on the skin, then incising the skin behind the ear, and exposing the temporal bone's surface. Next, the surgeon must drill out a bony bed for the BCI, calibrated to the appropriate BCI 601 or BCI 602 template. The next step is preparing a periosteal pocket behind the ear for the coil and demodulator of the device's implantable part, using the template. The BCI is then fixed in the bony bed with provided bone screws and the coil and demodulator placed in the periosteal pocket. Note that the demodulator does not need to be fixed, as two screws fixing the BCI are sufficient to hold the whole implant in place. Finally, the surgical wound is closed and sutured in layers, and a dressing is applied.

After surgery, the patient remains in the hospital for 2–3 days for observation. Sutures can be removed after 7–8 days; it is an outpatient procedure. Pain in the area behind the ear is a normal occurrence and will pass naturally. If needed, pain medications may be administered. When the wound is sufficiently healed, about 4–5 weeks after sutures' removal, the speech processor may be fitted and activated. In patients who meet the criteria for implantation, complications occur very rarely.

MIDDLE EAR IMPLANTS – SURGICAL TECHNIQUE

Vibrant Soundbridge (VSB)

The Vibrant Soundbridge MEI can be applied in different middle and outer ear pathologies in adults and children. Its operating principle consists in transmitting amplified sound information through the vibrations of the floating mass transducer (FMT) to a preserved mobile element of the middle ear anatomy.

The classic solution has been fixation to the long process of the incus. Today, the FMT can be fixed, using various couplers, in the following ways:

- To a mobile element of the middle ear: incus, malleus, or stapes in cases of congenital malformations, the incomplete formation of the inner ear or underdeveloped middle ear;

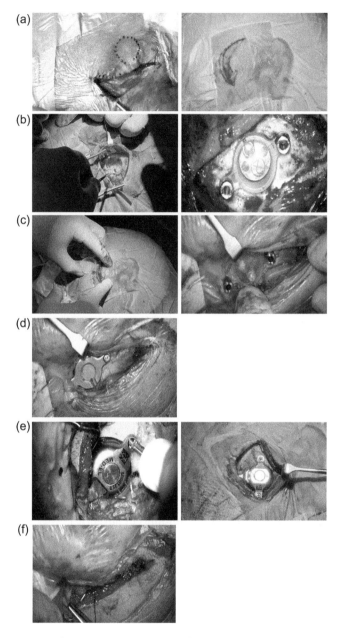

Figure 5.4 Surgical steps for the implantation of the internal part of the Bonebridge system – BCI: (a) planning the implant placement, skin incision, and exposure of the temporal bone surface, (b) drilling of the calibrated bed for the inner part of the implant according to the template, (c) preparing the periosteal pocket behind the ear, sized using the templates of the implant elements, (d) fixing of the implant element in the bone niche with screws, BCI 601 model, (e) fixing of the implant element in the bone niche with screws, BCI 602 model, (f) closing and suturing of the wound.

- To the mobile malleus or stapes after unsuccessful middle ear reconstruction surgeries (with couplers LP, SP, Bell, or Clip);
- To the incus, in cases of advanced otosclerosis, to reinforce the effects of stapedotomy (with coupler Symphonix or LP);
- To the mobile footplate of the stapes (coupler OW);
- To stimulate the round window membrane (without coupler, or RW or soft-RW couplers).

The surgical procedure for implanting the VSB with fixation to the ossicular chain's mobile elements comprises five steps, which are presented in Figure 5.5.

In the first step, the surgeon performs a retroauricular skin incision and elevates muscle and skin flap behind the pinna. The next step involves smoothing out the bone's surface and preparing the periosteal pocket for the implantable part of the implant. The surgeon then performs the limited conservative opening of the mastoid process and atticotomy or posterior tympanotomy to create access for vibroplasty. The surgeon then conducts the electrode from the implant's internal part and locks the coupler with titanium clamps to the middle ear's elected element. Finally, the implant's internal part is fixed with dedicated screws provided with the implant, and then, the wound is sutured in layers and dressing applied.

The patient remains in the hospital for 2–3 days after surgery. A visit to the clinic should be scheduled for 7–8 days after discharge to check the wound healing and remove sutures. Pain in the area behind the ear is a normal and passing occurrence; pain medication may be administered to relieve it.

The sound processor is fitted in a clinic about 4–5 weeks after removing stitches when the wound is healed.

Complications in patients who have been properly qualified according to the indications are rare.

VSB used in the round window stimulation

The FMT can be fixed in the round window niche to stimulate the round window membrane and transmit stimulation directly to the inner ear fluids. This solution is usually recommended in patients after radical middle ear surgeries.

Figure 5.6 shows the FMT round window placement options. The FMT may be placed on the round window membrane with a fragment of fascia between them, as proposed by Colletti et al. (2006). Later, Skarżyński has developed Colletti's idea to provide direct stimulation to the round window membrane in 2006 (Skarżyński et al. 2014c). The direct stimulation effects have proven to be better in the long term because it circumvents the problem of diminishing stimulation caused by gradual absorption of fascia placed between the FMT and the round window.

A crucial element of the procedure proposed by Skarżyński is preparation of the niche for the FMT to prevent its dislocation. This modification consists in a delicate reduction of the lateral lip of the round window niche with a diamond burr to optimize the FMT placement and ensure that it will be partially covered with a bony lip. The bed under the FMT should be evened out to provide good transmission of vibrations along the long axis of the FMT.

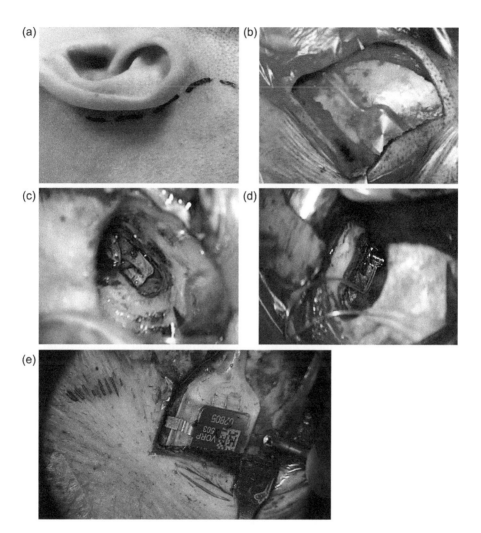

Figure 5.5 Surgical steps for the implantation of the Vibrant Soundbridge middle ear implant: (a) placement of the incision to lift the periosteal flap behind the pinna, (b) smoothing out of the bone surface and preparing the periosteal pocket for the implant elements, (c) limited conservative opening of the mastoid and atticotomy, or posterior tympanotomy to create good access to the long or short process of the incus, (d) laying of the electrode and crimping of the titanium coupler to the long or short process of the incus, (e) fixation of the implant with dedicated screws and closure of the wound with subcutaneous and skin sutures.

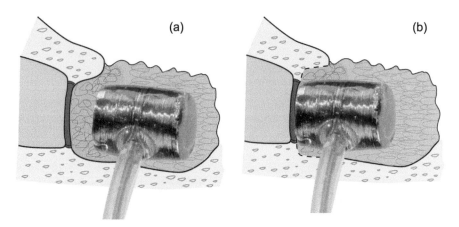

Figure 5.6 Stimulation of the round window membrane: (a) indirect according to Colletti, (b) direct according to Skarżyński.

Codacs® System

The Codacs implant comprises the implantable inner part fixed in the temporal bone, and a typical stapes prosthesis fitted on the vibrating rod and transmitting information directly to the inner ear fluids. A processor is placed behind an auricle together with a coil transmitting information through the skin to an implanted receiver.

Surgery for Codacs implantation is conducted in steps, which are shown in Figure 5.7. The first step is the S-shaped incision of the skin behind the pinna and exposure of the temporal bone surface. The second stage is a typical conservative antromastoidectomy and posterior tympanotomy to provide good visualization of the stapes suprastructure and footplate. Then, the surgeon must prepare the bed in the bone for the internal part of the implant. The implant is fastened in this bony bed with specially provided bone screws. Next, the stapes prosthesis is clamped to the actuator's rod and piston sealed with a clot of venal blood (Figure 5.7e shows the view from the external auditory meatus). Finally, the periosteal flap is placed back over the implanted device, sutured in layers, and dressed. If there was an additional approach made through the external auditory canal, packing should be applied inside the canal.

After surgery, the patient remains in the hospital for 2–3 days. A follow-up visit in a clinic should be scheduled 7–8 days later to check the wound healing and remove sutures. Pain in the area behind the ear is a normal occurrence. It will pass naturally after a few days. Pain relievers may be given as needed. The sound processor may be fitted and activated as soon as the wound is sufficiently healed, usually 4–5 weeks after removing sutures. Complications in patients who have been properly qualified for intervention according to the indications are rare.

MET®

The current generation (T2) MET MEI (Cochlear Ltd.) is a semi-implantable device consisting of an external audio processor and an internal implant – a coil, demodulator,

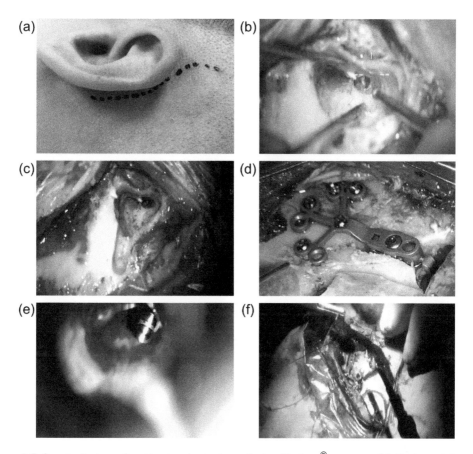

Figure 5.7 Surgical steps for the implantation of the Codacs® system: (a) S-shaped incision behind the pinna to expose the surface of the temporal bone squama,
(b) typical conservative antromastoidectomy and posterior tympanotomy with
good visualization of stapes suprastructure and footplate, (c) preparing of the
appropriate bone niche for good fixation of the internal part of the implant
in the bone, (d) fixing of the internal parts of the implant with bone screws,
(e) clamping of the stapes prosthesis to the actuator rod and sealing with the
clot of venal blood – seen from the direction of the external auditory meatus,
(f) covering of the implanted elements with periosteal flap and suturing in two
layers.

and an actuator that is fixed into the mastoid with a special bracket. In a typical application, the tip of the transducer is attached to the body of the incus.

Our clinical program of MET implants that started in 2014 has so far included
only classical cases of stimulation applied to the incus's body. In our program, the surgical procedure of MET implantation comprises six surgical steps, which are shown
in Figure 5.8.

First, the operating surgeon makes a C-shaped skin incision behind the pinna to
expose the temporal bone's surface. Then, he performs a typical conservative antromastoidotomy within limits set with the template. Good visualization of the short

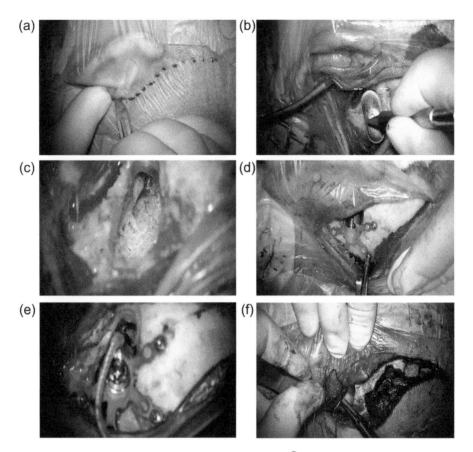

Figure 5.8 Surgical steps for the implantation of the MET® system: (a) C-shaped skin incision to expose the temporal bone surface, (b) typical conservative antromastoidectomy within the borders set using the template, (c) good visualization of the short process and body of the incus, depending on the pathology; in this step, it may be necessary to perform the posterior tympanotomy to visualize the stapes, stapes footplate, or the round window membrane, (d) preparation of the bone surface and fixing of the implant with dedicated bone screws, (e) verification of the positioning and final fastening of the actuator that directly stimulates the incus, (f) closing and suturing of the wound in two layers.

process and body of the incus is essential. Depending on the pathology, it may be necessary to perform also the posterior tympanotomy to visualize the stapes, stapes footplate, or the round window membrane. The next step involves preparing the bone's surface and fixing the implant's internal part with bone screws. The surgeon must then verify the placement and fix the actuator's rod to the incus's body. The last step is to suture the subcutaneous layer and skin to close the surgical wound and apply the dressing.

The patient remains in the hospital for 2–3 days after surgery. Sutures can be removed about 7–8 days later, in an outpatient setting. Pain in the area behind the ear is a normal occurrence and will pass naturally after a few days. Pain relievers may be given as needed.

The sound processor is fitted when the wound is sufficiently healed, typically 4–5 weeks after removing sutures. In patients who have been properly qualified for intervention according to the indications, complications are seldom encountered.

CONCLUSIONS

Our otosurgical program has been in place for nearly 20 years so far and encompassed a wide range of hearing implants. We have gained extensive surgical experience and follow-up results in an extended observation period. In the course of the program, new target groups of patients have been identified, adults as well as children, and indications for the application of bone conduction and MEIs have been expanded.

Application of a bone conduction or a MEI should always be preceded by a simulation trial to confirm that patient's benefit after implantation will be better than with classic HAs.

Our patients' results to date, with different types of hearing implants, prove that stable and satisfactory results are obtainable in different groups of patients under the condition of following all implantation criteria and indications.

Chapter 6

Hearing preservation classification according to Skarżyński et al. (2013)

Henryk Skarżyński, Artur Lorens and Piotr H. Skarżyński
Institute of Physiology and pathology of Hearing

CONTENTS

INTRODUCTION

Insertion of an electrode into the cochlea usually causes a certain degree of trauma to delicate cochlear structures (electrode insertion trauma, EIT), which may activate hair cell and ganglion cell death mechanisms, including necrosis and apoptosis. Damage to the inner ear's cochlear structures may lead to the degeneration of neural tissue and the reduction of the number of neural elements. A sufficient number of intact neural elements is crucial for a cochlear implant to provide good speech discrimination. It is generally assumed that the amount of EIT correlates with the level of postoperative hearing preservation (HP). Thus, the extent of HP is believed to serve as a good indicator of EIT's magnitude. Therefore, HP has become a standard cochlear implant surgical approach among the whole cochlear implant patient group, regardless of preoperative residual hearing level.

With an increasingly higher number of cochlear implant patients with preserved hearing, there is a need for a HP classification tool. There have been several attempts to classify HP after cochlear implantation. However, none of these schemes was independent of the initial hearing level, and classifications were suitable only for a limited group of subjects. Moreover, none of the existing classification schemes recognizes that HP in patients with substantial preoperative hearing is more valuable than in patients with poorer residual hearing.

The presence of these multiple systems has made it difficult to compare different studies' results. If a standard method is used, the reporting of surgical and device intervention results will improve, facilitating comparison studies and meta-analysis of results. The latter is particularly important in the hearing implant field, where conducting randomized, controlled double-blinded studies is impossible. The sample sizes are often small (usually ranging from case studies to small groups of 10–20 subjects), and the use of different HP classification systems handicaps a meta-analysis. A meta-analysis of data using the same HP classification system would allow us to pool data

DOI: 10.1201/9781003164876-6

for more potent evidence-based medicine. Consequently, we would be better able to support health technology assessment for reimbursement.

HEARRING GROUP HP CLASSIFICATION SYSTEM

A uniform HP classification aims to have a reliable method of classifying possible postoperative hearing loss in patients between different CI clinics and centers.

To remedy the current lack of an accepted HP classification standard, in 2013, on the initiative of Henryk Skarżyński, the Hearring group proposed a comprehensive HP Classification System that (1) is suitable for reporting the HP results of all HP surgery cases, (2) is independent of the user's preoperative hearing levels, and (3) considers the relative change of hearing thresholds (Skarżyński et al. 2013). The system classifies HP when using an intervention system which comprises all elements of surgery (round window, cochleostomy, drugs used, blood contamination, etc.), the electrode itself (contacts, atraumaticity, length, coated or not), trauma due to the electrode and the surgery, as well as the fact that the electrode is a space filler.

The Hearring group hopes clinicians put this system into practice not only because it clearly and accurately describes HP results but because the system will enable a more extensive overview of hearing and structural preservation. By making the results of different HP studies more comparable, the application of our standard will allow better meta-analysis of data, thereby resulting in better evidence-based practice in the field of cochlear implantation.

The classification uses the calculation of relative change of the mean hearing thresholds in relation to the primary value (preoperative):

$$\text{Relative change} = (PTApost - PTApre)/(PTAmax - PTApre)$$

where

PTApost is the pure tone average measured postoperatively
PTApre is the pure tone average measured preoperatively
PTAmax is the limit of the audiometer.

The equation presents the relative change as a percentage of hearing loss. The hearing loss is converted to preservation (PS) by calculating 100% – relative change in %:

$$PS = (1 - \text{relative change}) \times 100\%$$

Based on the PS percentage indicator, we determine the categorical scale of HP (Table 6.1).

The HP classification system is based on a routine audiogram. The selection of frequency for pure tone average determination is based on ASHA guidelines as they are the most commonly used of the several audiometric procedure standards. Hearing threshold levels should be obtained at octave intervals from 125–8,000 Hz. In addition, the implementation of inter-octave frequencies is recommended and provides a more

Table 6.1 Proposed HP classification scale

Preservation numerical scale	Categorical scale
100%–75%	Complete HP
75%–25%	Partial HP
<25%	Minimal HP
No measurable hearing	Loss of hearing

Table 6.2 Maximal detectable hearing measurable for each frequency

Frequency (Hz)	125	250	500	750	1k	1.5k	2k	3k	4k	6k	8k
Acoustic pressure levels HL (dB)	90	105	110	120	120	120	120	120	115	100	95

complete and accurate hearing profile. Missing inter-octaves are automatically inter-polated in the formula sheet https://www.hearring.com/hearring-tools.

The hearing threshold levels range from –10 to 120 dB HL, again based on the ASHA recommendation. However, one must consider the maximum output levels of the audiometer in the equation. The levels selected to fit the equation for all clinically available audiometers are presented in Table 6.2.

CONCLUSIONS

The practical advantages of the uniform HP classification system are:

- Availability of the system that enables retrospective and prospective observation and categorization of the degree of HP in particular clinics; graphic presentation of the results facilitates monitoring and comparison of changes in HP in various time intervals;
- Opportunity to conduct extensive research on large populations by integrating multiple results from numerous clinics; the multicenter data can be used for corre-lation analyses and constitute the basis for statistical inference.

The Hearring Group recommends using a HP classification system in clinical prac-tice because it describes the results of HP clearly and transparently and because its widespread use will enable the review of structural hearing preservation results from multiple clinics. The use of the proposed standard will create conditions for comparing the results of different clinical studies on hearing preservation after cochlear implan-tation. This, in turn, will enable meta-analyses to be carried out and   thus con-tribute to increasing knowledge in the practice of evidence-based medicine in the field of cochlear implants.

Chapter 7

Review of clinical material presented during demonstration surgeries

Piotr H. Skarżyński, Beata Dziendziel, Elżbieta Włodarczyk and Henryk Skarżyński
Institute of Physiology and Pathology of Hearing

CONTENTS

DOI: 10.1201/9781003164876-7

A. CHILDREN AGED 0–9 YEARS

I. Girl, II months – cochlear implant

Born at 42 weeks, cesarean section, first pregnancy. Apgar score 10, birth mass 3,450 g. A risk of birth asphyxia due to the poor progress of labor. Newborn hearing screening test result: bilaterally abnormal. First auditory brainstem response (ABR) test performed at 3 months of age: bilaterally no response for 0.5, 1 kHz, and for click (Figure 7.1.1).

Right ear		Left ear	
0,5 kHz	90 dB	0,5 kHz	95 dB
1 kHz	100 dB	1 kHz	100 dB
2 kHz	100 dB	2 kHz	95 dB
4 kHz	no response	4 kHz	95 dB

Figure 7.1.1 Auditory brainstem response (ABR).

CI right ear, Med-El CONCERTO FLEX28™ electrode

2. Boy, 12 months – cochlear implant

Born at 26 weeks, second pregnancy, cesarean section – premature birth, *breech* presentation. Apgar score 7, birth mass 910 g. Pregnancy complicated by premature rupture of membranes, urinary tract infection after swimming in a pool. Neonatal period – congenital pneumonia, necrotizing enterocolitis on the second day after birth, ototoxic drugs administration. Hearing screening test results – bilaterally normal. The first ABR test at 7 months of age: bilaterally 100 dB for click. Last ABR test at 8 months of age: right ear 100/90/80/75, left ear 85/80/70/70. Hearing aids since the age of 9 months, but with no good auditory results. Motor development: delayed (Figure 7.2.1).

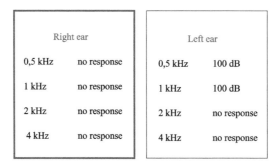

Right ear		Left ear	
0,5 kHz	no response	0,5 kHz	100 dB
1 kHz	no response	1 kHz	100 dB
2 kHz	no response	2 kHz	no response
4 kHz	no response	4 kHz	no response

Figure 7.2.1 Auditory brainstem response (ABR).

CI right ear, Med-El SYNCHRONY Standard electrode

3. Girl, 16 months – cochlear implant

Born at 38 weeks, cesarean section – breech presentation, first pregnancy. Apgar score 9, birth mass 3,280 g. Newborn hearing screening test result: abnormal in the right ear. First ABR test performed at 7 months of age: right ear 70 dB, left ear 20 dB for a click. The last ABR test performed at 9 months of age: no response for click in the right ear, left ear 20 dB (Figure 7.3.1).

Right ear		Left ear	
0,5 kHz	90 dB	0,5 kHz	40 dB
1 kHz	100 dB	1 kHz	20 dB
2 kHz	no response	2 kHz	20 dB
4 kHz	no response	4 kHz	20 dB

Figure 7.3.1 Auditory brainstem response (ABR).

CI right ear, Med-El SONATA FLEX28™ electrode

4. Boy, 2 years – cochlear implant

Born at 39 weeks, natural birth, first pregnancy. Apgar score 10, birth mass 3,280 g. Pregnancy and neonatal period without complications. Newborn hearing screening test result: bilaterally abnormal. First ABR test performed at 6 months of age: right ear 50 dB for click, left ear 95 dB for a click. Hearing aids since the age of 7 months. Motor development: delayed (Figure 7.4.1).

Right ear		Left ear	
0,5 kHz	50 dB	0,5 kHz	80 dB
1 kHz	40 dB	1 kHz	90 dB
2 kHz	40 dB	2 kHz	no response
4 kHz	30 dB	4 kHz	no response

Figure 7.4.1 Auditory brainstem response (ABR).

CI left ear, Med-El COCNCERTO FLEX28™ electrode

5. Girl, 2 years – cochlear implant

Born at 40 weeks, natural birth. Apgar score 10, birth mass 3,640 g. Pregnancy and neonatal period with no complications. Neonatal hearing screening test results normal. Hearing loss was noticed when the child was 4–5 months old, confirmed by ASSR (Auditory Steady-State Responses) and ABR tests at 6 months. In the medical history of hearing disorder: episodes of otitis with effusion – ventilation tube treatment. She had left-ear cochlear implantation (synchrony). The implant was activated when she was 13 months old. Hearing aid in the right ear used regularly. Head imaging: MRI – visible Arnold-Chiari malformation type 1, without pathology in the area of the VII and VIII cranial nerve (Figure 7.5.1).

Right ear		Left ear	
0,5 kHz	80 dB	0,5 kHz	70 dB
1 kHz	90 dB	1 kHz	80 dB
2 kHz	100 dB	2 kHz	no response
4 kHz	no response	4 kHz	no response

Figure 7.5.1 Auditory brainstem response (ABR).

Second CI, right ear, Med-El SYNCHRONY Standard electrode

6. Boy, 5 years – cochlear implant

Profound congenital bilateral sensorineural genetic hearing loss. Hearing aids: in both ears since 5 months of age. Due to profound hearing loss and the lack of rehabilitation progress, the patient was implanted in the right ear at the age of 12 months. Subjectively worse hearing in the right ear. Speech and auditory development after the first implantation: correct in view of the patient's age. Head imaging: MRI – no abnormalities (Figure 7.6.1).

Right ear		Left ear	
0,5 kHz	90 dB	0,5 kHz	80 dB
1 kHz	no response	1 kHz	90 dB
2 kHz	no response	2 kHz	100 dB
4 kHz	no response	4 kHz	no response

Figure 7.6.1 Auditory brainstem response (ABR).

CI left ear, Med-El CONCERTO FLEX28™ electrode

7. Boy, 7 years – cochlear implant

Born at 26 weeks, natural birth. Apgar score 6, birth mass 900 g. Neonatal period – resuscitation, intubation, respirator, placed in an incubator, intraventricular bleeding, chronic lung disease. Newborn hearing screening test result: bilaterally abnormal. ABR test: 90 dB thresholds bilaterally for a click. Hearing aids: used regularly since the age of 4. Before that, he had used hearing aids, but only occasionally. Hearing responses in hearing aids only to loud sounds. Congenital defects: microcephaly. The patient is fed through a gastric feeding tube (Figures 7.7.1–7.7.5).

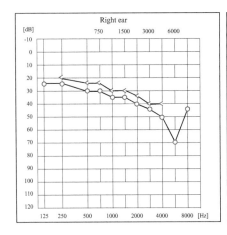
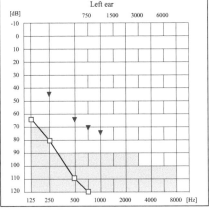

Figure 7.7.1 Preoperative pure-tone audiometry.

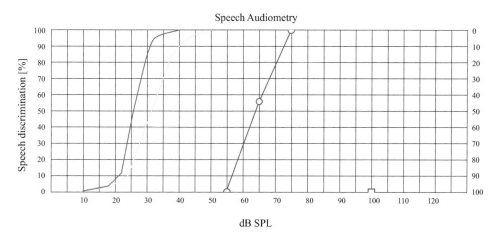

Figure 7.7.2 **Preoperative speech audiometry.**

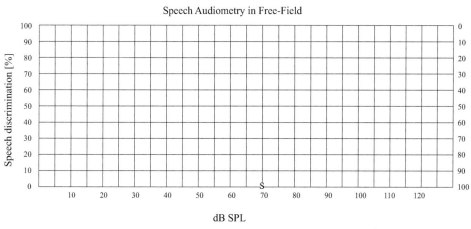

LEGEND:
S – left ear in hearing aid, right ear in passive masking

Figure 7.7.3 **Preoperative speech audiometry in free-field.**

PDT-ES, CI left ear, HiRes 90K™ Advantage C, Advanced Bionics electrode

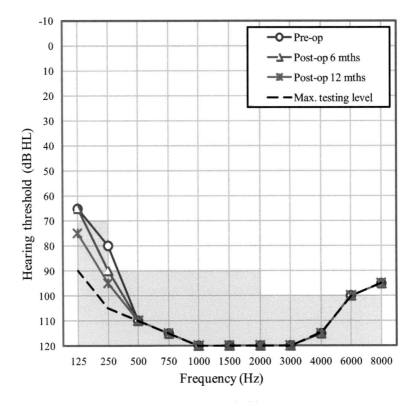

Figure 7.7.4 Pre- and postoperative hearing thresholds.

Hearing Preservation, Calculation in [%]			
Legend:		Follow-up	
S	Hearing Preservation	6 months	12 months
75-100%	Complete HP	S=80.0%	S=50.0%
26-74%	Partial HP		
1-25%	Minimal HP		
No detectable hearing	Loss of hearing		

Figure 7.7.5 Hearing preservation results.

8. Boy, 9 years – cochlear implant

Born at 40 weeks, natural birth. Apgar score 10, birth mass 2,500 g. Newborn hearing screening test result: bilaterally normal. Hearing loss diagnosed at the age of 6. Hearing aids: bilaterally since the age of 6. He has big problems with speech understanding (Figures 7.8.1–7.8.5).

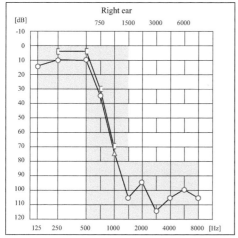
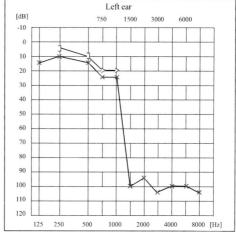

Figure 7.8.1 **Preoperative pure-tone audiometry.**

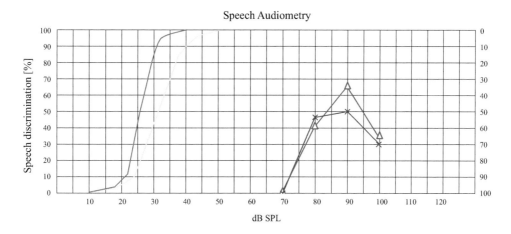

Figure 7.8.2 **Preoperative speech audiometry.**

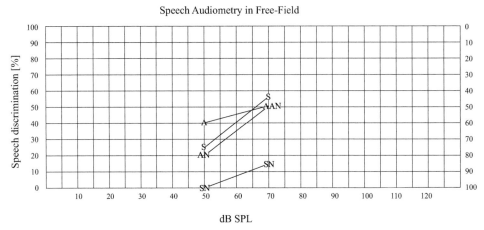

LEGEND:
A – right ear in hearing aid, left ear in passive masking
S – left ear in hearing aid, right ear in passive masking
AN – right ear in hearing aid, SNR + 10 dB, left ear in passive masking
SN – left ear in hearing aid, SNR + 10 dB, right ear in passive masking

Figure 7.8.3 Preoperative speech audiometry in free-field.

PDT-EC (from 500 Hz), CI right ear, Med-El CONCERTO FLEX24™ electrode

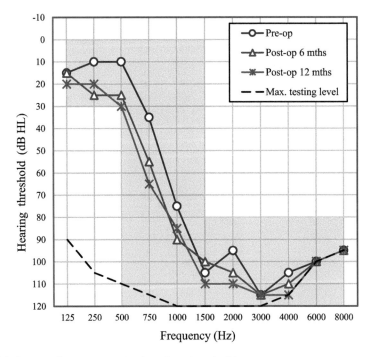

Figure 7.8.4 Pre- and postoperative hearing thresholds.

Hearing Preservation, Calculation in [%]			
Legend:		Follow-up	
S	Hearing Preservation	6 months	12 months
75 – 100%	Complete HP		
26 – 74%	Partial HP	S = 83.3%	S = 76.7%
1 – 25%	Minimal HP		
No detectable hearing	Loss of hearing		

Figure 7.8.5 Hearing preservation results.

9. Girl, 9 years – cochlear implant

Born at 40 weeks, cesarean section due to the risk of asphyxia. Apgar score 9, birth mass 3,065 g. Pregnancy and the neonatal period without complications. Newborn hearing screening test result: bilaterally abnormal. ABR test at the age of 8 months: right ear 70 dB, left ear 60 dB for click. Hearing aids: bilateral since the age of 3. Communicates verbally, speech is relatively well developed (Figures 7.9.1–7.9.5).

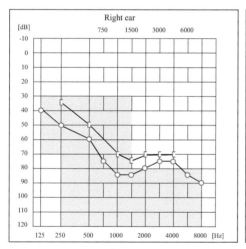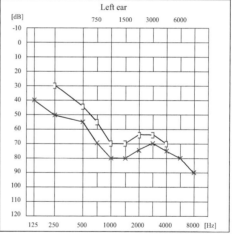

Figure 7.9.1 Preoperative pure-tone audiometry.

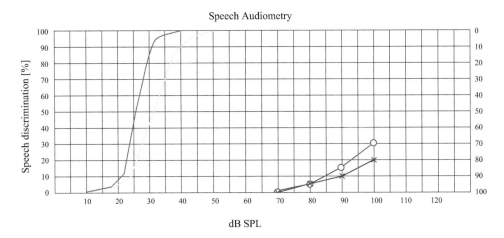

Figure 7.9.2 **Preoperative speech audiometry.**

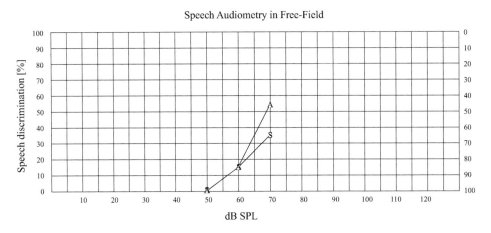

LEGEND:
A – right ear in hearing aid, left ear in passive masking
S – left ear in hearing aid, right ear in passive masking

Figure 7.9.3 **Preoperative speech audiometry in free-field.**

PDT-EAS, CI right ear, Med-El CONCERTO FLEX24™ electrode

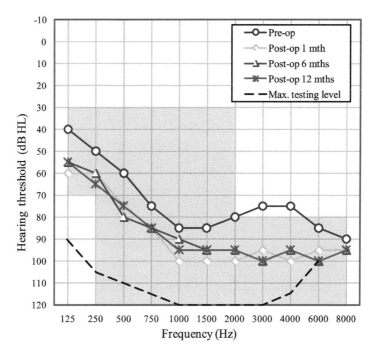

Figure 7.9.4 Pre- and postoperative hearing thresholds.

Hearing Preservation, Calculation in [%]				
Legend:		**Follow-up**		
S	**Hearing Preservation**	**1 month**	**6 months**	**12 months**
75 – 100%	Complete HP			
26 – 74%	Partial HP	S = 59.8%	S = 63.4%	S = 62.2%
1 – 25%	Minimal HP			
No detectable hearing	Loss of hearing			

Figure 7.9.5 Hearing preservation results.

10. Girl, 9 years – cochlear implant

She has a cochlear implant in the right ear (Med-El), activated when she was 7 years old. Hearing aid in the left ear used irregularly since the implantation. Cause of hearing loss: neuroblastoma treated with cisplatin when she was 1.5 years old. Parents observed significant progress in her auditory development after the first cochlear implantation (Figures 7.10.1–7.10.5).

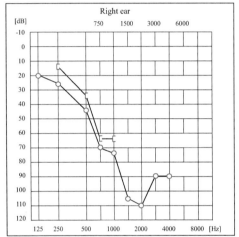 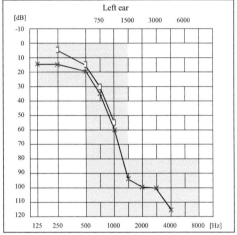

Figure 7.10.1 **Preoperative pure-tone audiometry.**

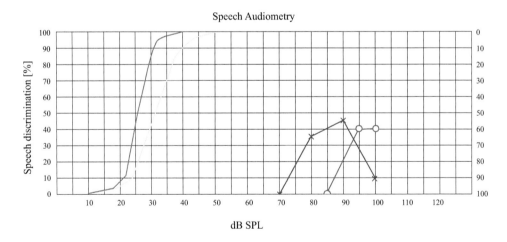

Figure 7.10.2 **Preoperative speech audiometry.**

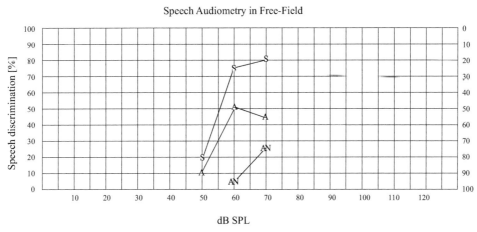

LEGEND:
S – right ear in hearing aid, left ear in passive masking
A – left ear in hearing aid, right ear in passive masking
AN – left ear in hearing aid, SNR + 10 dB, right ear in passive masking

Figure 7.10.3 Preoperative speech audiometry in free-field.

Second CI PDT-EC (from 500 Hz), CI left ear, Med-El SONATA FLEX20 electrode

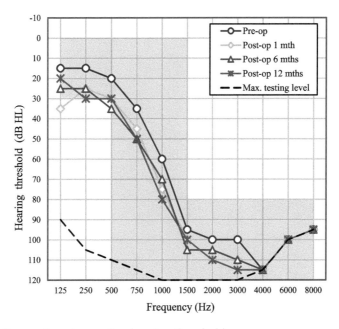

Figure 7.10.4 Pre- and postoperative hearing thresholds.

Hearing Preservation, Calculation in [%]					
Legend:		Follow-up			
S	Hearing Preservation	1 month	6 months	12 months
75 – 100%	Complete HP	S = 80.4%	S = 81.5%	S = 79.3%
26 – 74%	Partial HP			
1 – 25%	Minimal HP			
No detectable hearing	Loss of hearing			

Figure 7.10.5 Hearing preservation results.

B. CHILDREN AND YOUNG PEOPLE AGED 10–18 YEARS

11. Boy, 10 years – cochlear implant

Born at 37 weeks, natural birth. Apgar score 3–4–7–8, birth weight 2,240 g. Newborn hearing screening test result: normal. The neonatal period – pneumonia treated, among others, by Biodacin. Delayed motor development, cerebral palsy, began to walk at the age of 2. Hearing loss was noticed and confirmed by pure-tone audiometry at the age of 8. He has been using hearing aids since the age of 9, with a noticeable progress in auditory responses. Head imaging: MRI – visible periventricular leukomalacia associated with intrapartum hypoxia and ischemia; TK – no pathologies (Figures 7.11.1–7.11.5).

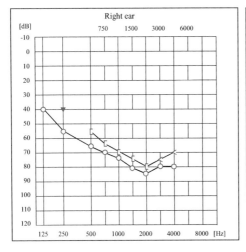 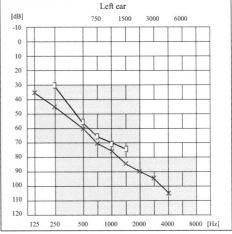

Figure 7.11.1 Preoperative pure-tone audiometry.

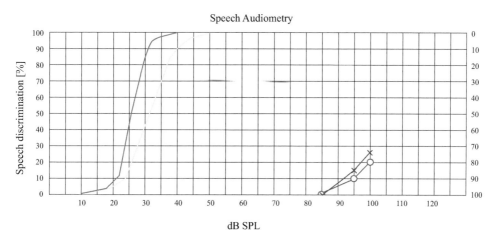

Figure 7.11.2 **Preoperative speech audiometry.**

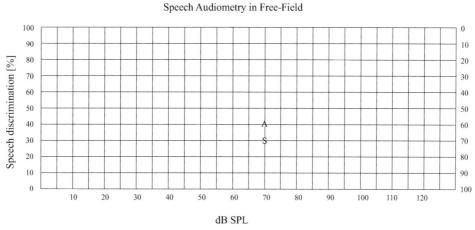

LEGEND:
A – right ear in hearing aid, left ear in passive masking
S – left ear in hearing aid, right ear in passive masking

Figure 7.11.3 **Preoperative speech audiometry in free-field.**

PDT-EAS, CI left ear, Med-El CONCERTO FLEX24™

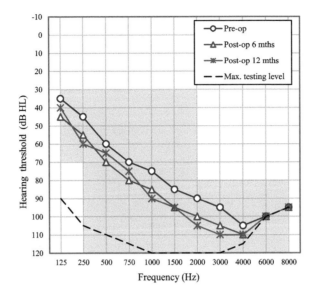

Figure 7.11.4 Pre- and postoperative hearing thresholds.

Hearing Preservation, Calculation in [%]			
Legend:		**Follow-up**	
S	**Hearing Preservation**	**6 months**	**12 months**
75 – 100%	Complete HP		
26 – 74%	Partial HP	S = 76.1%	S = 74.6%
1 – 25%	Minimal HP		
No detectable hearing	Loss of hearing		

Figure 7.11.5 Hearing preservation results.

12. Boy, 11 years – cochlear implant

Born at 41 weeks, cesarean section due to a risk of birth asphyxia, Apgar score of 9–10, birth weight of 2,500 g. Dysmorphia was diagnosed after birth, genetic tests performed, Hirschsprung's disease diagnosed. Newborn hearing screening test result: abnormal. Hearing loss was confirmed at the age of 3 months by the ABR test. Hearing aids: uses regularly on both sides since the age of 4 months. Motor development: delayed, he began to walk when he was 2.5 years old, and he is still undergoing rehabilitation. Other diseases: lactose and fructose intolerance, allergy, mild mental retardation (Figures 7.12.1–7.12.5).

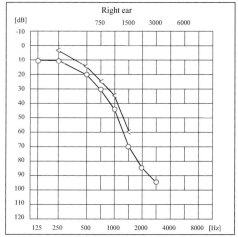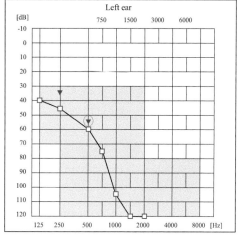

Figure 7.12.1 Preoperative pure-tone audiometry.

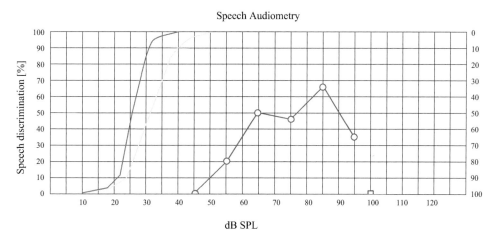

Figure 7.12.2 Preoperative speech audiometry.

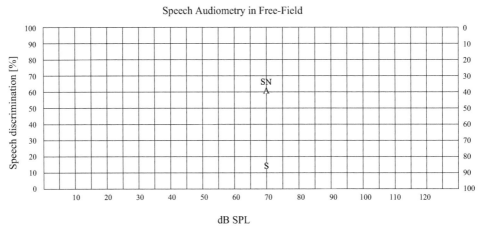

LEGEND:
A – right ear in hearing aid, left ear in passive masking
S – left ear in hearing aid, right ear in passive masking
SN – right and left ear in hearing aid

Figure 7.12.3 **Preoperative speech audiometry in free-field.**

PDT-EAS, CI left ear, Advanced Bionics HiFocus™ SlimJ

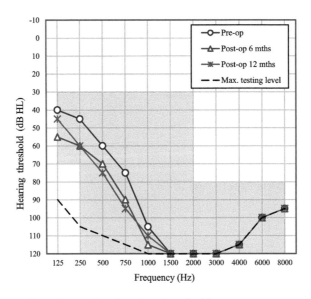

Figure 7.12.4 **Pre- and postoperative hearing thresholds.**

Hearing Preservation, Calculation in [%]			
Legend:		Follow-up	
S	Hearing Preservation	6 months	12 months
75 – 100%	Complete HP	S = 69.8%	S = 72.1%
26 – 74%	Partial HP		
1 – 25%	Minimal HP		
No detectable hearing	Loss of hearing		

Figure 7.12.5 Hearing preservation results.

13. Girl, 12 years – cochlear implant

Cochlear implant user in left ear since the age of 4. Since implantation, significant progress in auditory and speech development. She rejected using the hearing aid on the right ear approximately 2 years after implantation. Chronic diseases: sight defect, neonatal brachial plexus palsy (right-sided). Head imaging: CT – no pathologies (Figures 7.13.1–7.13.5).

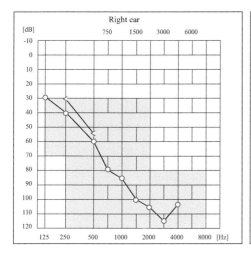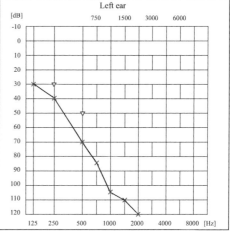

Figure 7.13.1 Preoperative pure-tone audiometry.

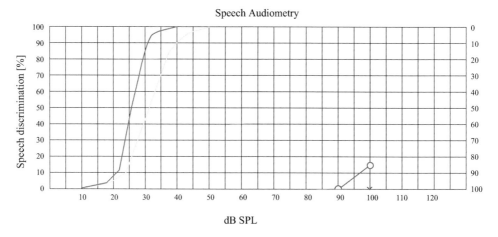

Figure 7.13.2 **Preoperative speech audiometry.**

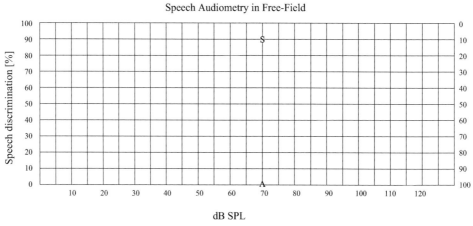

LEGEND:
A – right ear in hearing aid, left ear in passive masking
S – left ear in cochlear implant, right ear in passive masking

Figure 7.13.3 **Preoperative speech audiometry in free-field.**

PDT-EAS, second CI, right ear, Med-El CONCERTO FLEX24™

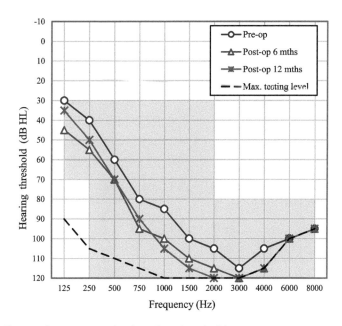

Figure 7.13.4 Pre- and postoperative hearing thresholds.

Hearing Preservation, Calculation in [%]			
Legend:		Follow-up	
S	Hearing Preservation	6 months	12 months
75 – 100%	Complete HP		
26 – 74%	Partial HP	S = 64.4%	S = 66.1%
1 – 25%	Minimal HP		
No detectable hearing	Loss of hearing		

Figure 7.13.5 Hearing preservation results.

14. Girl, 14 years – bone conduction implant

Congenital malformation of the right outer ear in the form of microtia and atresia. The patient did not decide to undergo auricular reconstruction. Head imaging: CT of the temporal bone – anatomical conditions enable Bonebridge (BB) implantation in the right ear with the use of lifts (Figures 7.14.1–7.14.4).

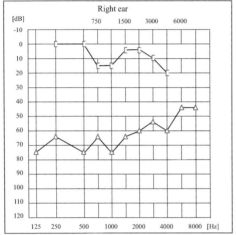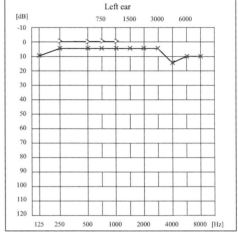

Figure 7.14.1 **Preoperative pure-tone audiometry.**

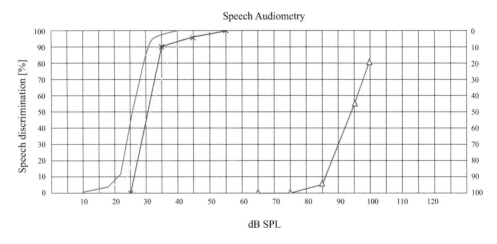

Figure 7.14.2 **Preoperative speech audiometry.**

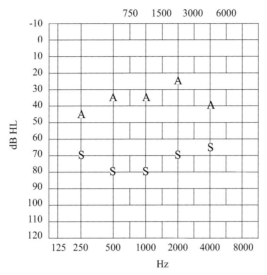

Pure-Tone Audiometry in Free-Field

LEGEND:

A – implant (contralateral ear actinely masked)

S – implant (contralateral ear actinely masked)

Figure 7.14.3 Pure-tone audiometry in a free-field for aided (A) and unaided (S) conditions after 3-month follow-up.

Med-El Bonebridge (BB) BCI602, right ear

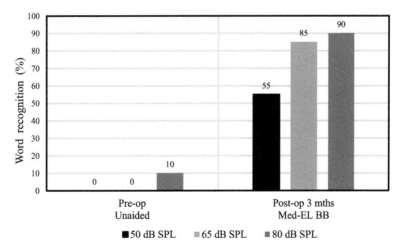

Figure 7.14.4 Word recognition score unaided and aided in quiet at 50, 65, and 80 dB SPL after 3-month follow-up. Non-implanted ear in active masking.

15. Boy, 16 years – cochlear implant

Hearing loss since the age of 2 due to meningitis. Right-ear cochlear implantation at the age of 7. Since the age of 2, he used a hearing aid on the left ear, but he stopped using it 1 year after implantation. Head imaging: CT – no pathologies (Figures 7.15.1–7.15.5).

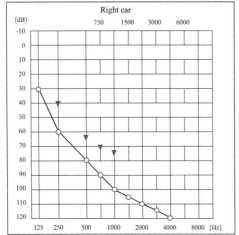 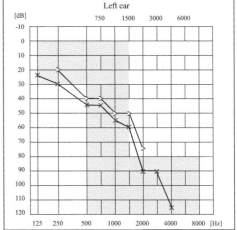

Figure 7.15.1 **Preoperative pure-tone audiometry.**

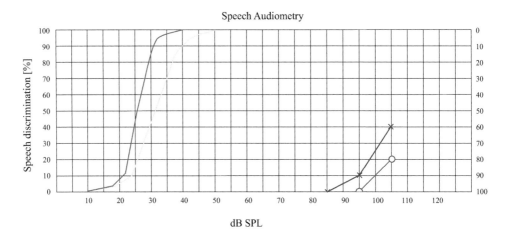

Figure 7.15.2 **Preoperative speech audiometry.**

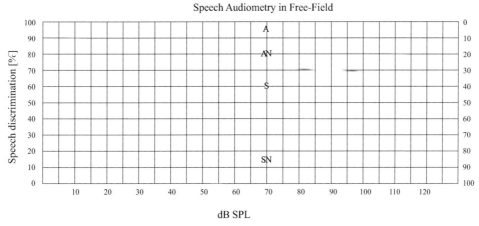

Figure 7.15.3 Preoperative speech audiometry in free-field.

PDT-EC (up to 250 Hz), second CI, left ear, Med-El SONATA FLEX24™

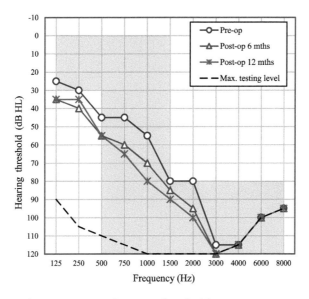

Figure 7.15.4 Pre- and postoperative hearing thresholds.

Hearing Preservation, Calculation in [%]			
Legend:		**Follow-up**	
S	**Hearing Preservation**	**6 months**	**12 months**
75 – 100%	Complete HP		
26 – 74%	Partial HP	**S = 80.0%**	**S = 75.3%**
1 – 25%	Minimal HP		
No detectable hearing	Loss of hearing		

Figure 7.15.5 Hearing preservation results.

16. Boy, 16 years – bone conduction implant

Congenital malformation of the outer and middle ear on the right side. Head imaging – CT, right side – mastoid cells are pneumatized; bony external ear canal narrow on its entire length (smallest cross-section about 1.7 × 3.2 mm), mostly filled with soft tissue; middle-ear cavities aerated; hypoplastic head of the malleus, in its inferior part, adhering to the body of the incus; absent manubrium of the malleus; long process of the incus shortened and deformed; stapes developed, in the typical location; bony labyrinth normal; mastoid part of the facial nerve channel displaced anteriorly by 3–5 mm; also the first segment of its tympanic part protrudes a little into the tympanic cavity. Due to the location of the sigmoid sinus, marginal anatomical conditions for BB implantation are kept if the 2 mm lift is used. Left side – no abnormalities (Figures 7.16.1–7.16.4).

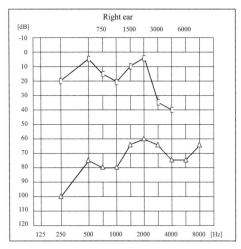 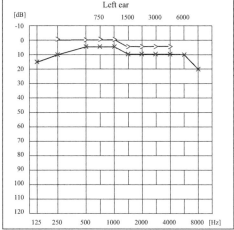

Figure 7.16.1 Preoperative pure-tone audiometry.

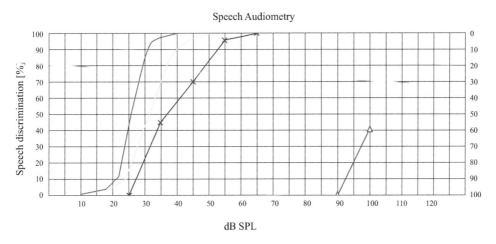

Figure 7.16.2 Preoperative speech audiometry.

Implant Med-El Bonebridge (BB) BCI601, right ear

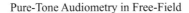

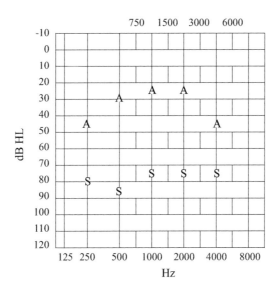

LEGEND:

A – implant (contralateral ear actinely masked)

S – unaided (contralateral ear actinely masked)

Figure 7.16.3 Pure-tone audiometry in a free-field for aided (A) and unaided (S) conditions after 12-month follow-up.

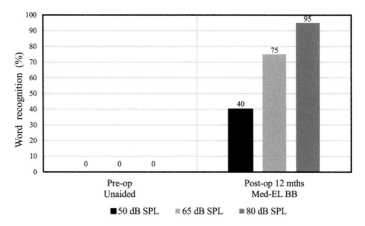

Figure 7.16.4 Word recognition score for unaided and aided conditions in quiet at 50, 65, and 80 dB SPL after 12-month follow-up. Non-implanted ear in passive masking.

17. Boy, 16 years – bone conduction implant

Bilateral congenital ear malformation – microtia with atresia. Baha implanted on the right side at the age of 6. Recurrent inflammations around the abutment. He underwent a three-stage functional reconstruction of the left auricle. Head imaging: CT of left temporal bone – bony labyrinth within anatomical norm; mastoid relatively small, built of diploë; round and oval window present; middle ear aerated, significantly smaller hypo- and mesotympanum; malformed ossicular chain: stapes present, not connected to the rest of the ossicles, incus and malleus dysplastic, fixed to one another and the lateral wall; facial nerve displaced inferiorly in the tympanic segment, anteriorly by 3 mm in the mastoid segment, otherwise typical topography; no external auditory canal; middle cranial fossa deepened, sigmoid sinus displaced laterally (Figures 7.17.1–7.17.4).

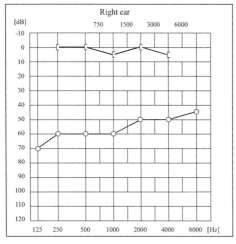
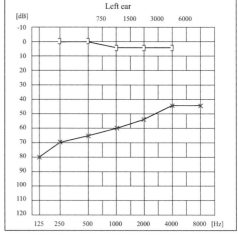

Figure 7.17.1 Preoperative pure-tone audiometry.

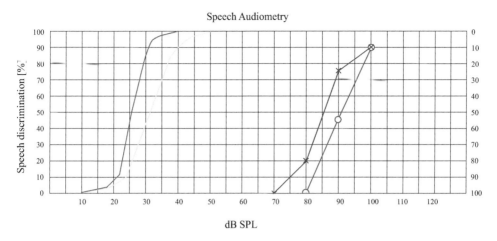

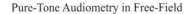

Figure 7.17.2 Preoperative speech audiometry.

Second implant, Cochlear Baha® Attract, left ear

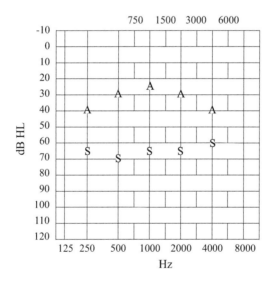

LEGEND:

A – implant (contralateral ear passively masked)

S – unaided (contralateral ear passively masked)

Figure 7.17.3 Pure-tone audiometry in a free-field for aided (A) and unaided (S) conditions after 12-month follow-up.

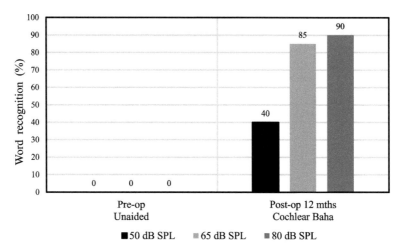

Figure 7.17.4 Word recognition score for unaided and aided conditions in quiet at 50, 65, and 80 dB SPL after 12-month follow-up. Non-implanted ear in passive masking.

18. Boy, 16 years – cochlear implant

Bilateral prelingual hearing loss, probably due to an ototoxic drug (gentamicin) administered shortly after birth. Hearing aids – bilaterally but not used due to the lack of hearing benefits. Head imaging: CT – no pathologies (Figures 7.18.1–7.18.5).

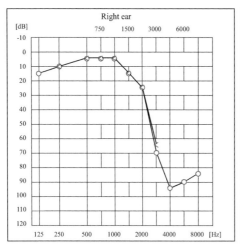
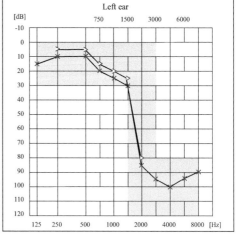

Figure 7.18.1 Preoperative pure-tone audiometry.

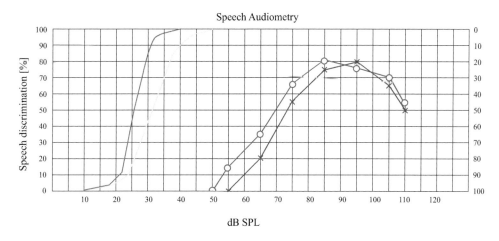

Figure 7.18.2 **Preoperative speech audiometry.**

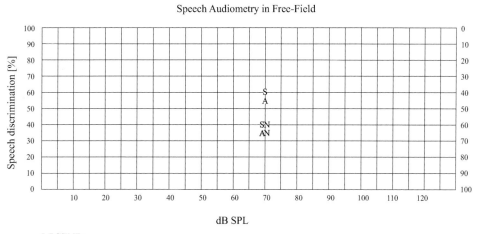

LEGEND:
A – right ear in hearing aid, left ear in passive masking
S – left ear in hearing aid, right ear in passive masking
AN – right ear in hearing aid, SNR + 10 dB, left ear in passive masking
SN – left ear in hearing aid, SNR + 10 dB, right ear in passive masking

Figure 7.18.3 **Preoperative speech audiometry in free-field.**

PDT-ENS, CI left ear, Med-El CONCERTO FLEX20

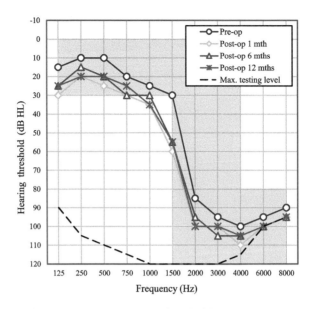

Figure 7.18.4 **Pre- and postoperative hearing thresholds.**

Hearing Preservation, Calculation in [%]				
Legend:		Follow-up		
S	Hearing Preservation	1 month	6 months	12 months
75 – 100%	Complete HP			
26 – 74%	Partial HP	S = 79.5%	S = 84.3%	S = 83.5%
1 – 25%	Minimal HP			
No detectable hearing	Loss of hearing			

Figure 7.18.5 **Hearing preservation results.**

19. Girl, 16 years – bone conduction implant

Chronic otitis media in childhood. Previous ear surgeries: left-ear tympanoplasty (another clinic) complicated by peripheral paresis of the left facial nerve (at the age of 7), left-ear ossiculoplasty (at the age of 10) and then myringoplasty (at the age of 12). Surgeries in the right ear: epitympanotomy with middle-ear lesion removal and myringoplasty (at the age of 13), re-myringoossiculoplasty with the right-ear lesion removal (at the age of 14), right-ear exploratory tympanotomy with lesion removal, second-look surgery (at the age of 15). Right-ear pulsing tinnitus, compatible with the pulse and a feeling of blockage. Hearing aids: not used (Figures 7.19.1–7.19.4).

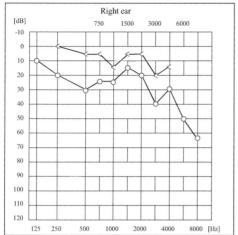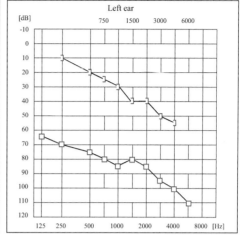

Figure 7.19.1 Preoperative pure-tone audiometry.

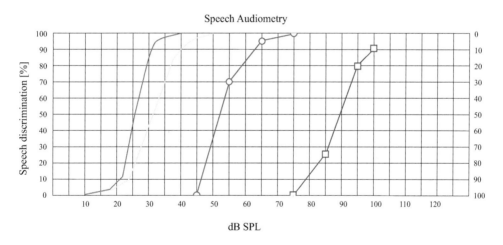

Figure 7.19.2 Preoperative speech audiometry.

Oticon Medical Ponto, left ear

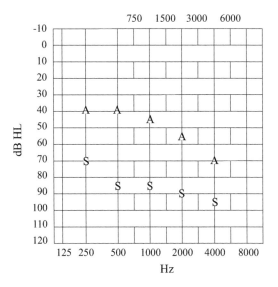

Figure 7.19.3 Pure-tone audiometry in a free-field for aided (A) and unaided (S) conditions after 12-month follow-up.

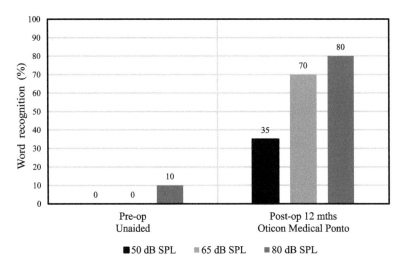

Figure 7.19.4 Word recognition score for unaided and aided conditions in quiet at 50, 65, and 80 dB SPL after 12-month follow-up. Non-implanted ear in passive masking.

C. ADULTS AGED 18–69 YEARS

20. Male, 19 years – bone conduction implant

Congenital malformation of the left external and middle ear. Reconstructive surgery of the left pinna. Hearing aids impossible to use due to the outer ear malformation. Head imaging: CT scan of the temporal bones. Left ear: aplasia of the external ear canal. Significant hypoplasia of the base of the temporal bone pyramid. The low position of the meninges of the middle cranial fossa. Mastoid process correctly formed, slightly smaller than the right one, mostly of diploic structure with single apneumatic cells in the lower part. Significant tympanic hypoplasia: without epitympanum, mesotympanum, and hypotympanum separated from each other, residual mesotympanum filled with soft-tissue mass or fluid, hypotympanum filled with air. Residual auditory ossicles. Sclerotic oval window. Round window correctly formed, narrower compared to the right side. Also, the bony labyrinth without noticeable changes. The hypoplastic labyrinthine part of the facial nerve canal. Aplasia of the remaining parts of the facial nerve canal. The anteroposterior dimension of the left mastoid process at the level corresponding to the middle part of the right-ear canal ca. 18 mm, the thickness of the bone between the sigmoid sinus and the external surface of the temporal bone ca. 12 mm, the thickness of the cortical bone ca. 1.2–2.1 mm – sufficient to implant a BB transducer, possibly with a lift (Figures 7.20.1–7.20.4).

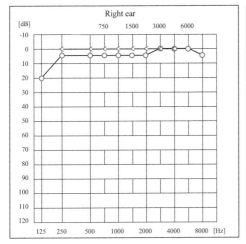
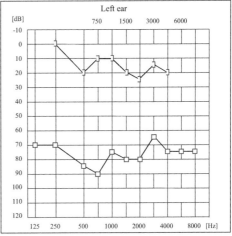

Figure 7.20.1 Preoperative pure-tone audiometry.

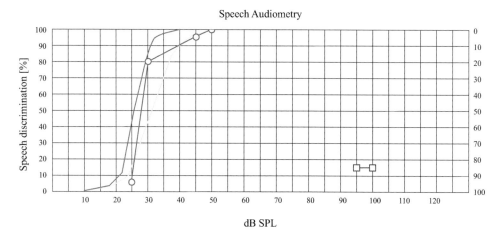

Figure 7.20.2 Preoperative speech audiometry.

Med-El Bonebridge (BB) BCI601, left ear

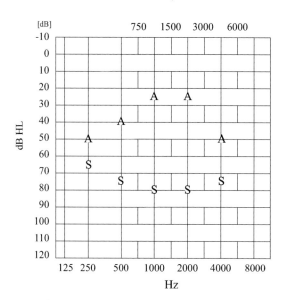

LEGEND:

A – implant (contralateral ear actively masked)

S – implant (contralateral ear actively masked)

Figure 7.20.3 Pure-tone audiometry in free-field for aided (A) and unaided (S) conditions after 3-month follow-up.

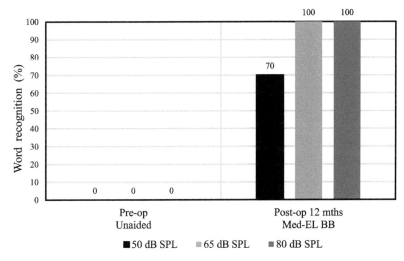

Figure 7.20.4 Word recognition score in free-field for unaided and aided conditions in quiet at 50, 65, and 80 dB SPL after 12-month follow-up. Non-implanted ear in active masking.

21. Male, 20 years – cochlear implant

Sudden idiopathic hearing loss in the right ear at the age of 18, no treatment. Since then, constant tinnitus in the right ear, no vertigo. Uses a hearing aid in the right ear – subjectively poor hearing benefits. Head imaging: MRI with contrast and CT – no pathologies (Figures 7.21.1–7.21.5).

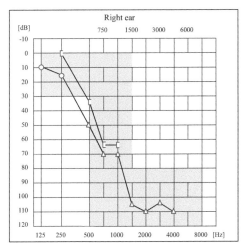
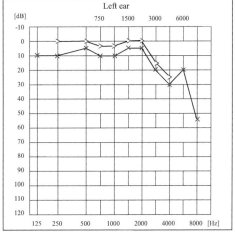

Figure 7.21.1 Preoperative pure-tone audiometry.

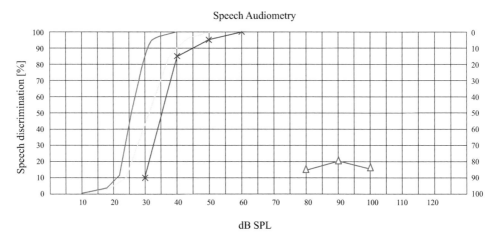

Figure 7.21.2 **Preoperative speech audiometry.**

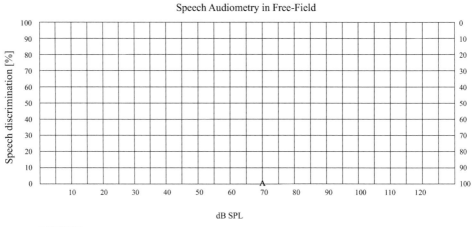

LEGEND:
A – right ear in hearing aid, left ear in active masking

Figure 7.21.3 **Preoperative speech audiometry in free-field.**

PDT-EC (up to 250 Hz), CI right ear, Med-El SYNCHRONY FLEX24™

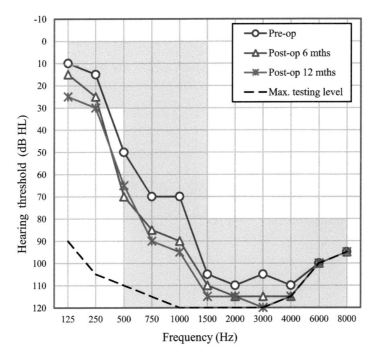

Figure 7.21.4 Pre- and postoperative hearing thresholds.

Hearing Preservation, Calculation in [%]			
Legend:		**Follow-up**	
S	**Hearing Preservation**	**6 months**	**12 months**
75 – 100%	Complete HP		
26 – 74%	Partial HP	**S = 74.3%**	**S = 66.2%**
1 – 25%	Minimal HP		
No detectable hearing	Loss of hearing		

Figure 7.21.5 Hearing preservation results.

22. Female, 27 years – cochlear implant

Bilateral progressive hearing loss since early childhood. Speech development: normal. From around the age of 25, the patient has significant problems with understanding speech. Subjectively worse hearing in the right ear. Due to limited hearing benefits, she does not use hearing aids (Figures 7.22.1–7.22.5).

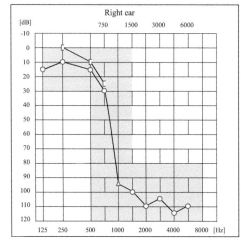
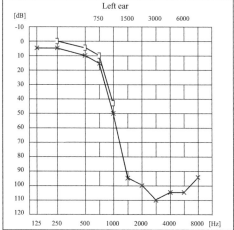

Figure 7.22.1 **Preoperative pure-tone audiometry.**

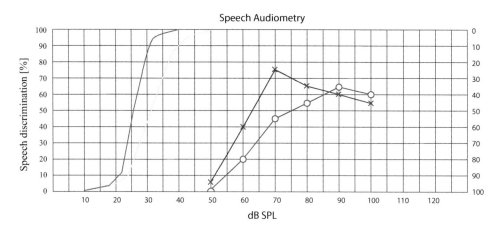

Figure 7.22.2 **Preoperative speech audiometry.**

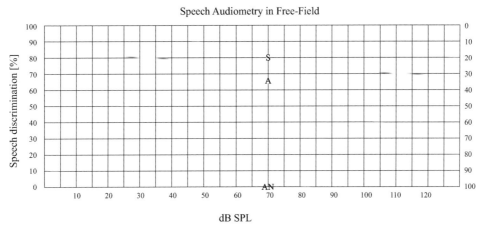

Speech Audiometry in Free-Field

LEGEND:
A – right ear in hearing aid, left ear in passive masking
S – left ear in hearing aid, right ear in passive masking
AN – right ear in hearing aid, SNR + 10 dB, left ear in passive masking
SN – left ear in hearing aid, SNR + 10 dB, right ear in passive masking

Figure 7.22.3 Preoperative speech audiometry in free-field.

PDT-EC (up to 750 Hz), CI right ear, Med-El SONATA FLEX20

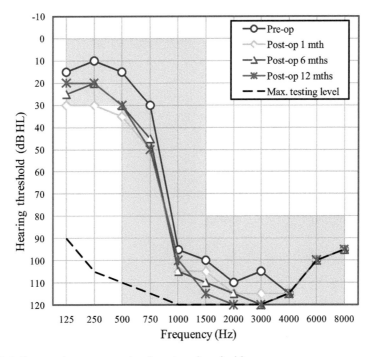

Figure 7.22.4 Pre- and postoperative hearing thresholds.

Hearing Preservation, Calculation in [%]				
Legend:		**Follow-up**		
S	Hearing Preservation	1 month	6 months	12 months
75 – 100%	Complete HP	S = 75.0%	S = 78.6%	S = 77.4%
26 – 74%	Partial HP			
1 – 25%	Minimal HP			
No detectable hearing	Loss of hearing			

Figure 7.22.5 Hearing preservation results.

23. Female, 29 years – cochlear implant

Bilateral progressive hearing loss for several years. There are no episodes of otitis media with effusion in the history of the disease. Bilateral, periodic tinnitus. Periodic vertigo. Hearing aids: not used due to the lack of hearing benefits. Head imaging: MRI – no pathologies (Figures 7.23.1–7.23.5).

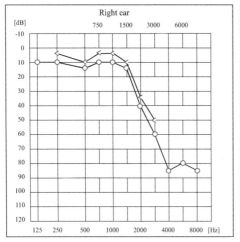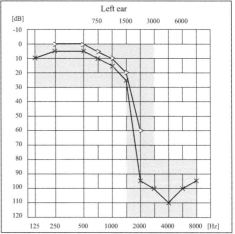

Figure 7.23.1 Preoperative pure-tone audiometry.

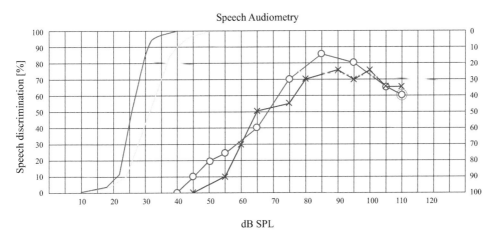

Figure 7.23.2 **Preoperative speech audiometry.**

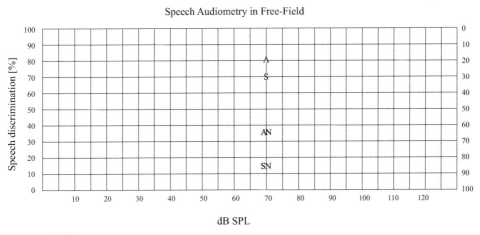

LEGEND:
A – right ear in hearing aid, left ear in passive masking
S – left ear in hearing aid, right ear in passive masking
AN – right ear in hearing aid, SNR + 10 dB, left ear in passive masking
SN – left ear in hearing aid, SNR + 10 dB, right ear in passive masking

Figure 7.23.3 **Preoperative speech audiometry in free-field.**

PDT-ENS, CI left ear, Med-El SONATA FLEX20

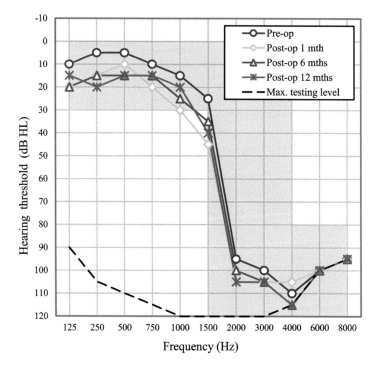

Figure 7.23.4 Pre- and postoperative hearing thresholds.

Hearing Preservation, Calculation in [%]				
Legend:		**Follow-up**		
S	**Hearing Preservation**	**1 month**	**6 months**	**12 months**
75 – 100%	Complete HP			
26 – 74%	Partial HP	S = 88.3%	S = 89.1%	S = 88.3%
1 – 25%	Minimal HP			
No detectable hearing	Loss of hearing			

Figure 7.23.5 Hearing preservation results.

24. Female, 29 years – cochlear implant

Sudden idiopathic hearing loss in the left ear at the age of 21. Severe tinnitus on the left side since the episode of sudden deafness. No vertigo. Hearing aids used regularly since the age of 22. For left ear – little hearing benefits. Head imaging: MRI – no pathologies (Figures 7.24.1–7.24.5).

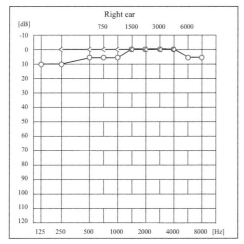
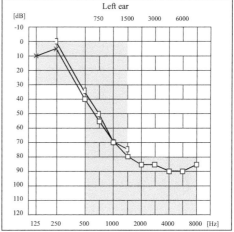

Figure 7.24.1 Preoperative pure-tone audiometry.

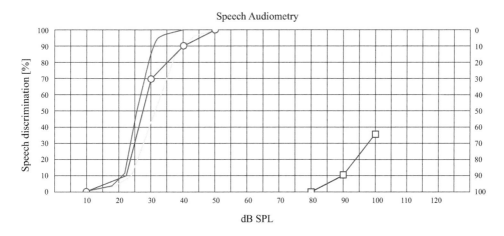

Figure 7.24.2 Preoperative speech audiometry.

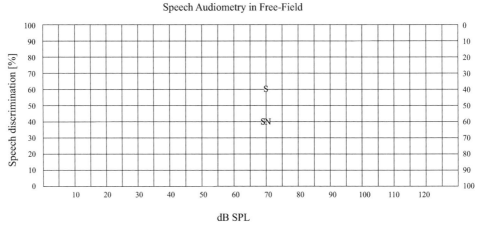

LEGEND:
S – left ear in hearing aid, right ear in active masking
SN – left ear in hearing aid, SNR + 10 dB, right ear in active masking

Figure 7.24.3 **Preoperative speech audiometry in free-field.**

PDT-EC (up to 250 Hz), CI left ear, Med-El SONATA FLEX24™

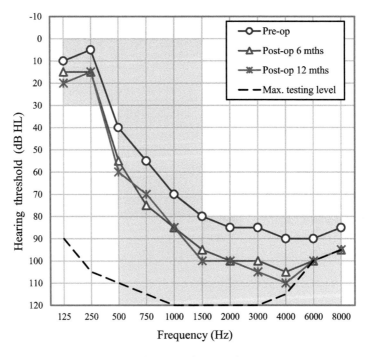

Figure 7.24.4 **Pre- and postoperative hearing thresholds.**

Hearing Preservation, Calculation in [%]			
Legend:		**Follow-up**	
S	**Hearing Preservation**	**6 months**	**12 months**
75 – 100%	Complete HP		
26 – 74%	Partial HP	S = 71.8%	S = 68.0%
1 – 25%	Minimal HP		
No detectable hearing	Loss of hearing		

Figure 7.24.5 Hearing preservation results.

25. Female, 33 years – cochlear implant

Bilateral sudden hearing loss at the age of 28 due to pneumonia caused by *Streptococcus pyogenes*, complicated by septic shock with acute respiratory distress syndrome and thrombosis of the venous sinuses of the brain. She was in a pharmacological coma for 3 weeks. A user of a cochlear implant in the left ear since the age of 30. Periodic right-sided tinnitus. She does not use a hearing aid in the right ear – subjectively no hearing benefits. Head imaging: MRI with contrast – slight residual changes after venous thrombosis, otherwise no pathologies (Figures 7.25.1–7.25.5).

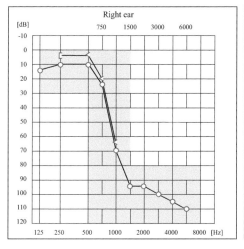 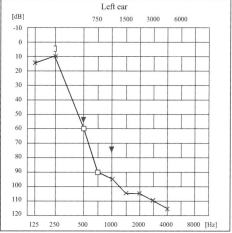

Figure 7.25.1 Preoperative pure-tone audiometry.

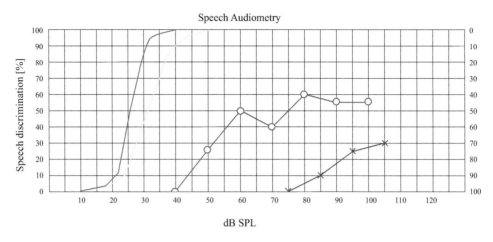

Figure 7.25.2 Preoperative speech audiometry.

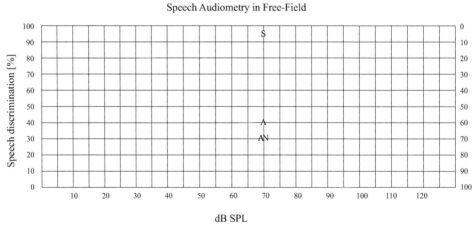

LEGEND:
A – right ear in hearing aid, left ear in passive masking
AN – right ear in hearing aid, SNR + 10 dB, left ear in passive masking
S – left ear in cochlear implant, right ear in passive masking

Figure 7.25.3 Preoperative speech audiometry in free-field.

PDT-EC (up to 750 Hz), second CI, right ear, Med-El SONATA FLEX24™

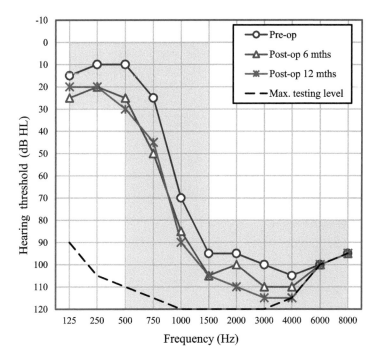

Figure 7.25.4 **Pre- and postoperative hearing thresholds.**

Hearing Preservation, Calculation in [%]			
Legend:		**Follow-up**	
S	**Hearing Preservation**	**6 months**	**12 months**
75 – 100%	Complete HP	S = 78.6%	S = 74.5%
26 – 74%	Partial HP		
1 – 25%	Minimal HP		
No detectable hearing	Loss of hearing		

Figure 7.25.5 **Hearing preservation results.**

26. Male, 35 years – cochlear implant

Hearing loss in the right ear since the age of 19 – sudden hearing loss due to infection. Hearing loss in the left ear since childhood. Ossiculoplasty and re-ossiculoplasty of the left ear. Bilateral tinnitus. No vertigo. Hearing aids: he uses the BICROS system. Head imaging: MRI – no pathologies (Figures 7.26.1–7.26.5).

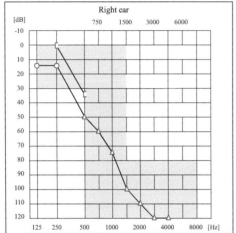
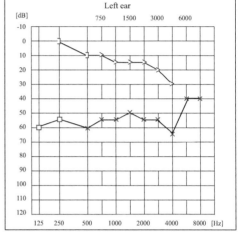

Figure 7.26.1 Preoperative pure-tone audiometry.

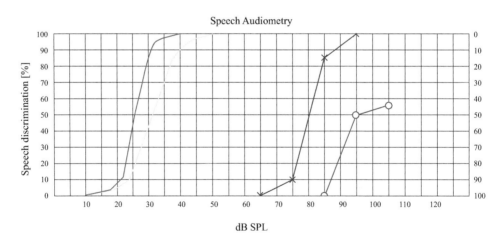

Figure 7.26.2 Preoperative speech audiometry.

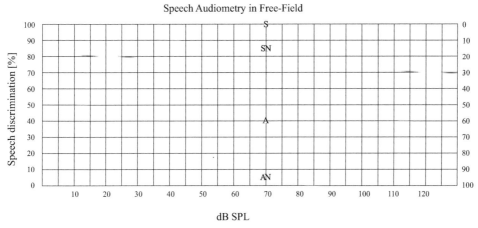

LEGEND:
A – right ear in hearing aid, left ear in active masking
S – left ear in hearing aid, right ear in passive masking
AN – right ear in hearing aid, SNR + 10 dB, left ear in active masking
SN – left ear in hearing aid, SNR + 10 dB, right ear in passive masking

Figure 7.26.3 Preoperative speech audiometry in free-field.

PDT-EC (up to 250 Hz), CI right ear, Med-El SONATA FLEX24™

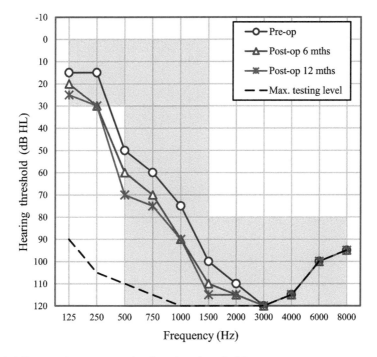

Figure 7.26.4 Pre- and postoperative hearing thresholds.

Hearing Preservation, Calculation in [%]			
Legend:		Follow-up	
S	Hearing Preservation	6 months	12 months
75 – 100%	Complete HP		
26 – 74%	Partial HP	S = 80.3%	S = 73.2%
1 – 25%	Minimal HP		
No detectable hearing	Loss of hearing		

Figure 7.26.5 Hearing preservation results.

27. Female, 36 years – cochlear implant

Bilateral sensorineural hearing loss at the age of 6, faster hearing loss progression in the right ear. The etiology of the hearing loss is unknown. No episodes of otitis media in medical history. No vertigo or tinnitus. Head imaging: MRI with contrast – no pathologies (Figures 7.27.1–7.27.5).

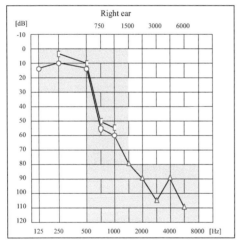 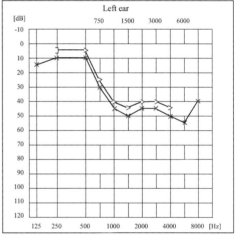

Figure 7.27.1 Preoperative pure-tone audiometry.

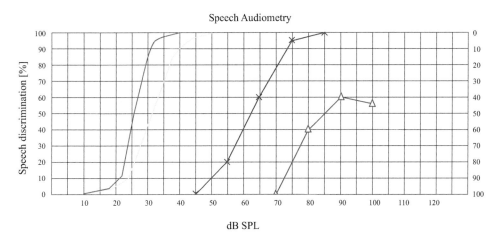

Figure 7.27.2 **Preoperative speech audiometry.**

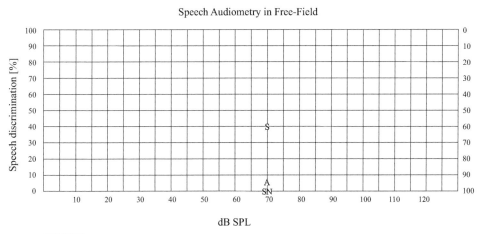

LEGEND:
A – right ear in hearing aid, left ear in active masking
S – left ear in hearing aid, right ear in passive masking
SN – left ear in hearing aid, SNR + 10 dB, right ear in passive masking

Figure 7.27.3 **Preoperative speech audiometry in free-field.**

PDT-EC (up to 500 Hz), CI right ear, Med-El SONATA FLEX24™

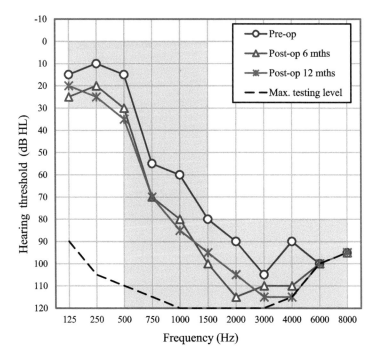

Figure 7.27.4 Pre- and postoperative hearing thresholds.

Hearing Preservation, Calculation in [%]			
Legend:		**Follow-up**	
S	**Hearing Preservation**	**6 months**	**12 months**
75 – 100%	Complete HP		
26 – 74%	Partial HP	**S = 71.7%**	**S = 70.7%**
1 – 25%	Minimal HP		
No detectable hearing	Loss of hearing		

Figure 7.27.5 Hearing preservation results.

28. Female, 38 years – bone conduction implant

Severe right-sided hearing loss since early childhood – the patient does not remember if she could ever hear with her right ear. Etiology of hearing loss unknown. Periodic vertigo. Hearing aids never due to no apparent hearing benefits. Head imaging: CT of the temporal bone – no pathologies (Figures 7.28.1–7.28.3).

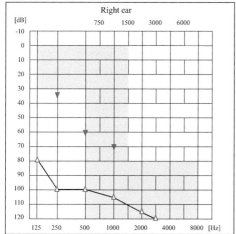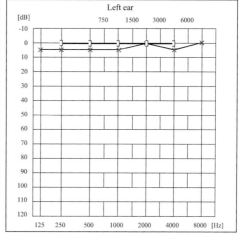

Figure 7.28.1 **Preoperative pure-tone audiometry.**

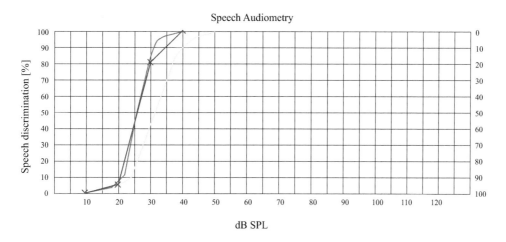

Figure 7.28.2 **Preoperative speech audiometry.**

Med-El Bonebridge (BB) BCI601, right ear – single-sided deafness, SSD

Polish sentence Matrix test	
Unaided	SRT = 3,2
Med-El BB (SSD)	SRT = 0,8

Figure 7.28.3 Speech reception thresholds, SRT in noise, assessed on the basis of the *Polish Sentence Matrix Test* before surgery and after 12 months of follow-up; noise level at 65 dB SPL.

29. Female, 39 years – cochlear implant

Bilateral hearing loss since birth. Born from a twin pregnancy, forceps delivery, birth weight of 2,380 g. Patient with cerebral palsy, moderate intellectual, and motor disability. Rehabilitation allowed her to move independently. He uses hearing aids on both sides since the age of 15. Communicates verbally using simple sentences and supports herself with lip reading (Figures 7.29.1–7.29.5).

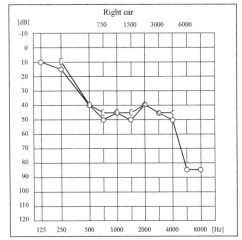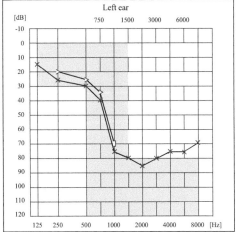

Figure 7.29.1 **Preoperative pure-tone audiometry.**

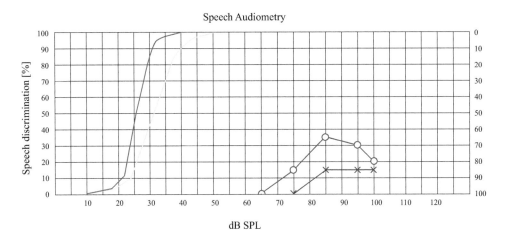

Figure 7.29.2 **Preoperative speech audiometry.**

Speech Audiometry in Free-Field

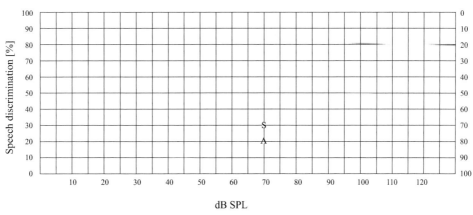

LEGEND:
S – right ear in hearing aid, left ear in active masking
A – left ear in hearing aid, right ear in passive masking

Figure 7.29.3 Preoperative speech audiometry in free-field.

PDT-EC (up to 500 Hz), CI left ear, Med-El CONCERTO FLEX24™

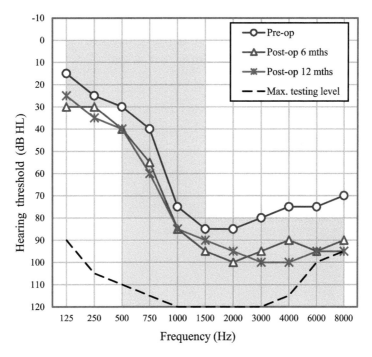

Figure 7.29.4 Pre- and postoperative hearing thresholds.

Hearing Preservation, Calculation in [%]			
Legend:		**Follow-up**	
S	**Hearing Preservation**	**6 months**	**12 months**
75 – 100%	Complete HP		
26 – 74%	Partial HP	S = 73.0%	S = 70.3%
1 – 25%	Minimal HP		
No detectable hearing	Loss of hearing		

Figure 7.29.5 Hearing preservation results.

30. Female, 40 years – cochlear implant

Hearing problems since the age of 25. The patient reports that hearing loss and tinnitus started after she gave birth to her baby. Since the age of 27, she uses hearing aids on both sides – subjectively no improvement in speech understanding. The patient complains primarily on problems with speech understanding. Subjectively worse hearing in the left ear. Bilateral tinnitus started simultaneously with hearing loss. Head imaging: CT – no pathologies (Figures 7.30.1–7.30.5).

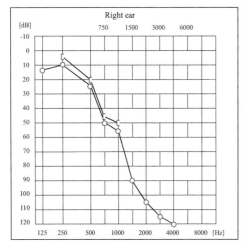 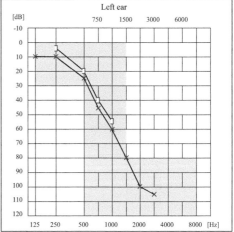

Figure 7.30.1 Preoperative pure-tone audiometry.

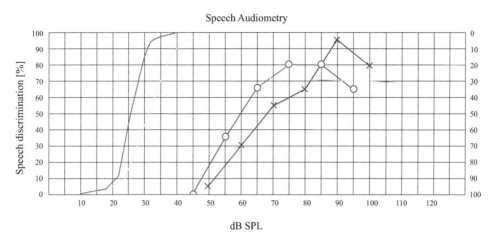

Figure 7.30.2 **Preoperative speech audiometry.**

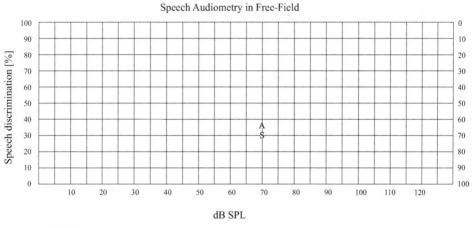

LEGEND:
A – right ear in hearing aid, left ear in passive masking
S – left ear in hearing aid, right ear in passive masking

Figure 7.30.3 **Preoperative speech audiometry in free-field.**

PDT-EC (up to 500 Hz), CI left ear, Med-El SONATA FLEX24™

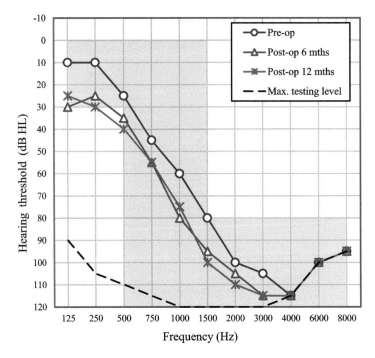

Figure 7.30.4 Pre- and postoperative hearing thresholds.

Hearing Preservation, Calculation in [%]			
Legend:		**Follow-up**	
S	**Hearing Preservation**	**6 months**	**12 months**
75 – 100%	Complete HP		
26 – 74%	Partial HP	**S = 77.4%**	**S = 75.3%**
1 – 25%	Minimal HP		
No detectable hearing	Loss of hearing		

Figure 7.30.5 Hearing preservation results.

31. Female, 40 years – cochlear implant

Bilateral progressive hearing loss since the age of 28. Subjectively worse hearing in the left ear. Bilateral tinnitus. Hearing aids on both sides since the age of 30 – subjectively limited hearing benefit. Chronic conditions: monitored for any signs of multiple sclerosis or Susac syndrome. Head imaging: MRI – no pathologies (Figures 7.31.1–7.31.5).

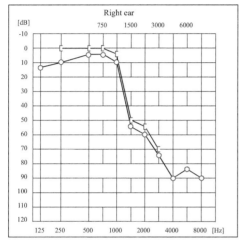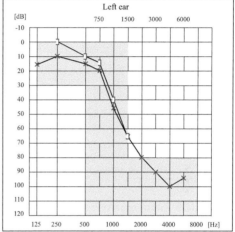

Figure 7.31.1 **Preoperative pure-tone audiometry.**

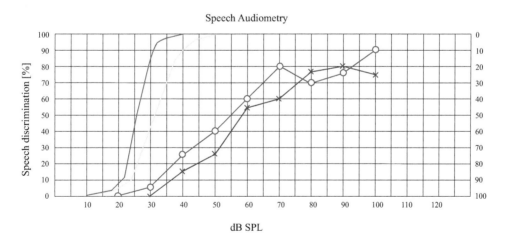

Figure 7.31.2 **Preoperative speech audiometry.**

Speech Audiometry in Free-Field

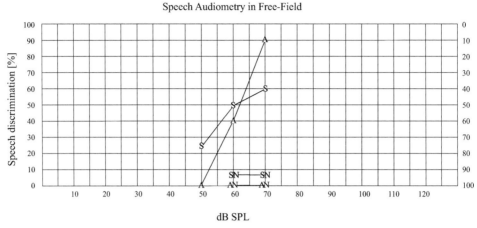

dB SPL

LEGEND:
A – right ear in hearing aid, left ear in passive masking
S – left ear in hearing aid, right ear in passive masking
AN – right ear in hearing aid, SNR + 10 dB, left ear in passive masking
SN – left ear in hearing aid, SNR + 10 dB, right ear in passive masking

Figure 7.31.3 Preoperative speech audiometry in free-field.

PDT-EC (up to 750 Hz), CI left ear, Med-El SONATA FLEX24™

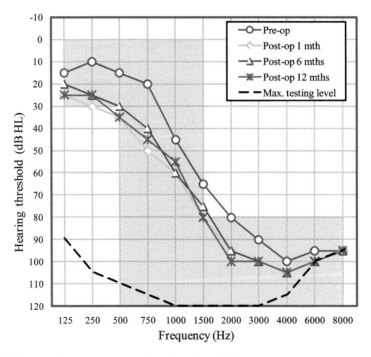

Figure 7.31.4 Pre- and postoperative hearing thresholds.

Hearing Preservation, Calculation in [%]				
Legend:		**Follow-up**		
S	**Hearing Preservation**	**1 month**	**6 months**	**12 months**
75 – 100%	Complete HP			
26 – 74%	Partial HP	S = 75.0 %	S = 80.2%	S = 76.7%
1 – 25%	Minimal HP			
No detectable hearing	Loss of hearing			

Figure 7.31.5 Hearing preservation results.

32. Male, 40 years – cochlear implant

Bilateral progressive hearing loss since the age of 6. There have been episodes of otitis media with effusion in the history of the disease. Bilateral tinnitus since about 25 years of age. He used hearing aids on both sides at the age of 27. Due to the lack of hearing benefits, he stopped using the hearing aid in the right ear after 3 years, and in the left ear – after 10 years. Head imaging: CT without contrast – no pathologies (Figures 7.32.1–7.32.5).

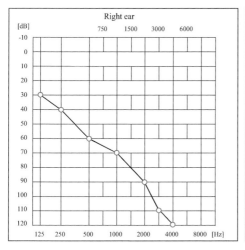 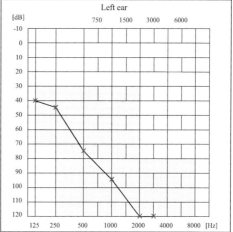

Figure 7.32.1 Preoperative pure-tone audiometry.

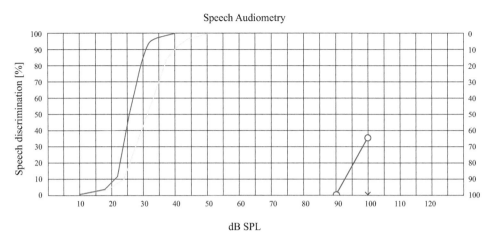

Figure 7.32.2 Preoperative speech audiometry.

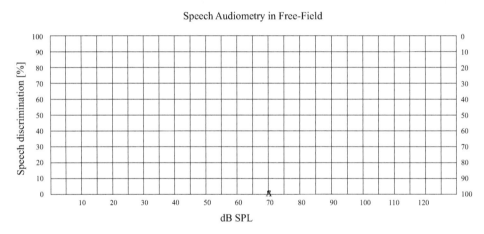

LEGEND:
A – right ear in hearing aid, left ear in passive masking
S – left ear in hearing aid, right ear in passive masking

Figure 7.32.3 Preoperative speech audiometry in free-field.

PDT-EAS, CI left ear, Oticon NEURO Zti EVO

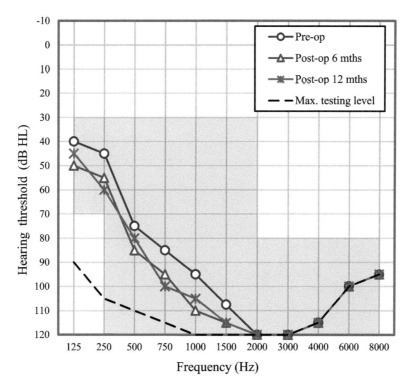

Figure 7.32.4 Pre- and postoperative hearing thresholds.

Hearing Preservation, Calculation in [%]			
Legend:		Follow-up	
S	Hearing Preservation	6 months	12 months
75 – 100%	Complete HP		
26 – 74%	Partial HP	S = 70.6%	S = 72.9%
1 – 25%	Minimal HP		
No detectable hearing	Loss of hearing		

Figure 7.32.5 Hearing preservation results.

33. Male, 41 years – middle-ear implant

Bilateral, progressive hearing loss since the age of 10. In medical history: episodes of otitis media in childhood. No tinnitus and vertigo. Despite repeated attempts to use hearing aids, he did not use any hearing prosthesis due to the increased occlusion effect (Figures 7.33.1–7.33.4).

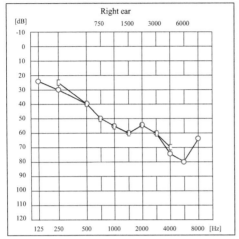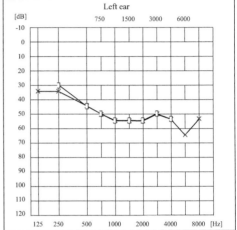

Figure 7.33.1 **Preoperative pure-tone audiometry.**

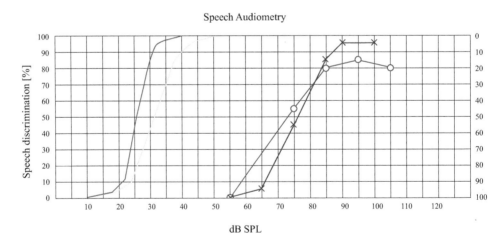

Figure 7.33.2 **Preoperative speech audiometry.**

Med-El Vibrant Soundbridge (VSB) with LP-coupler, right ear

Pure-Tone Audiometry in Free-Field

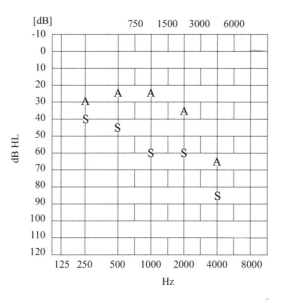

LEGEND:

A – implant (contralateral ear passively masked)

S – unaided (contralateral ear passively masked)

Figure 7.33.3 Pure-tone audiometry in a free-field for aided (A) and unaided (S) conditions after 12-month follow-up.

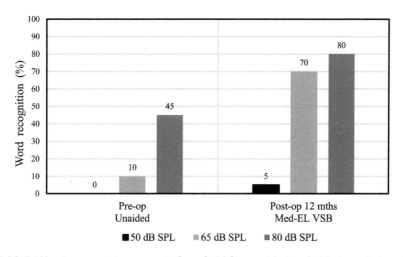

Figure 7.33.4 Word recognition score in free-field for unaided and aided conditions in quiet at 50, 65, and 80 dB SPL after 12-month follow-up. Non-implanted ear in passive masking.

34. Male, 41 years – bone conduction implant

Chronic otitis media associated with cholesteatoma. Numerous ear surgeries, including bilateral modified radical surgery and subsequent reoperations. At the age of 39, reconstruction surgery of the left middle-ear postoperative cavity was performed with the reconstruction of the posterior wall of the external auditory canal using the BonAlive bioactive glass. He uses a hearing aid in the right ear. Periodic left-sided tinnitus (Figures 7.34.1–7.34.4).

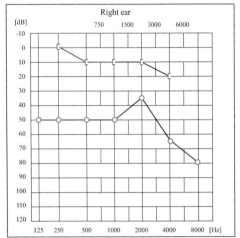
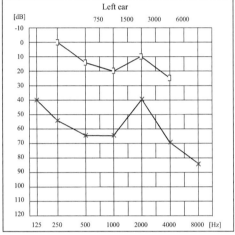

Figure 7.34.1 **Preoperative pure-tone audiometry.**

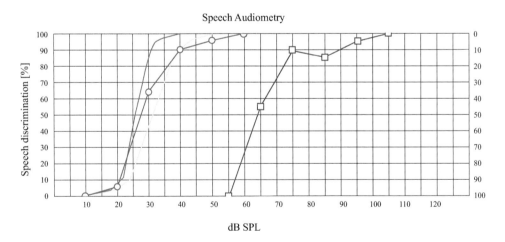

Figure 7.34.2 **Preoperative speech audiometry.**

Implant Med-El Bonebridge (BB) BCI601, left ear

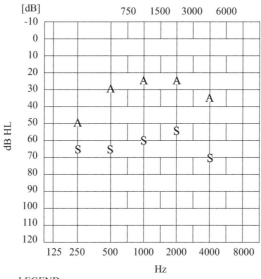

Figure 7.34.3 Pure-tone audiometry in a free-field for aided (A) and unaided (S) conditions after 12-month follow-up.

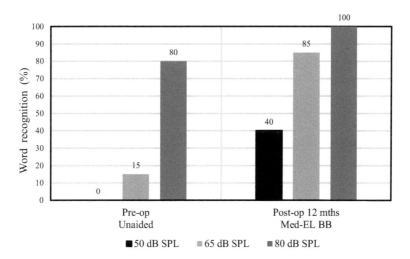

Figure 7.34.4 Word recognition score in free-field for unaided and aided conditions in quiet at 50, 65, and 80 dB SPL after 12-month follow-up. Non-implanted ear in passive masking.

35. Female, 43 years – cochlear implant

Bilateral hearing loss since early childhood, probably after gentamicin treatment. Children's cerebral palsy – involuntary body movements, spastic muscle movements. She has been using hearing aids on both sides since the age of 32 (Figures 7.35.1–7.35.5).

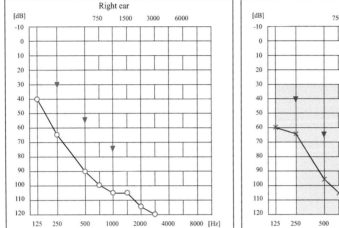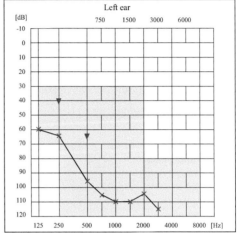

Figure 7.35.1 **Preoperative pure-tone audiometry.**

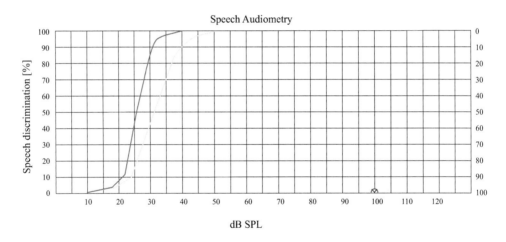

Figure 7.35.2 **Preoperative speech audiometry.**

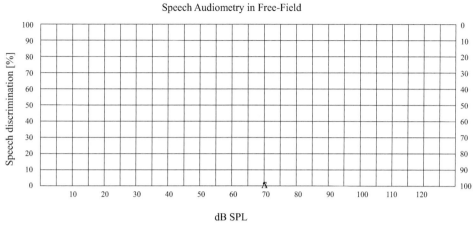

LEGEND:
A – right ear in hearing aid, left ear in passive masking
S – left ear in hearing aid, right ear in passive masking

Figure 7.35.3 Preoperative speech audiometry in free-field.

PDT-EAS, CI left ear, Cochlear Nucleus® Straight Research Array (SRA)

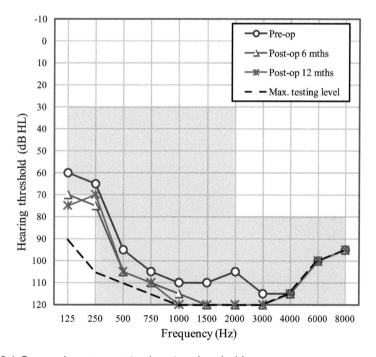

Figure 7.35.4 Pre- and postoperative hearing thresholds.

Hearing Preservation, Calculation in [%]			
Legend:		Follow-up	
S	Hearing Preservation	6 months	12 months
75 – 100%	Complete HP	S = 48.1%	S = 44.4%
26 – 74%	Partial HP		
1 – 25%	Minimal HP		
No detectable hearing	Loss of hearing		

Figure 7.35.5 Hearing preservation results.

36. Female, 43 years – bone conduction implant

Bilateral hearing loss since childhood due to otitis media. Numerous ear operations: myringoplasty, myringoossiculoplasty, and reoperations. At the age of 33, she had stapedotomy in the left ear. After that surgery, she had a short-lived improvement in hearing. Bilateral tinnitus. She does not use hearing aids due to effusion because of the closure of the external auditory canal (Figures 7.36.1–7.36.4).

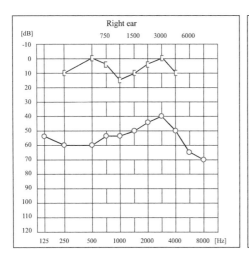
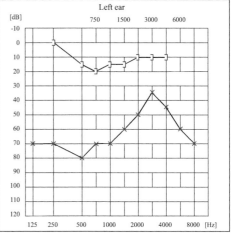

Figure 7.36.1 Preoperative pure-tone audiometry.

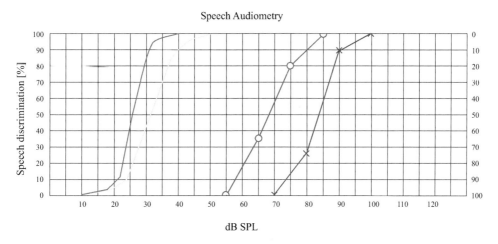

Figure 7.36.2 Preoperative speech audiometry.

Cochlear™ Baha® Attract, left ear

Pure-Tone Audiometry in Free-Field

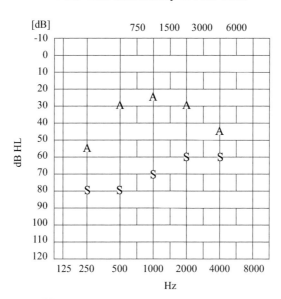

LEGEND:

A – implant (contralateral ear passively masked)

S – unaided (contralateral ear passively masked)

Figure 7.36.3 Pure-tone audiometry in a free-field for aided (A) and unaided (S) conditions after 12-month follow-up.

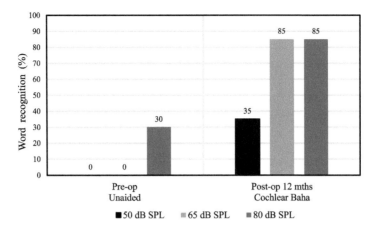

Figure 7.36.4 Word recognition score for unaided and aided conditions in quiet at 50, 65, and 80 dB SPL after 12-month follow-up. Non-implanted ear in passive masking.

37. Female, 44 years – bone conduction implant

Recurrent chronic otitis media since early childhood. Bilateral myringoossiculoplasty at the age of 40. Based on the intraoperative image of the left ear, it was found that it could not be reconstructed due to active inflammations, advanced tympanosclerosis, complete immobilization of the residual stapes with sclerotic masses (Figures 7.37.1–7.37.4).

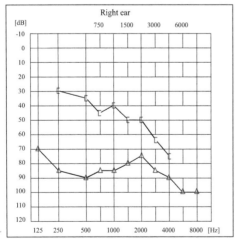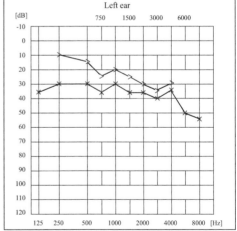

Figure 7.37.1 Preoperative pure-tone audiometry.

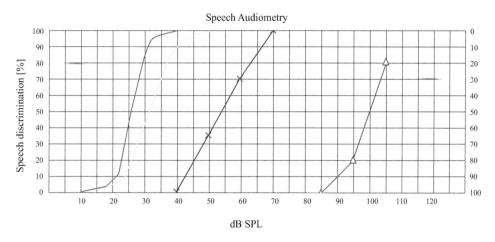

Figure 7.37.2 Preoperative speech audiometry.

Oticon Medical Ponto, right ear

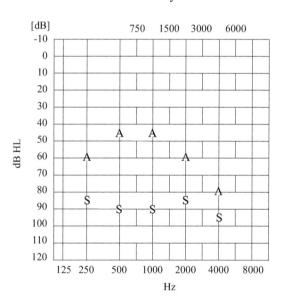

LEGEND:

A – implant (contralateral ear actively masked)

S – unaided (contralateral ear actively masked)

Figure 7.37.3 Pure-tone audiometry in a free-field for aided (A) and unaided (S) conditions after 12-month follow-up.

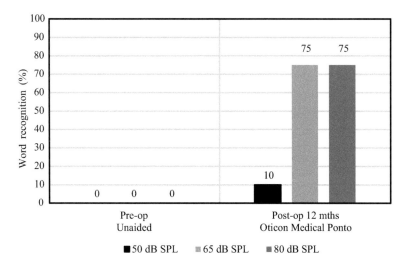

Figure 7.37.4 Word recognition score for unaided and aided conditions in quiet at 50, 65, and 80 dB SPL after 12-month follow-up. Non-implanted ear in active masking.

38. Female, 44 years – cochlear implant

Bilateral, progressive hearing loss from the age of 27. Subjectively worse hearing in the right ear. No vertigo or tinnitus. Hearing aids: do not use due to a subjective lack of hearing benefits and occlusion (Figures 7.38.1–7.38.5).

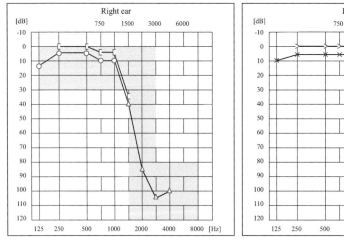
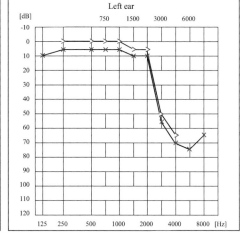

Figure 7.38.1 Preoperative pure-tone audiometry.

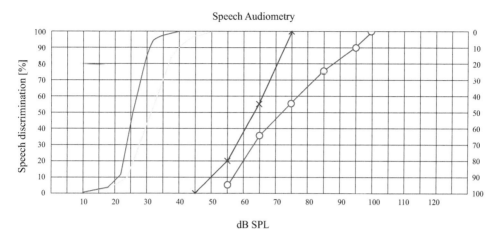

Figure 7.38.2 **Preoperative speech audiometry.**

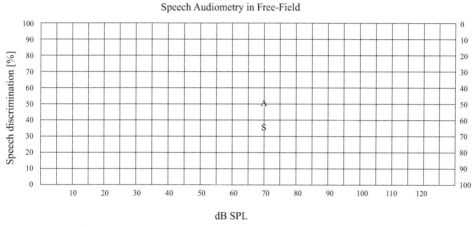

LEGEND:
A – right ear in hearing aid, left ear in active masking
S – right ear unaided, left ear in active masking

Figure 7.38.3 **Preoperative speech audiometry in free-field.**

PDT-ENS, CI right ear, Med-El SYNCHRONY FLEX20

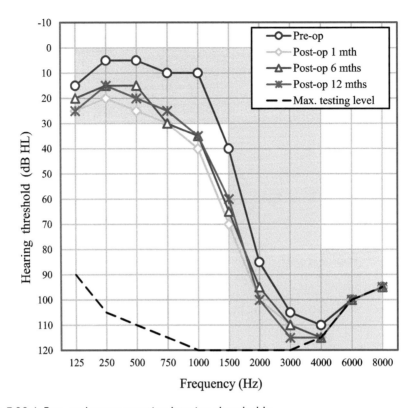

Figure 7.38.4 Pre- and postoperative hearing thresholds.

Hearing Preservation, Calculation in [%]				
Legend:		**Follow-up**		
S	**Hearing Preservation**	**1 month**	**6 months**	**12 months**
75 – 100%	Complete HP			
26 – 74%	Partial HP	**S = 76.2%**	**S = 81.7%**	**S = 80.2%**
1 – 25%	Minimal HP			
No detectable hearing	Loss of hearing			

Figure 7.38.5 Hearing preservation results.

39. Female, 44 years – cochlear implant

Bilateral progressive hearing loss since the age of 25. Bilateral tinnitus, recently inten-
sifying. Periodic vertigo. She is using a cochlear implant in the right ear since the age
of 36 and a hearing aid in left ear since the age of 33 (Figures 7.39.1–7.39.5).

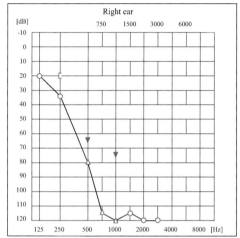
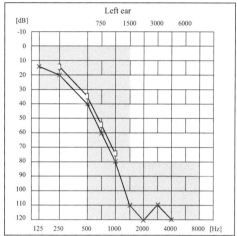

Figure 7.39.1 **Preoperative pure-tone audiometry.**

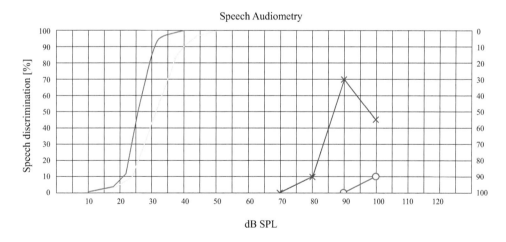

Figure 7.39.2 **Preoperative speech audiometry.**

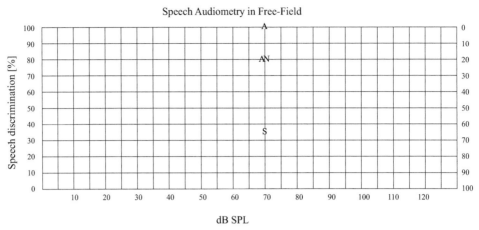

Figure 7.39.3 Preoperative speech audiometry in free-field.

PDT-EC (up to 250 Hz), second CI, left ear, Med-El SONATA FLEX24™

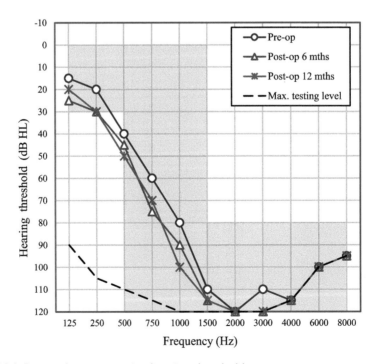

Figure 7.39.4 Pre- and postoperative hearing thresholds.

Hearing Preservation, Calculation in [%]			
Legend:		**Follow-up**	
S	**Hearing Preservation**	**6 months**	**12 months**
75 – 100%	Complete HP		
26 – 74%	Partial HP	S = 81.2%	S = 79.7%
1 – 25%	Minimal HP		
No detectable hearing	Loss of hearing		

Figure 7.39.5 Hearing preservation results.

40. Female, 46 years – cochlear implant

Bilateral gradually progressive hearing loss of unknown etiology since the age of 25. User of a cochlear implant in the right ear since the age of 30. Does not use a hearing aid in the left ear due to the lack of hearing benefits. Bilateral (compensated) tinnitus. No vertigo (Figures 7.40.1–7.40.5).

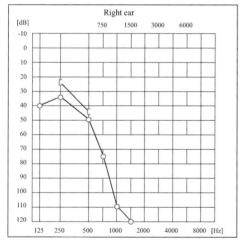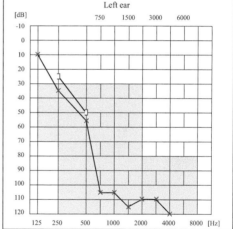

Figure 7.40.1 Preoperative pure-tone audiometry.

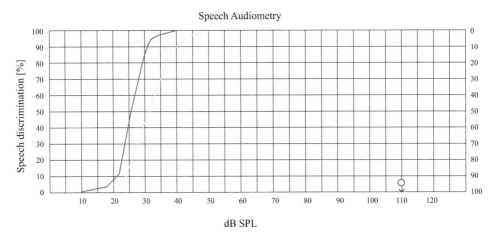

Figure 7.40.2 **Preoperative speech audiometry.**

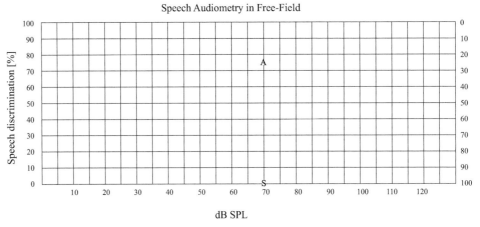

LEGEND:
A – right ear in cochlear implant, left ear in passive masking
S – left ear in hearing aid, right ear in passive masking

Figure 7.40.3 **Preoperative speech audiometry in free-field.**

PDT-EAS, second CI, left ear, Med-El SONATA FLEX28™

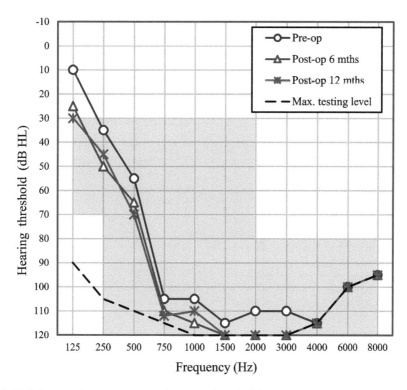

Figure 7.40.4 Pre- and postoperative hearing thresholds.

Hearing Preservation, Calculation in [%]			
Legend:		**Follow-up**	
S	**Hearing Preservation**	**6 months**	**12 months**
75 – 100%	Complete HP		
26 – 74%	Partial HP	**S = 68.6%**	**S = 67.8%**
1 – 25%	Minimal HP		
No detectable hearing	Loss of hearing		

Figure 7.40.5 Hearing preservation results.

41. Male, 46 years – cochlear implant

Sudden idiopathic hearing loss in the left ear at the age of 32. Since then, constant tinnitus. No hearing improvement after treatment. He did not use hearing aids due to the lack of hearing benefits. Heard imaging: CT of the temporal bones and MRI – no pathologies (Figures 7.41.1–7.41.5).

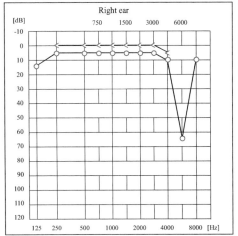
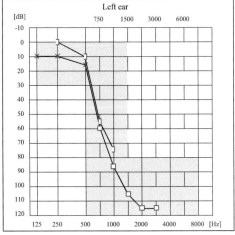

Figure 7.41.1 **Preoperative pure-tone audiometry.**

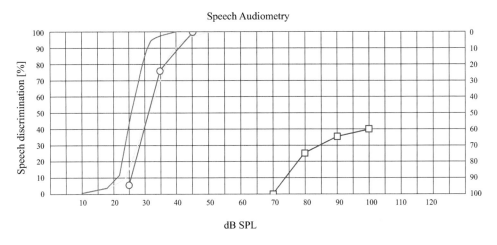

Figure 7.41.2 **Preoperative speech audiometry.**

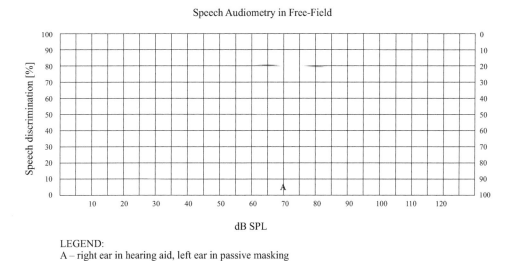

LEGEND:
A – right ear in hearing aid, left ear in passive masking

Figure 7.41.3 Preoperative speech audiometry in free-field.

PDT-EC (up to 500 Hz), CI left ear, Med-El SONATA FLEX24™

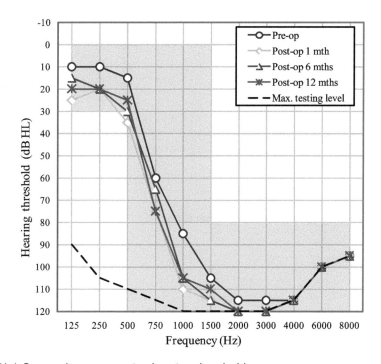

Figure 7.41.4 Pre- and postoperative hearing thresholds.

Hearing Preservation, Calculation in [%]				
Legend:		**Follow-up**		
S	**Hearing Preservation**	**1 month**	**6 months**	**12 months**
75 – 100%	Complete HP			
26 – 74%	Partial HP	S = 72.7%	S = 80.5%	S = 79.2%
1 – 25%	Minimal HP			
No detectable hearing	Loss of hearing			

Figure 7.41.5 Hearing preservation results.

42. Female, 47 years – cochlear implant

Bilateral gradually progressive hearing loss of unknown etiology since the age of 17. No history of otitis media with effusion. Bilateral tinnitus. No vertigo. Hearing aids since the age of 25, but used irregularly due to the lack of hearing benefits. Head imaging: CT with contrast – no pathologies (Figures 7.42.1–7.42.5).

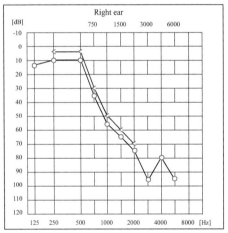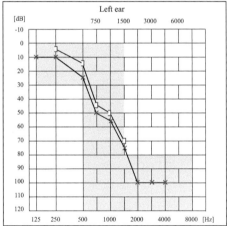

Figure 7.42.1 Preoperative pure-tone audiometry.

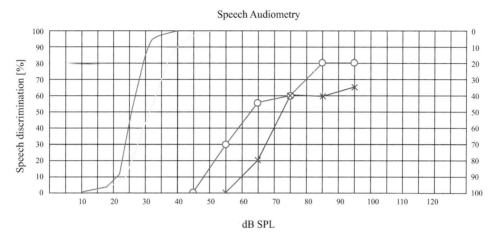

Figure 7.42.2 Preoperative speech audiometry.

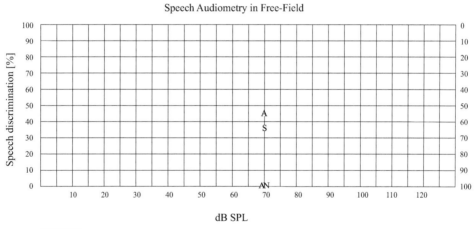

LEGEND:
A – right ear in hearing aid, left ear in passive masking
S – left ear in hearing aid, right ear in passive masking
AN – right ear in hearing aid, SNR + 10 dB, left ear in passive masking

Figure 7.42.3 Preoperative speech audiometry in free-field.

PDT-EC (up to 500 Hz), CI left ear, Med-El CONCERTO FLEX24™

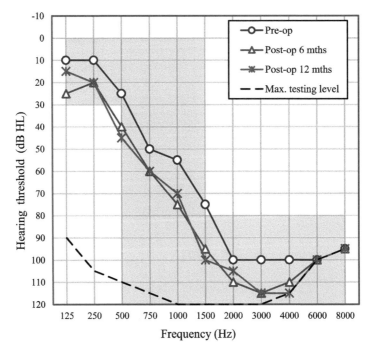

Figure 7.42.4 Pre- and postoperative hearing thresholds.

Hearing Preservation, Calculation in [%]			
Legend:		Follow-up	
S	Hearing Preservation	6 months	12 months
75 – 100%	Complete HP		
26 – 74%	Partial HP	S = 74.5%	S = 75.5%
1 – 25%	Minimal HP		
No detectable hearing	Loss of hearing		

Figure 7.42.5 Hearing preservation results.

43. Female, 48 years – middle-ear implant

Bilateral hearing loss due to chronic otitis media mainly in childhood. Previous ear surgeries: bilateral myringoossiculoplasty and reoperations. Never used hearing aids (Figures 7.43.1–7.43.4).

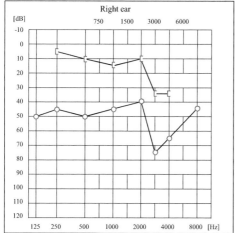
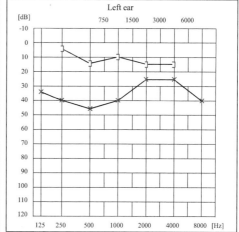

Figure 7.43.1 Preoperative pure-tone audiometry.

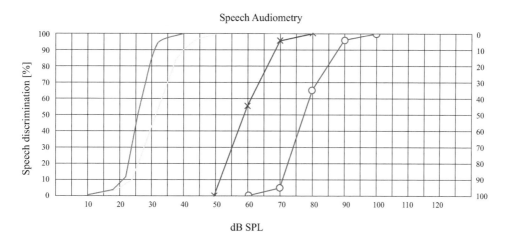

Figure 7.43.2 Preoperative speech audiometry.

Implant Med-El Vibrant Soundbridge (VSB), right ear

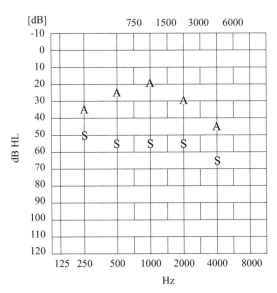

Figure 7.43.3 Pure-tone audiometry in a free-field for aided (A) and unaided (S) conditions after 12-month follow-up.

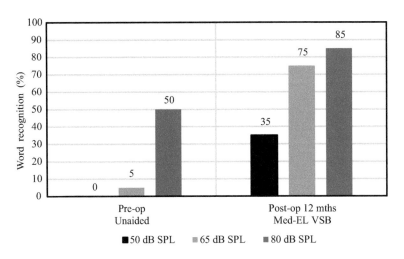

Figure 7.43.4 Word recognition score for unaided and aided conditions in quiet at 50, 65, and 80 dB SPL after 12-month follow-up. Non-implanted ear in passive masking.

44. Female, 48 years – middle-ear implant

Bilateral hearing loss since the age of 20 but it progresses very slowly. She stopped using hearing aids after 3 months due to the occlusion effect. Head imaging: CT – no pathologies (Figures 7.44.1–7.44.4).

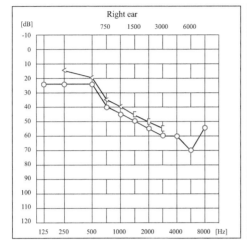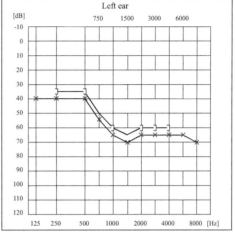

Figure 7.44.1 Preoperative pure-tone audiometry.

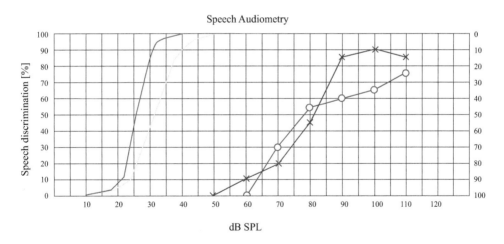

Figure 7.44.2 Preoperative speech audiometry.

Cochlear™ MET® system, left ear

Pure-Tone Audiometry in Free-Field

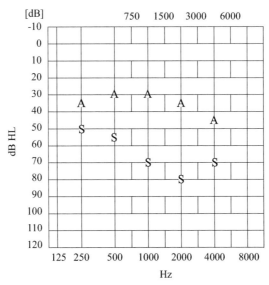

LEGEND:

A – implant (contralateral ear passively masked)

S – unaided (contralateral ear passively masked)

Figure 7.44.3 Pure-tone audiometry in a free-field for aided (A) and unaided (S) conditions after 3-month follow-up.

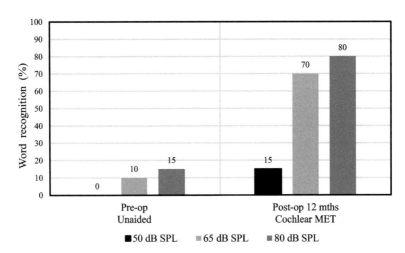

Figure 7.44.4 Word recognition score for unaided and aided conditions in quiet at 50, 65, and 80 dB SPL after 12-month follow-up. Non-implanted ear in passive masking.

45. Female, 49 years – bone conduction implant

Hearing problems since around the age of 31 due to otitis media. Numerous previous ear surgeries: vent tube, ossiculoplasty, myringoossiculoplasty, and reoperations. She used a hearing aid in her right ear but she stopped after about a year due to severe condition of otitis media with effusion (Figures 7.45.1–7.45.4).

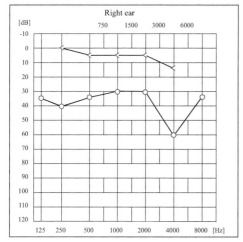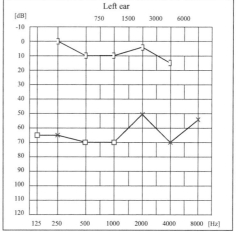

Figure 7.45.1 Preoperative pure-tone audiometry.

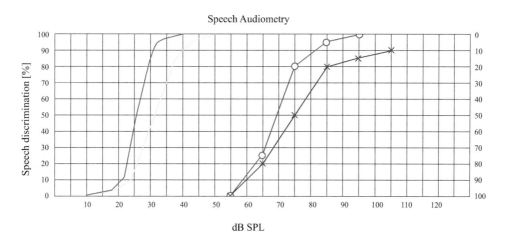

Figure 7.45.2 Preoperative speech audiometry.

Med-El Bonebridge (BB) BCI602, left ear

Pure-Tone Audiometry in Free-Field

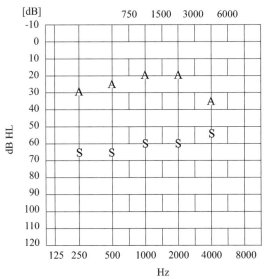

LEGEND:

A – implant (contralateral ear passively masked)

S – unaided (contralateral ear passively masked)

Figure 7.45.3 Pure-tone audiometry in a free-field for aided (A) and unaided (S) conditions after 3-month follow-up.

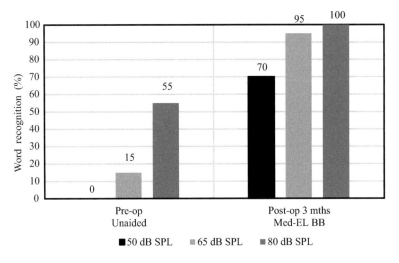

Figure 7.45.4 Word recognition score for unaided and aided conditions in quiet at 50, 65, and 80 dB SPL after 3-month follow-up. Non-implanted ear in passive masking.

46. Female, 50 years – cochlear implant

Bilateral gradually progressive hearing loss of unknown etiology since the age of 35. She worked in noise for many years. Sudden hearing loss at the age of 56, hearing improvement after pharmacological treatment. Bilateral tinnitus. Vertigo: a feeling of spinning. Hearing aids for both ears since the age of 36. She stopped using the hearing aid in her right ear after 6 years due to the lack of hearing benefits. Head imaging: MRI with contrast – no pathologies (Figures 7.46.1–7.46.5).

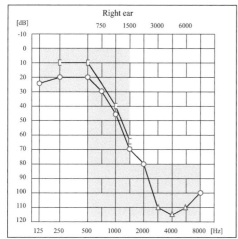
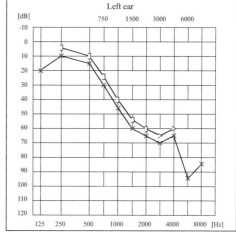

Figure 7.46.1 Preoperative pure-tone audiometry.

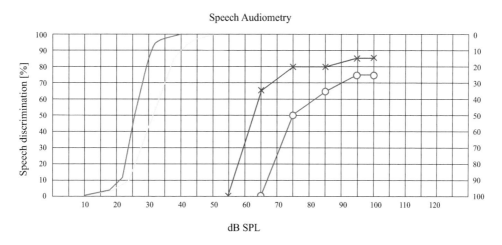

Figure 7.46.2 Preoperative speech audiometry.

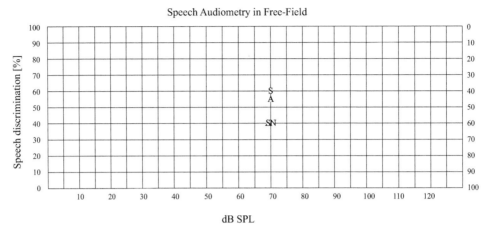

Speech Audiometry in Free-Field

LEGEND:
A – right ear in hearing aid, left ear in passive masking
S – left ear in hearing aid, right ear in passive masking
AN – right ear in hearing aid, SNR + 10 dB, left ear in passive masking
SN – left ear in hearing aid, SNR + 10 dB, right ear in passive masking

Figure 7.46.3 Preoperative speech audiometry in free-field.

PDT-EC (up to 750 Hz), CI right ear, Med-El SONATA FLEX24™

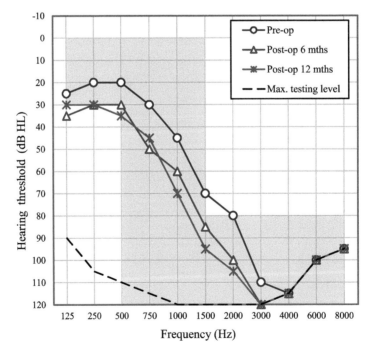

Figure 7.46.4 Pre- and postoperative hearing thresholds.

Hearing Preservation, Calculation in [%]			
Legend:		**Follow-up**	
S	**Hearing Preservation**	**6 months**	**12 months**
75 – 100%	Complete HP		
26 – 74%	Partial HP	**S = 78.0%**	**S = 74.0%**
1 – 25%	Minimal HP		
No detectable hearing	Loss of hearing		

Figure 7.46.5 Hearing preservation results.

47. Female, 50 years – cochlear implant

Hearing problems since the age of 27 due to otosclerosis. Bilateral stapedotomy at the age of 30 and 35 and restapedotomy of the right ear. Left-sided tinnitus. Hearing aid in the left ear since the age of 35 (Figures 7.47.1–7.47.5).

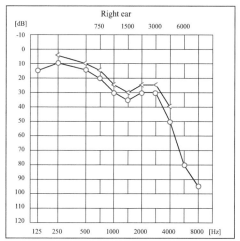
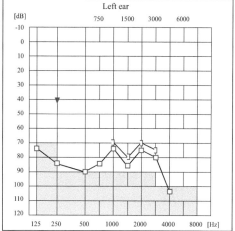

Figure 7.47.1 Preoperative pure-tone audiometry.

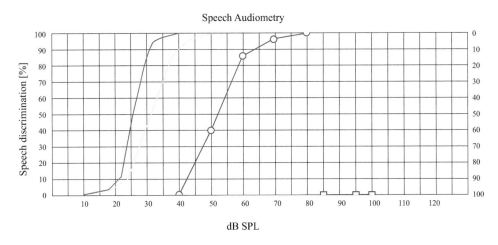

Figure 7.47.2 **Preoperative speech audiometry.**

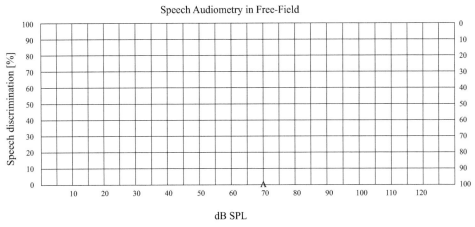

LEGEND:
A – left ear in hearing aid, right ear in active masking

Figure 7.47.3 **Preoperative speech audiometry in free-field.**

PDT-ES, CI left ear, Cochlear™ Nucleus® CI522

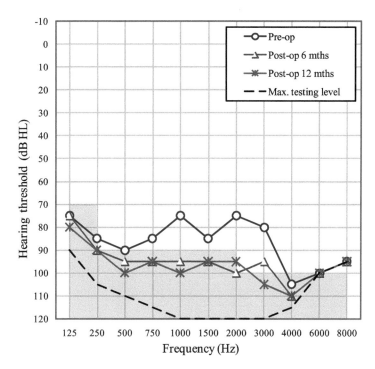

Figure 7.47.4 Pre- and postoperative hearing thresholds.

Hearing Preservation, Calculation in [%]			
Legend:		**Follow-up**	
S	**Hearing Preservation**	**6 months**	**12 months**
75 – 100%	Complete HP		
26 – 74%	Partial HP	S = 63.5%	S = 55.8%
1 – 25%	Minimal HP		
No detectable hearing	Loss of hearing		

Figure 7.47.5 Hearing preservation results.

48. Female, 51 years – middle-ear implant

Bilateral congenital defect of the middle and outer ear. Left middle-ear implant user since the age of 9. Since the age of 41, she has been using a bone conduction hearing aid (mounted in a spectacle frame). She uses it systematically, but there are major problems with feedback. No otitis media in the history of the disease. No tinnitus or vertigo (Figures 7.48.1–7.48.4).

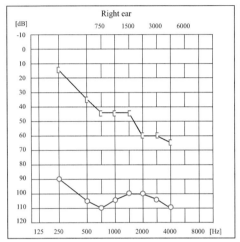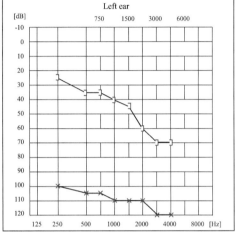

Figure 7.48.1 Preoperative pure-tone audiometry.

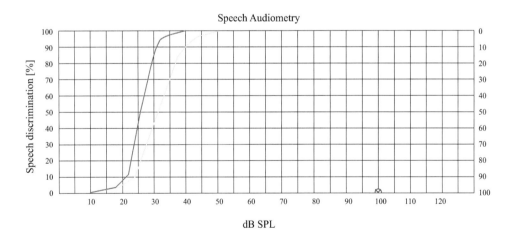

Figure 7.48.2 Preoperative speech audiometry.

Second implant, Med-El Vibrant Soundbridge (VSB) with SP-coupler, right ear

Pure-Tone Audiometry in Free-Field

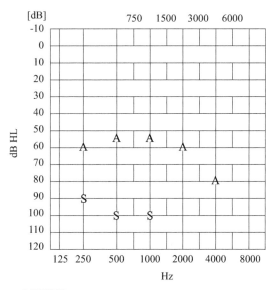

LEGEND:

A – implant (contralateral ear passively masked)

S – unaided (contralateral ear passively masked)

Figure 7.48.3 Pure-tone audiometry in a free-field for aided (A) and unaided (S) conditions after 12-month follow-up.

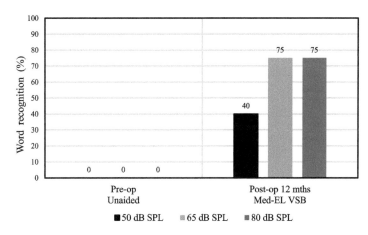

Figure 7.48.4 Word recognition score for unaided and aided conditions in quiet at 50, 65, and 80 dB SPL after 12-month follow-up. Non-implanted ear in passive masking.

49. Male, 51 years – cochlear implant

Bilateral hearing loss of unknown etiology diagnosed at the age of 35. Previous ear surgeries: ossiculoplasty of the left ear and two reoperations but no hearing improvement. Hearing aids never used. Head imaging: MR – no pathologies (Figures 7.49.1–7.49.5).

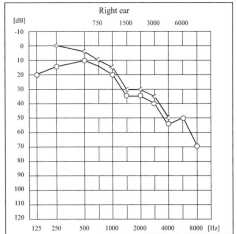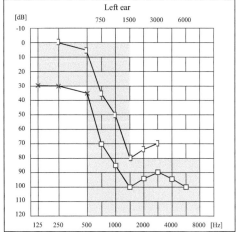

Figure 7.49.1 **Preoperative pure-tone audiometry.**

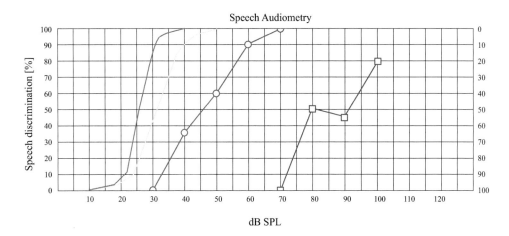

Figure 7.49.2 **Preoperative speech audiometry.**

Speech Audiometry in Free-Field

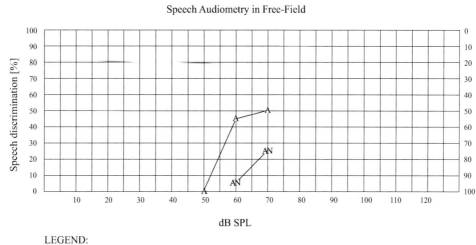

LEGEND:
A – left ear in hearing aid, right ear in active masking
AN – left ear in hearing aid, SNR + 10 dB, right ear in active masking

Figure 7.49.3 Preoperative speech audiometry in free-field.

PDT-EC (up to 250 Hz), CI left ear, Med-El SONATA FLEX24™

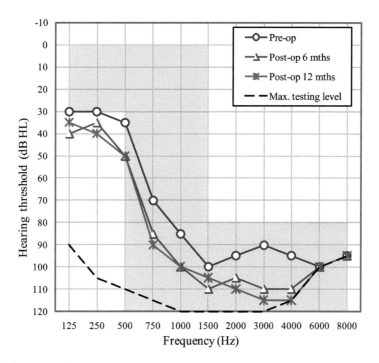

Figure 7.49.4 Pre- and postoperative hearing thresholds.

Hearing Preservation, Calculation in [%]			
Legend:		**Follow-up**	
S	**Hearing Preservation**	**6 months**	**12 months**
75 – 100%	Complete HP		
26 – 74%	Partial HP	**S = 70.1%**	**S = 66.2%**
1 – 25%	Minimal HP		
No detectable hearing	Loss of hearing		

Figure 7.49.5 Hearing preservation results.

50. Female, 52 years – cochlear implant

Sudden hearing loss of unknown etiology in the right ear with tinnitus at the age of 54. Hearing loss was accompanied by vertigo. No improvement in hearing and tinnitus after pharmacological treatment. No episodes of otitis media with effusing in medical history. Hearing aids: tried to use the CROS system and a conventional hearing aid but no hearing benefits. Head imaging: MRI with contrast – no pathologies (Figures 7.50.1–7.50.5).

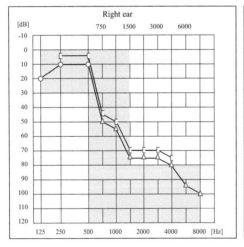 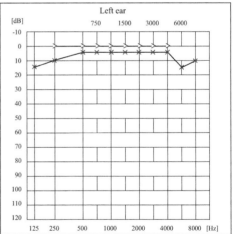

Figure 7.50.1 Preoperative pure-tone audiometry.

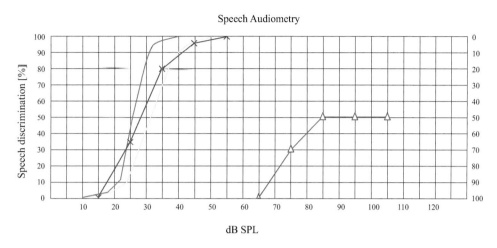

Figure 7.50.2 **Preoperative speech audiometry.**

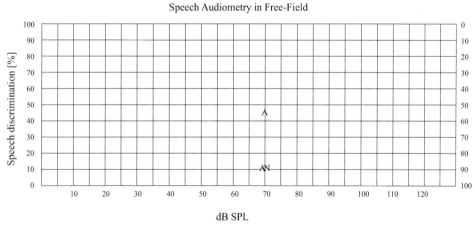

LEGEND:
A – right ear in hearing aid, left ear in active masking
AN – right ear in hearing aid, SNR + 10 dB, left ear in active masking

Figure 7.50.3 **Preoperative speech audiometry in free-field.**

PDT-EC (up to 500 Hz), CI right ear, Med-El CONCERTO FLEX24™

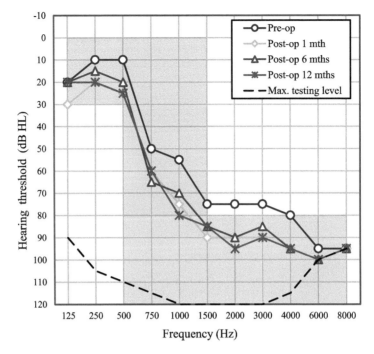

Figure 7.50.4 **Pre- and postoperative hearing thresholds.**

Hearing Preservation, Calculation in [%]				
Legend:		**Follow-up**		
S	**Hearing Preservation**	**1 month**	**6 months**	**12 months**
75 – 100%	Complete HP			
26 – 74%	Partial HP	S = 77.2%	S = 82.5%	S = 78.1%
1 – 25%	Minimal HP			
No detectable hearing	Loss of hearing			

Figure 7.50.5 **Hearing preservation results.**

51. Male, 52 years – cochlear implant

Sudden hearing loss in the left ear at the age of 45 as a result of a head injury, in CT – no fractures in the temporal bone. No improvement in hearing after treatment. Left-sided tinnitus. He does not use a hearing aid in the left ear due to the lack of hearing benefits. Head imaging: MRI with contrast – no pathologies (Figures 7.51.1–7.51.5).

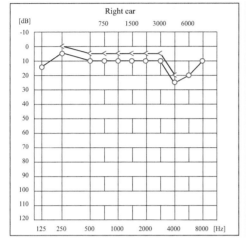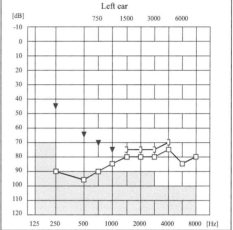

Figure 7.51.1 **Preoperative pure-tone audiometry.**

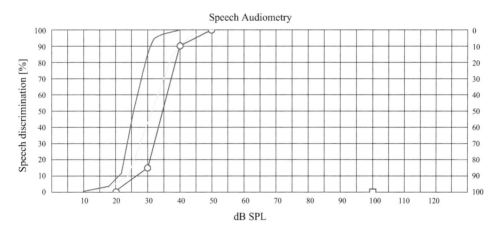

Figure 7.51.2 **Preoperative speech audiometry.**

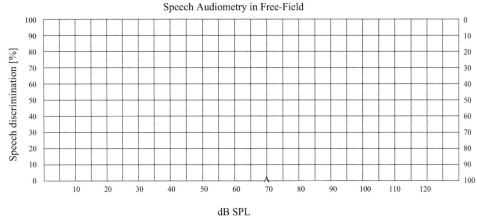

LEGEND:
A – left in hearing aid, right ear in active masking

Figure 7.51.3 Preoperative speech audiometry in free-field.

PDT-ES, CI left ear, Advanced Bionics HiRes 90K™ Advantage

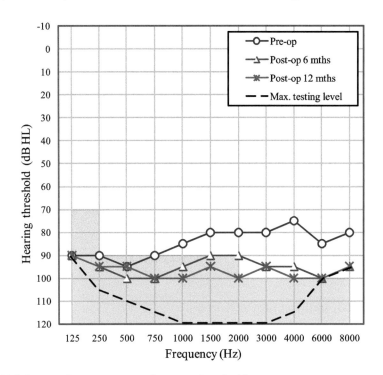

Figure 7.51.4 Pre- and postoperative hearing thresholds.

Hearing Preservation, Calculation in [%]			
Legend:		Follow-up	
S	Hearing Preservation	6 months	12 months
75 – 100%	Complete HP	S = 58.9%	S = 51.8%
26 – 74%	Partial HP		
1 – 25%	Minimal HP		
No detectable hearing	Loss of hearing		

Figure 7.51.5 Hearing preservation results.

52. Male, 53 years – cochlear implant

Sudden hearing loss in the right ear at the age of 49 after head injury and fracture of the right occipital and temporal bone (transverse fracture), complicated by subdural hematoma, hemorrhage in the left frontal lobe, with a contusion of the left cerebellar hemisphere. Right-sided tinnitus. Chronic vertigo. Hearing aids CROS test – subjectively hearing impressions unfavorable. Imaging diagnostics: CT of the temporal bones – comminuted fractures on the occipital, the fracture goes through the temporal bone, a transverse fracture from the posterior part of the temporal bone pyramid through the upper part of the semicircular canals and through the bottom of the lateral edge of the inner auditory canal. Head imaging: MRI – the continuity of the right auditory nerve is preserved (Figures 7.52.1–7.52.5).

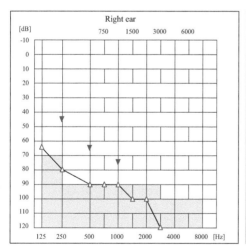
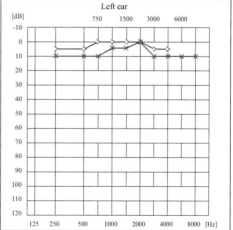

Figure 7.52.1 Preoperative pure-tone audiometry.

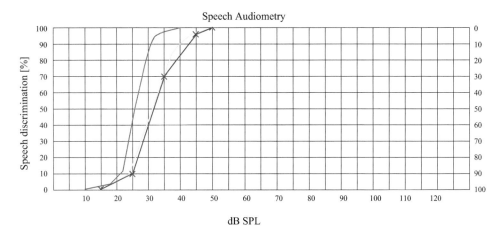

Figure 7.52.2 **Preoperative speech audiometry.**

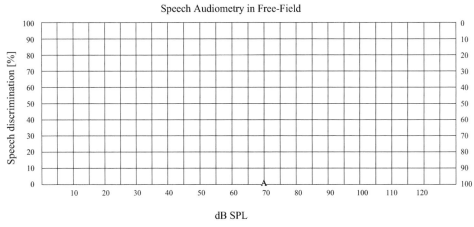

LEGEND:
A – right ear in hearing aid, left ear in active masking

Figure 7.52.3 **Preoperative speech audiometry in free-field.**

PDT-ES, CI right ear, Cochlear™ Nucleus® Straight Research Array (SRA)

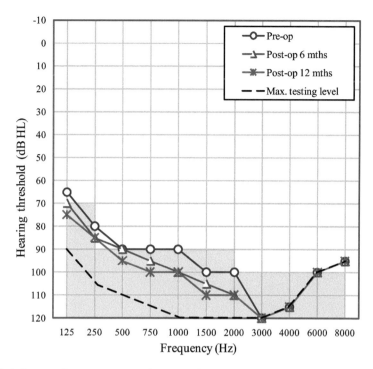

Figure 7.52.4 Pre- and postoperative hearing thresholds.

Hearing Preservation, Calculation in [%]			
Legend:		Follow-up	
S	Hearing Preservation	6 months	12 months
75 – 100%	Complete HP		
26 – 74%	Partial HP	S = 75.8%	S = 63.6%
1 – 25%	Minimal HP		
No detectable hearing	Loss of hearing		

Figure 7.52.5 Hearing preservation results.

53. Male, 54 years – cochlear implant

Bilateral gradually progressive hearing loss since about 30 years of age. Bilateral tinnitus; no vertigo. Hearing aid in the right ear since the age of 46. Chronic conditions: Crohn's disease (Figures 7.53.1–7.53.5).

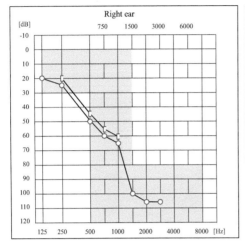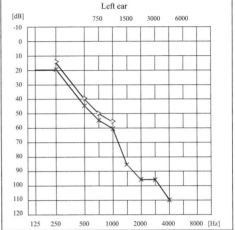

Figure 7.53.1 **Preoperative pure-tone audiometry.**

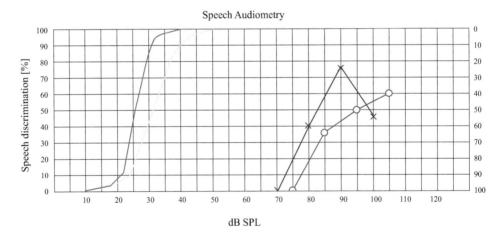

Figure 7.53.2 **Preoperative speech audiometry.**

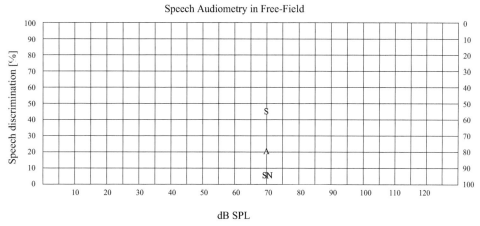

Speech Audiometry in Free-Field

LEGEND:
A – right ear in hearing aid, left ear in passive masking
S – left ear in hearing aid, right ear in passive masking
SN – left ear in hearing aid, SNR + 10 dB, right ear in passive masking

Figure 7.53.3 Preoperative speech audiometry in free-field.

PDT-EC (from 250 Hz), CI right ear, Med-El SONATA FLEX24™

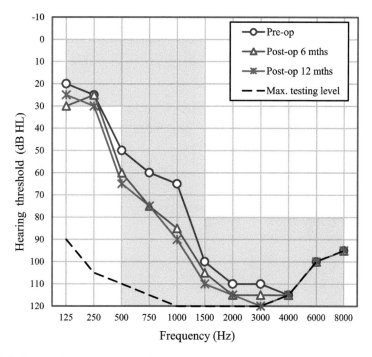

Figure 7.53.4 Pre- and postoperative hearing thresholds.

Hearing Preservation, Calculation in [%]			
Legend:		**Follow-up**	
S	**Hearing Preservation**	**6 months**	**12 months**
75 – 100%	Complete HP		
26 – 74%	Partial HP	S = 80.6%	S = 75.0%
1 – 25%	Minimal HP		
No detectable hearing	Loss of hearing		

Figure 7.53.5 Hearing preservation results.

54. Female, 55 years – cochlear implant

Bilateral hearing loss probably since birth as a result of treatment with ototoxic drugs in the perinatal period. Developed speech. No prior ear surgeries. No tinnitus. Occasional vertigo, mainly in stressful situations. There was an attempt of the hearing-aid fitting, but no success due to the occlusion effect (Figures 7.54.1–7.54.5).

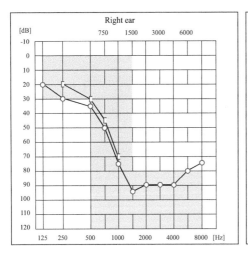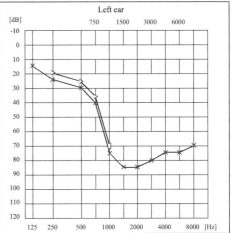

Figure 7.54.1 Preoperative pure-tone audiometry.

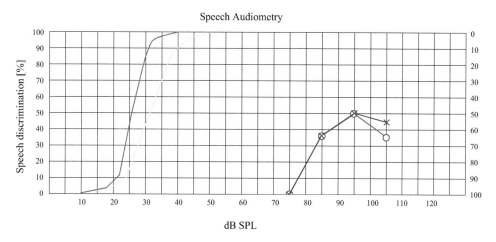

Figure 7.54.2 **Preoperative speech audiometry.**

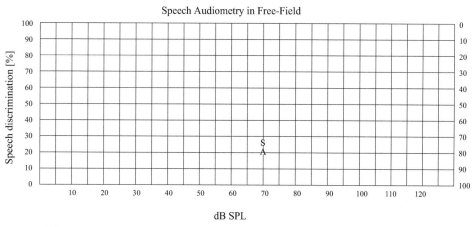

LEGEND:
A – right ear in hearing aid, left ear in passive masking
S – left ear in hearing aid, right ear in passive masking

Figure 7.54.3 **Preoperative speech audiometry in free-field.**

PDT-EC (from 250 Hz), CI right ear, Med-El SONATA FLEX20

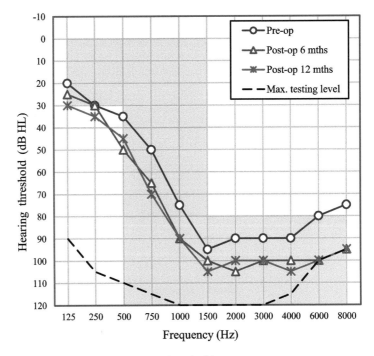

Figure 7.54.4 Pre- and postoperative hearing thresholds.

Hearing Preservation, Calculation in [%]			
Legend:		Follow-up	
S	Hearing Preservation	6 months	12 months
75 – 100%	Complete HP	S = 72.9%	S = 69.8%
26 – 74%	Partial HP		
1 – 25%	Minimal HP		
No detectable hearing	Loss of hearing		

Figure 7.54.5 Hearing preservation results.

55. Male, 55 years – cochlear implant

Bilateral gradually progressive hearing loss since childhood. Meningitis at the age of 7, treated with ototoxic drugs. Moreover, for about 15–17 years, he worked in noise. He has never used hearing aids – no hearing benefit when trying to fit devices. Bilateral worsening tinnitus for many years. Head imaging: MRI with contrast – without pathology in the area of the VII and VIII cranial nerves on both sides, a slightly elongated AICA loop on the left side, no signs of adherence to the auditory nerve (Figures 7.55.1–7.55.5).

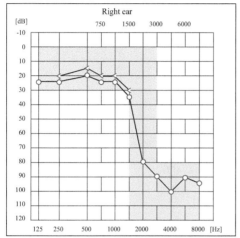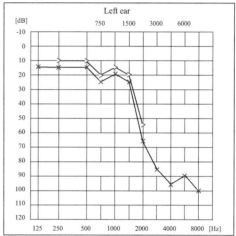

Figure 7.55.1 **Preoperative pure-tone audiometry.**

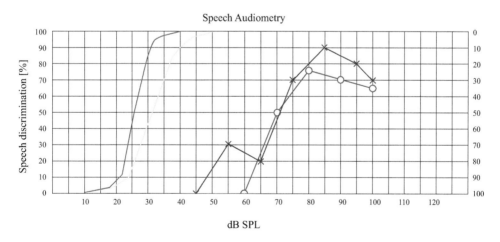

Figure 7.55.2 **Preoperative speech audiometry.**

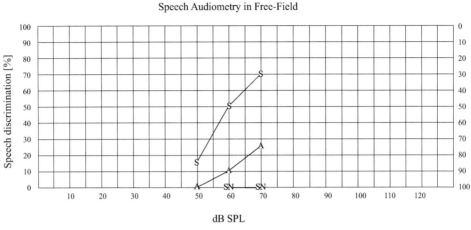

Figure 7.55.3 Preoperative speech audiometry in free-field.

PDT-ENS, CI right ear, Med-El SONATA FLEX20

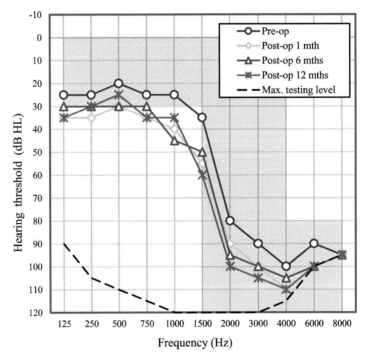

Figure 7.55.4 Pre- and postoperative hearing thresholds.

Hearing Preservation, Calculation in [%]				
Legend:		Follow-up		
S	Hearing Preservation	1 months	6 months	12 months
75 – 100%	Complete HP			
26 – 74%	Partial HP	S = 80.8%	S = 83.3%	S = 80.0%
1 – 25%	Minimal HP			
No detectable hearing	Loss of hearing			

Figure 7.55.5 Hearing preservation results.

56. Female, 56 years – cochlear implant

Bilateral gradually progressive hearing loss of unknown etiology since the age of 47. No tinnitus or vertigo. She does not use hearing aids due to the lack of improvement in speech understanding. Head imaging: CT – no pathologies (Figures 7.56.1–7.56.5).

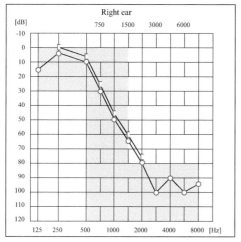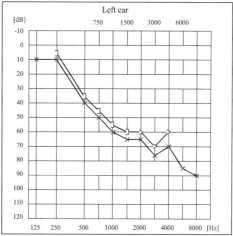

Figure 7.56.1 Preoperative pure-tone audiometry.

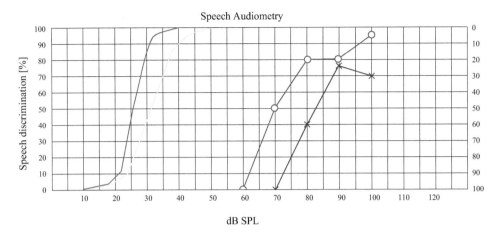

Figure 7.56.2 **Preoperative speech audiometry.**

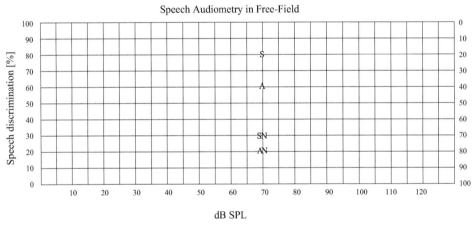

LEGEND:
A – right ear in hearing aid, left ear in passive masking
S – left ear in hearing aid, right ear in passive masking
AN – right ear in hearing aid, SNR + 10 dB, left ear in passive masking
SN – left ear in hearing aid, SNR + 10 dB, right ear in passive masking

Figure 7.56.3 **Preoperative speech audiometry in free-field.**

PDT-EC (from 750 Hz), CI right ear, Med-El SYNCHRONY FLEX24™

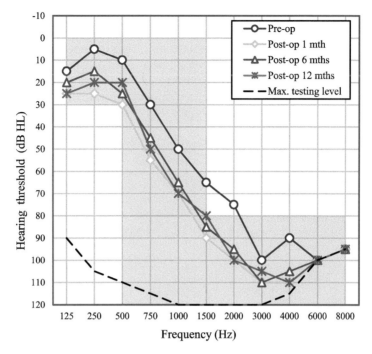

Figure 7.56.4 Pre- and postoperative hearing thresholds.

Hearing Preservation, Calculation in [%]				
Legend:		Follow-up		
S	Hearing Preservation	1 months	6 months	12 months
75 – 100%	Complete HP			
26 – 74%	Partial HP	S = 69.6%	S = 78.3%	S = 75.7%
1 – 25%	Minimal HP			
No detectable hearing	Loss of hearing			

Figure 7.56.5 Hearing preservation results.

57. Male, 56 years – bone conduction implant

Bilateral hearing loss since around 30 years of age due to recurrent otitis media with effusion. Right ear: removal of a brain abscess in the left temporal lobe. Left ear: condition following surgery to remove a brain abscess in the left temporal lobe, revision radical surgery, and reoperation. The anatomical conditions make it impossible to perform reconstructive surgery. Occasional right-sided tinnitus. He has used a hearing aid in his right ear since the age of 48 (Figures 7.57.1–7.57.4).

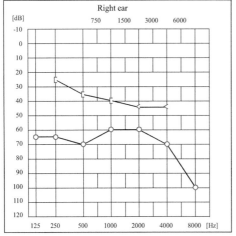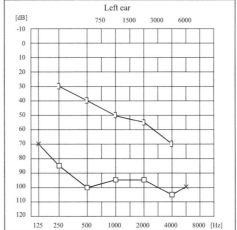

Figure 7.57.1 Preoperative pure-tone audiometry.

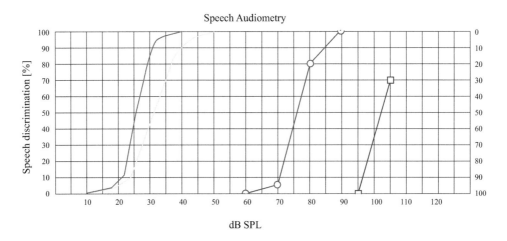

Figure 7.57.2 Preoperative speech audiometry.

Oticon Medical Ponto, left ear

Pure-Tone Audiometry in Free-Field

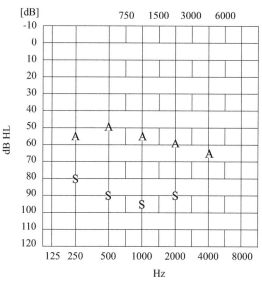

LEGEND:

A – implant (contralateral ear passively masked)

S – implant (contralateral ear passively masked)

Figure 7.57.3 Pure-tone audiometry in a free-field for aided (A) and unaided (S) conditions after 12-month follow-up.

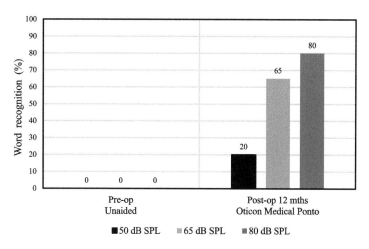

Figure 7.57.4 Word recognition score for unaided and aided conditions in quiet at 50, 65, and 80 dB SPL after 12-month follow-up. Non-implanted ear in passive masking.

58. Male, 57 years – bone conduction implant

Chronic otitis media in the right ear since childhood. Left-ear tympanoplasty at the age of 47 (performed in another clinic) complicated by peripheral paresis of the left facial nerve. Left-ear ossiculoplasty at the age of 52, followed by left-ear myringoplasty, which resulted in hearing improvement. Right-ear epitympanotomy with middle-ear lesion removal at the age of 53 and then myringoplasty and re-myringo-ossiculoplasty. Second-look surgery 2 years later. Right-ear pulsing tinnitus, compatible with the pulse and a feeling of blockage. Hearing aids never used (Figures 7.58.1–7.58.4).

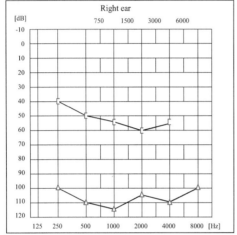
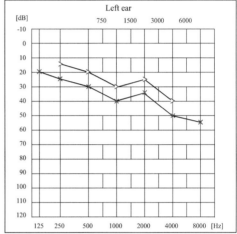

Figure 7.58.1 Preoperative pure-tone audiometry.

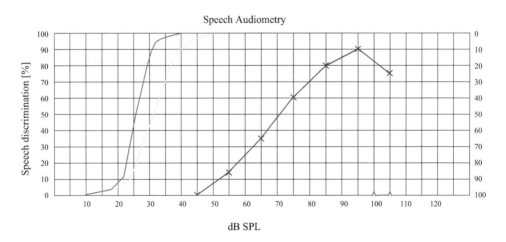

Figure 7.58.2 Preoperative speech audiometry.

Oticon Medical Ponto, right ear

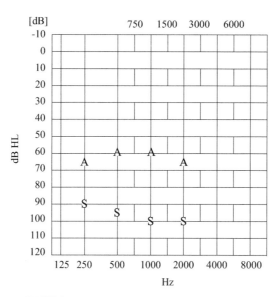

Pure-Tone Audiometry in Free-Field

LEGEND:

A – implant (contralateral ear actively masked)

S – implant (contralateral ear actively masked)

Figure 7.58.3 Pure-tone audiometry in a free-field for aided (A) and unaided (S) conditions after 12-month follow-up.

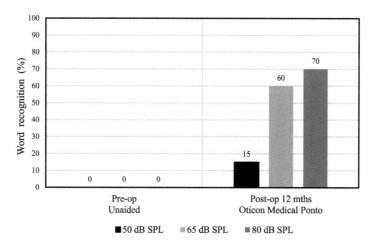

Figure 7.58.4 Word recognition score for unaided and aided conditions in quiet at 50, 65, and 80 dB SPL after 12-month follow-up. Non-implanted ear in active masking.

59. Male, 57 years – cochlear implant

Sudden bilateral hearing loss at the age of 39. Hearing improved after pharmacological treatment. Another episode of sudden hearing loss with significant hearing deterioration in the right ear one year later. Bilateral tinnitus since the age of 39. Hearing aid on the left ear since the age of 41. There was an attempt of the hearing-aid fitting on the right ear, but no benefits. Head imaging: MRI – no pathologies (Figures 7.59.1–7.59.5).

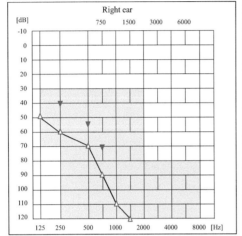
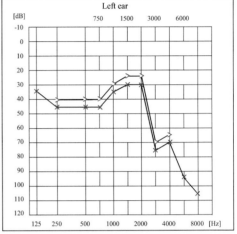

Figure 7.59.1 **Preoperative pure-tone audiometry.**

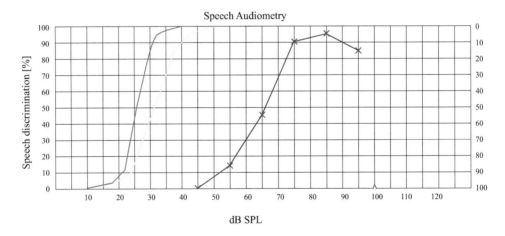

Figure 7.59.2 **Preoperative speech audiometry.**

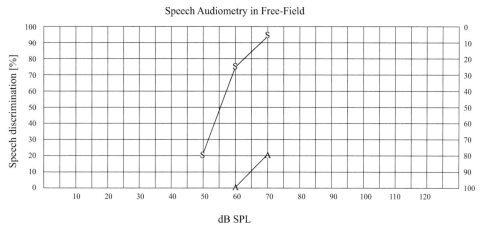

Speech Audiometry in Free-Field

LEGEND:
A – right ear in hearing aid, left ear in active masking
S – left ear in hearing aid, right ear in passive masking

Figure 7.59.3 Preoperative speech audiometry in free-field.

PDT-EAS, CI right ear, Oticon NEURO Zti EVO

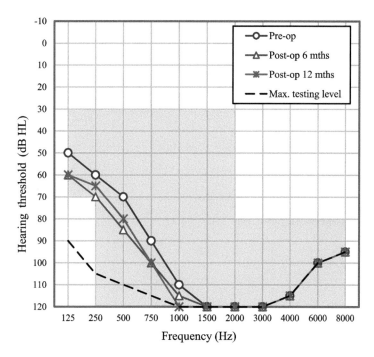

Figure 7.59.4 Pre- and postoperative hearing thresholds.

Hearing Preservation, Calculation in [%]			
Legend:		Follow-up	
S	Hearing Preservation	6 months	12 months
75 – 100%	Complete HP		
26 – 74%	Partial HP	S = 68.8%	S = 71.9%
1 – 25%	Minimal HP		
No detectable hearing	Loss of hearing		

Figure 7.59.5 Hearing preservation results.

60. Female, 58 years – cochlear implant

Progressive hearing loss in the left ear from the age of 50. Sudden idiopathic hearing loss in the right ear at the age of 54. Lack of improvement in hearing after treatment. She uses hearing aids on the left ear since the age of 51 and on the right ear since the age of 55. Head imaging: MRI – no pathologies (Figures 7.60.1–7.60.5).

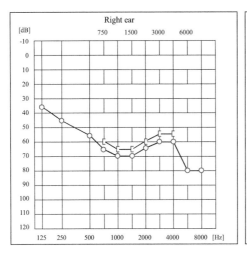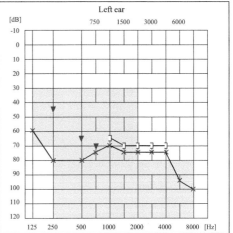

Figure 7.60.1 Preoperative pure-tone audiometry.

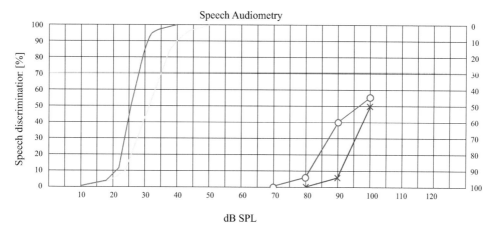

Figure 7.60.2 **Preoperative speech audiometry.**

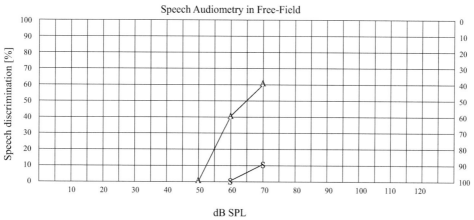

LEGEND:
A – right ear in hearing aid, left ear in passive masking
S – left ear in hearing aid, right ear in passive masking

Figure 7.60.3 **Preoperative speech audiometry in free-field.**

PDT-EAS, CI left ear, Oticon NEURO Zti EVO

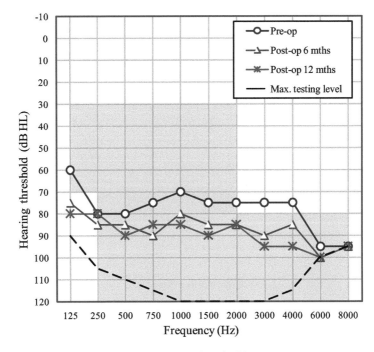

Figure 7.60.4 **Pre- and postoperative hearing thresholds.**

Hearing Preservation, Calculation in [%]			
Legend:		**Follow-up**	
S	**Hearing Preservation**	**6 months**	**12 months**
75 – 100%	Complete HP		
26 – 74%	Partial HP	**S = 71.8%**	**S = 64.8%**
1 – 25%	Minimal HP		
No detectable hearing	Loss of hearing		

Figure 7.60.5 **Hearing preservation results.**

61. Male, 59 years – cochlear implant

Gradually progressive hearing loss in the right ear since the age of 49. Bilateral sudden deafness at the age of 55. Hearing loss was accompanied by vertigo. No improvement in hearing after pharmacological treatment. Since hearing loss, he has suffered from persistent, bothersome tinnitus. Since the age of 56, he has been using a hearing aid on the left ear systematically. He does not use a hearing aid on the right ear due to the lack of hearing benefits, although there was an attempt of the hearing-aid fitting on that ear (Figures 7.61.1–7.61.5).

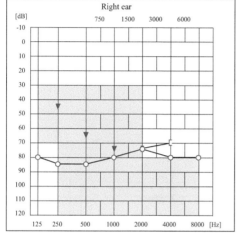
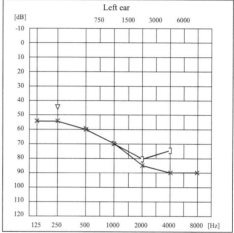

Figure 7.61.1 **Preoperative pure-tone audiometry.**

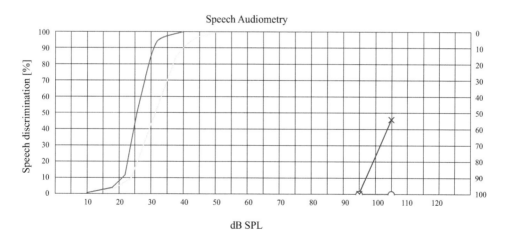

Figure 7.61.2 **Preoperative speech audiometry.**

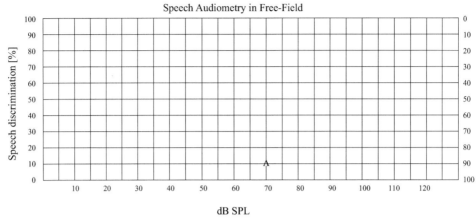

LEGEND:
A – right ear in hearing aid, left ear in passive masking

Figure 7.61.3 Preoperative speech audiometry in free-field.

PDT-EAS, CI right ear, Oticon NEURO Zti EVO

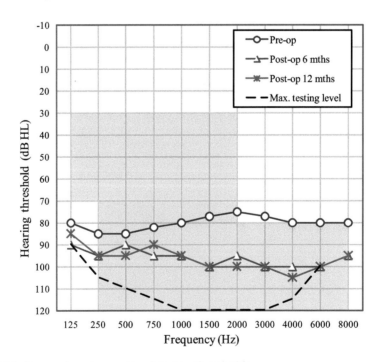

Figure 7.61.4 Pre- and postoperative hearing thresholds.

Hearing Preservation, Calculation in [%]			
Legend:		**Follow-up**	
S	**Hearing Preservation**	**6 months**	**12 months**
75 – 100%	Complete HP		
26 – 74%	Partial HP	**S = 47.1%**	**S = 45.6%**
1 – 25%	Minimal HP		
No detectable hearing	Loss of hearing		

Figure 7.61.5 Hearing preservation results.

62. Female, 60 years – cochlear implant

Right-sided progressive hearing loss from the age of 48. Sudden idiopathic deafness in the left ear at the age of 54 accompanied by tinnitus and vertigo. No hearing improvement after pharmacological treatment. Annoying tinnitus in the left ear. There was an attempt of the hearing-aid fitting on the left ear, but no benefits. Head imaging: MRI and CT – no pathologies (Figures 7.62.1–7.62.5).

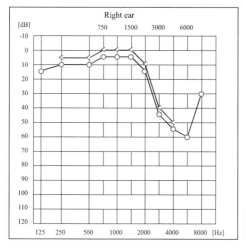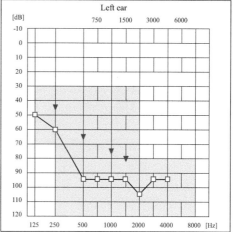

Figure 7.62.1 Preoperative pure-tone audiometry.

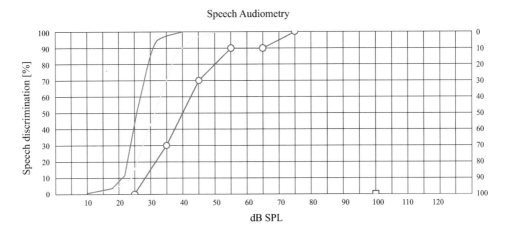

Figure 7.62.2 **Preoperative speech audiometry.**

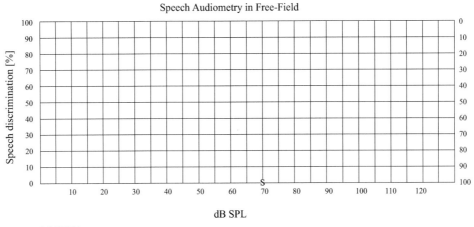

LEGEND:
S – left ear in hearing aid, right ear in active masking

Figure 7.62.3 **Preoperative speech audiometry in free-field.**

PDT-EAS, CI left ear, Cochlear™ Nucleus® CI422

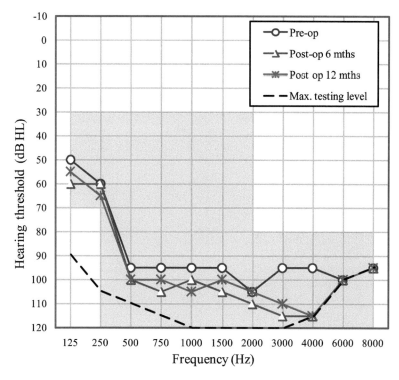

Figure 7.62.4 Pre- and postoperative hearing thresholds.

Hearing Preservation, Calculation in [%]			
Legend:		**Follow-up**	
S	**Hearing Preservation**	**6 months**	**12 months**
75 – 100%	Complete HP		
26 – 74%	Partial HP	**S = 63.0%**	**S = 69.6%**
1 – 25%	Minimal HP		
No detectable hearing	Loss of hearing		

Figure 7.62.5 Hearing preservation results.

63. Male, 60 years – middle-ear implant

Bilateral, chronic otitis media in childhood. Hearing loss was noticed at the age of 17. Previous ear surgeries: bilateral myringoossiculoplasty (in another clinic), radical modified right-ear surgery. He tried to use hearing aids, but he quit due to pain and discomfort and a feeling of wetness in the external ear canals (Figures 7.63.1–7.63.4).

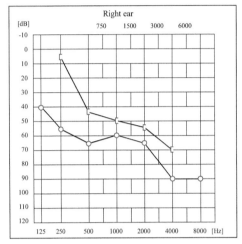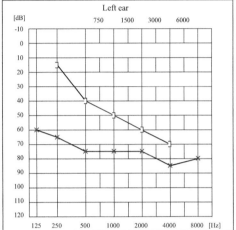

Figure 7.63.1 **Preoperative pure-tone audiometry.**

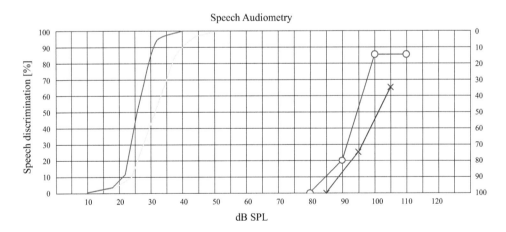

Figure 7.63.2 **Preoperative speech audiometry.**

Cochlear™ MET® system, left ear

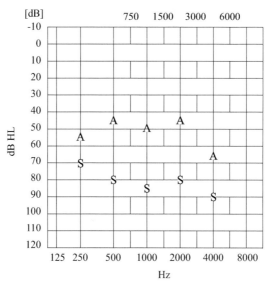

Figure 7.63.3 Pure-tone audiometry in a free-field for aided (A) and unaided (S) conditions after 12-month follow-up.

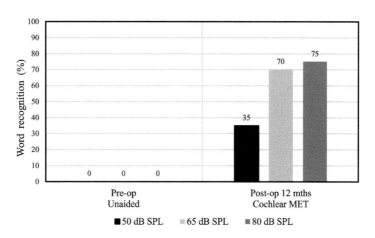

Figure 7.63.4 Word recognition score for unaided and aided conditions in quiet at 50, 65, and 80 dB SPL after 12-month follow-up. Non-implanted ear in passive masking.

64. Male, 60 years – cochlear implant

Bilateral gradually progressive hearing loss from the age of 30. From the age of 39, he has used a hearing aid on the right ear systematically, and between the age of 45 and 56, he had used hearing aids bilaterally, but at the age of 56, he stopped using it on the left ear due to the lack of hearing benefit (Figures 7.64.1–7.64.5).

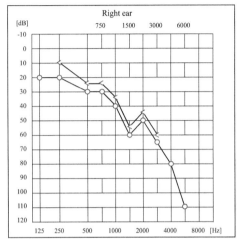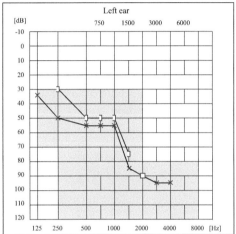

Figure 7.64.1 **Preoperative pure-tone audiometry.**

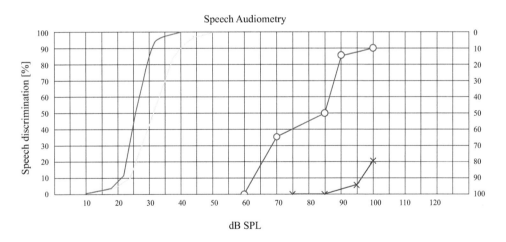

Figure 7.64.2 **Preoperative speech audiometry.**

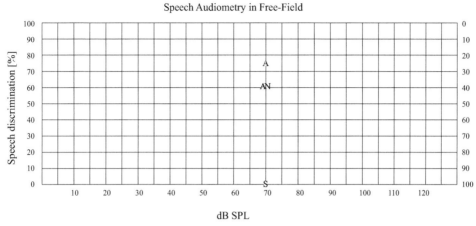

Figure 7.64.3 Preoperative speech audiometry in free-field.

PDT-EAS, CI left ear, Med-El CONCERTO FLEX24™

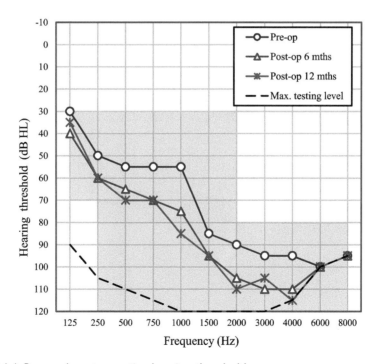

Figure 7.64.4 Pre- and postoperative hearing thresholds.

Hearing Preservation, Calculation in [%]			
Legend:		**Follow-up**	
S	**Hearing Preservation**	**6 months**	**12 months**
75 – 100%	Complete HP		
26 – 74%	Partial HP	S = 70.4%	S = 66.7%
1 – 25%	Minimal HP		
No detectable hearing	Loss of hearing		

Figure 7.64.5 Hearing preservation results.

65. Male, 61 years – cochlear implant

Sudden idiopathic deafness in the right ear at the age of 56 – no hearing improvement after pharmacological treatment. Hearing loss was accompanied by vertigo and right-sided tinnitus present until implantation. There was an attempt of the hearing-aid fitting, but subjectively no benefits. Head imaging: CT without contrast – no pathologies (Figures 7.65.1–7.65.5).

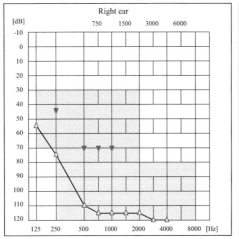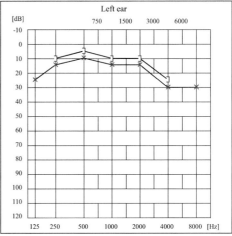

Figure 7.65.1 Preoperative pure-tone audiometry.

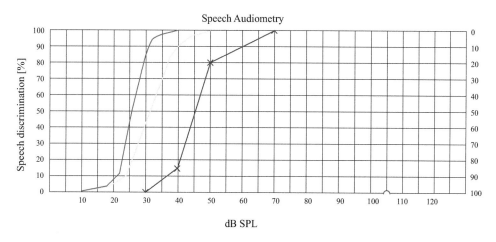

Figure 7.65.2 **Preoperative speech audiometry.**

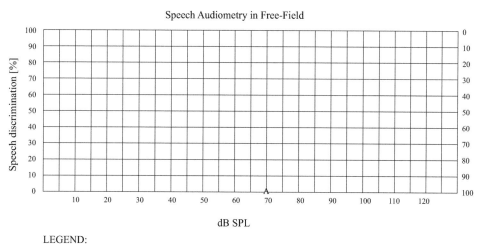

LEGEND:
A – right ear in hearing aid, left ear in active masking

Figure 7.65.3 **Preoperative speech audiometry in free-field.**

PDT-EAS, CI right ear, Advanced Bionics HiFocus™ SlimJ

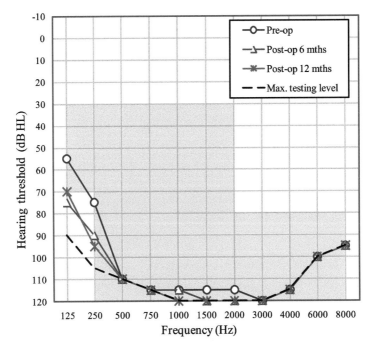

Figure 7.65.4 Pre- and postoperative hearing thresholds.

Hearing Preservation, Calculation in [%]			
Legend:		**Follow-up**	
S	**Hearing Preservation**	**6 months**	**12 months**
75 – 100%	Complete HP		
26 – 74%	Partial HP	S = 43.8%	S = 37.5%
1 – 25%	Minimal HP		
No detectable hearing	Loss of hearing		

Figure 7.65.5 Hearing preservation results.

66. Female, 62 years – middle-ear implant

Bilateral gradually progressive hearing loss since the age of 30 due to otosclerosis. Previous ear surgeries: bilateral stapedotomy and restapedotomy in the right ear. Since the age of 42, she has used hearing aids on both sides. After 11 years, she stopped using her right-ear hearing aid due to the lack of hearing benefits. Right-sided tinnitus for many years (Figures 7.66.1–7.66.4).

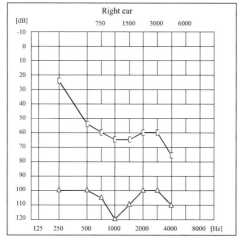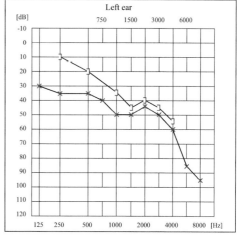

Figure 7.66.1 **Preoperative pure-tone audiometry.**

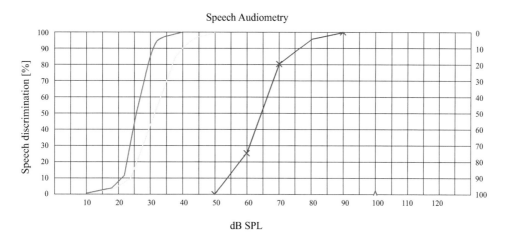

Figure 7.66.2 **Preoperative speech audiometry.**

Cochlear™ Codacs®, right ear

Pure-Tone Audiometry in Free-Field

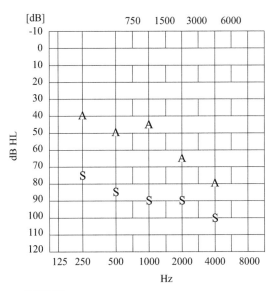

LEGEND:

A – implant (contralateral ear actively masked)

S – unaided (contralateral ear actively masked)

Figure 7.66.3 Pure-tone audiometry in a free-field for aided (A) and unaided (S) conditions after 12-month follow-up.

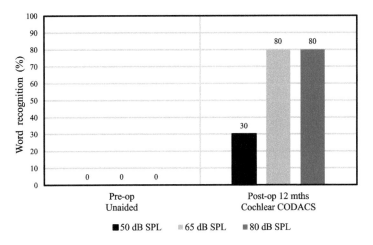

Figure 7.66.4 Word recognition score for unaided and aided conditions in quiet at 50, 65, and 80 dB SPL after 12-month follow-up. Non-implanted ear in active masking.

67. Female, 62 years – middle-ear implant

Bilateral gradually progressive hearing loss since the age of 50. In childhood, otitis media mainly the right ear. After a few months of using a hearing aid on the right ear, she stopped using it due to pain and recurrent otitis with effusion (Figures 7.67.1–7.67.4).

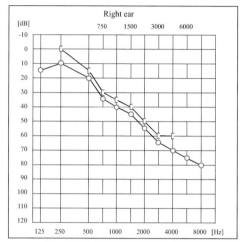
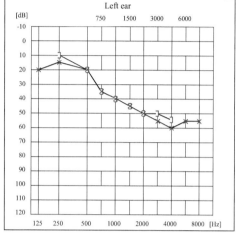

Figure 7.67.1 **Preoperative pure-tone audiometry.**

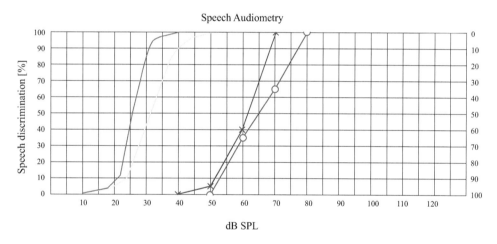

Figure 7.67.2 **Preoperative speech audiometry.**

Med-El Vibrant Soundbridge (VSB), right ear

Pure-Tone Audiometry in Free-Field

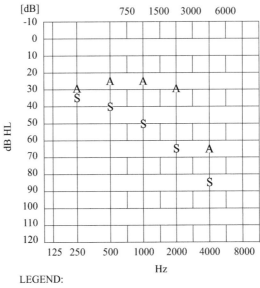

LEGEND:

A – implant (contralateral ear passively masked)

S – unaided (contralateral ear passively masked)

Figure 7.67.3 Pure-tone audiometry in a free-field for aided (A) and unaided (S) conditions after 12-month follow-up.

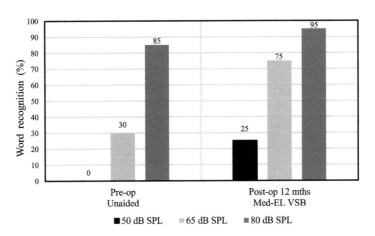

Figure 7.67.4 Word recognition score for unaided and aided conditions in quiet at 50, 65, and 80 dB SPL after 12-month follow-up. Non-implanted ear in passive masking.

68. Male, 62 years – cochlear implant

Sudden right-ear idiopathic hearing loss at the age of 46 – no hearing improvement after pharmacological treatment. Constant, bothersome right-sided tinnitus since the incident of sudden deafness. Gradually progressive hearing loss in the left ear since the age of 40. He has used a hearing aid on the left ear since the age of 45 (Figures 7.68.1–7.68.5).

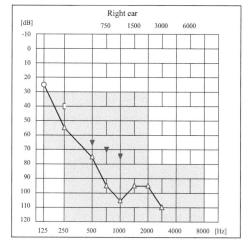
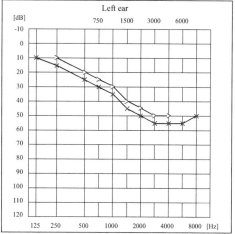

Figure 7.68.1 **Preoperative pure-tone audiometry.**

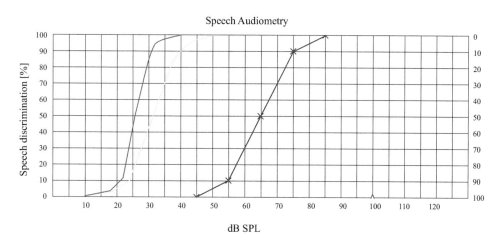

Figure 7.68.2 **Preoperative speech audiometry.**

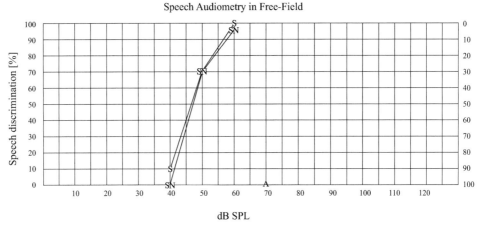

LEGEND:
A – right ear in hearing aid, left ear in active masking
S – left ear in hearing aid, right ear in passive masking
SN – left ear in hearing aid, SNR + 10 dB, right ear in passive masking

Figure 7.68.3 Preoperative speech audiometry in free-field.

PDT-EAS, CI right ear, Cochlear™ Nucleus® Straight Research Array (SRA)

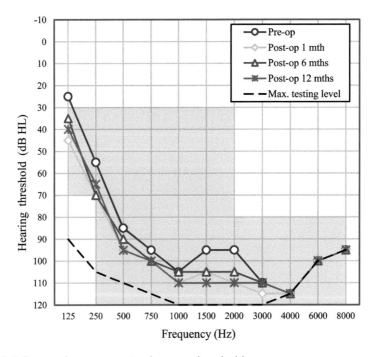

Figure 7.68.4 Pre- and postoperative hearing thresholds.

Hearing Preservation, Calculation in [%]				
Legend:		**Follow-up**		
S	**Hearing Preservation**	**1 month**	**6 months**	**12 months**
75 – 100%	Complete HP			
26 – 74%	Partial HP	S = 63.8 %	S = 76.6 %	S = 68.1 %
1 – 25%	Minimal HP			
No detectable hearing	Loss of hearing			

Figure 7.68.5 Hearing preservation results.

69. Male, 62 years – cochlear implant

Hearing problems since the age of 22, probably due to acoustic trauma (charge explosion during military exercises). Subjectively worse hearing in the right ear. Recurrent otitis with effusion mostly in winter. Bilateral tinnitus. Four episodes of intense vertigo after a fall. He does not use hearing aids due to the strong occlusion effect. Head imaging: CT – no pathologies (Figures 7.69.1–7.69.5).

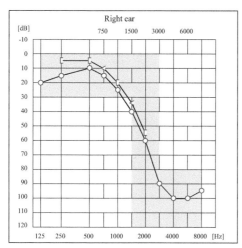
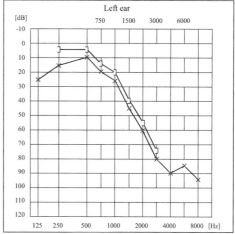

Figure 7.69.1 Preoperative pure-tone audiometry.

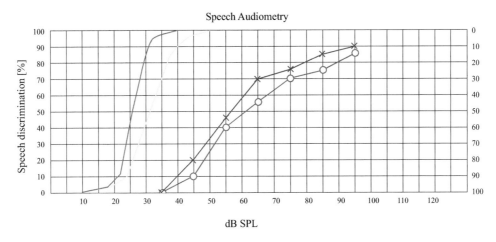

Figure 7.69.2 Preoperative speech audiometry.

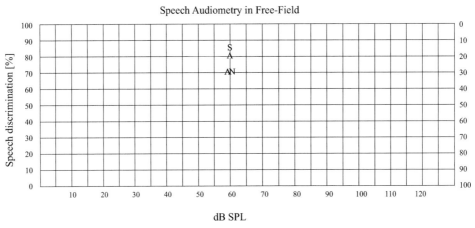

LEGEND:
A – right ear in hearing aid, left ear in passive masking
S – left ear in hearing aid, right ear in passive masking
AN – right and left ear unaided

Figure 7.69.3 Preoperative speech audiometry in free-field.

PDT-ENS, CI right ear, Med-El SONATA FLEX20

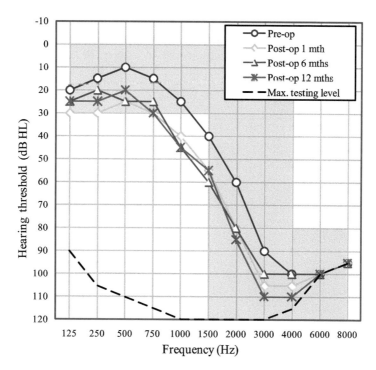

Figure 7.69.4 **Pre- and postoperative hearing thresholds.**

Hearing Preservation, Calculation in [%]				
Legend:		Follow-up		
S	Hearing Preservation	1 month	6 months	12 months
75-100%	Complete HP			
26-74%	Partial HP	S=80.5%	S=83.6%	S=79.7%
1-25%	Minimal HP			
No detectable hearing	Loss of hearing			

Figure 7.69.5 **Hearing preservation results.**

70. Male, 63 years – cochlear implant

Bilateral gradually progressive hearing loss since the age of 50. Bilateral tinnitus but not very annoying. He had a few episodes of vertigo in the past. He has used hearing aids on the right ear since the age of 59, on the left ear since the age of 57 (Figures 7.70.1–7.70.5).

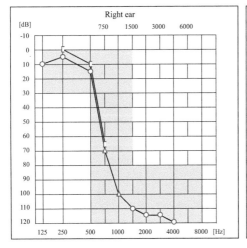
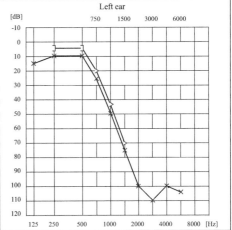

Figure 7.70.1 Preoperative pure-tone audiometry.

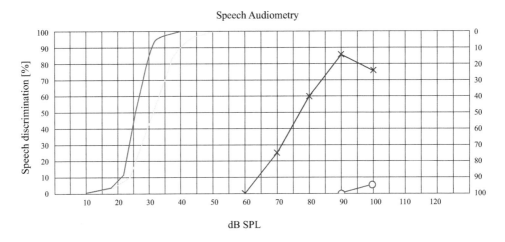

Figure 7.70.2 Preoperative speech audiometry.

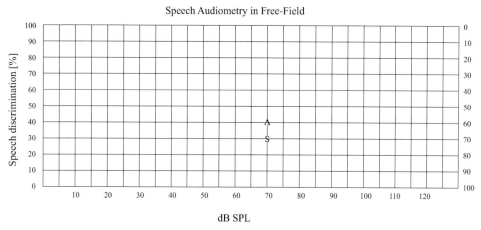

LEGEND:
A – left ear in hearing aid, right ear in passive masking
S – right ear in hearing aid, left ear in passive masking

Figure 7.70.3 Preoperative speech audiometry in free-field.

PDT-EC (from 500 Hz), CI right ear, Med-El CONCERTO FLEX24™

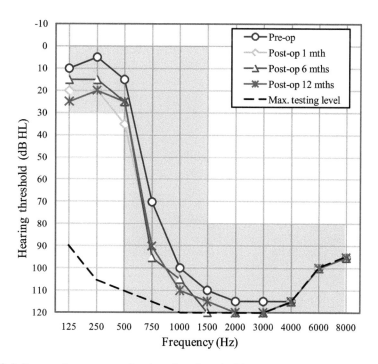

Figure 7.70.4 Pre- and postoperative hearing thresholds.

Hearing Preservation, Calculation in [%]				
Legend:		Follow-up		
S	Hearing Preservation	1 month	6 months	12 months
75 – 100%	Complete HP			
26 – 74%	Partial HP	S = 75.0%	S = 79.2%	S = 76.4%
1 – 25%	Minimal HP			
No detectable hearing	Loss of hearing			

Figure 7.70.5 Hearing preservation results.

71. Female, 64 years – cochlear implant

Bilateral gradually progressive hearing loss since the age of 53. Bilateral tinnitus for many years. Hearing aids: on the right ear since the age of 55, on the left ear since the age of 61. Subjectively, limited hearing benefits from using hearing aids. Head imaging: MRI with contrast – no pathologies (Figures 7.71.1–7.71.5).

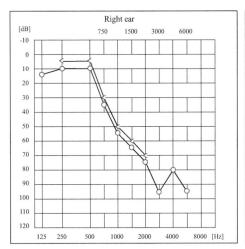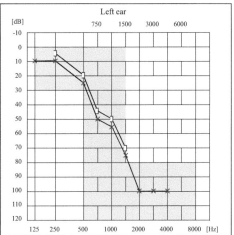

Figure 7.71.1 Preoperative pure-tone audiometry.

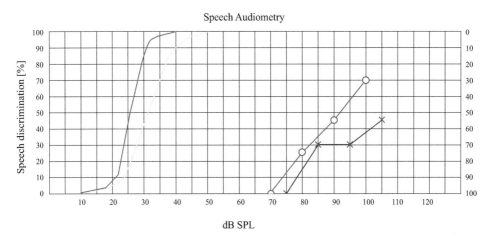

Figure 7.71.2 **Preoperative speech audiometry.**

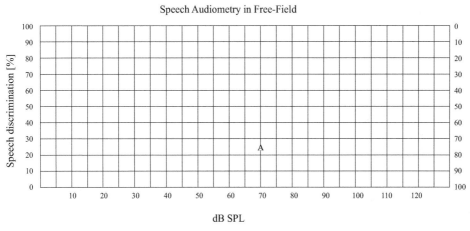

LEGEND:
A – left ear in hearing aid, right ear in passive masking

Figure 7.71.3 **Preoperative speech audiometry in free-field.**

PDT-EC (from 500 Hz), CI left ear, Med-El SONATA FLEX24™

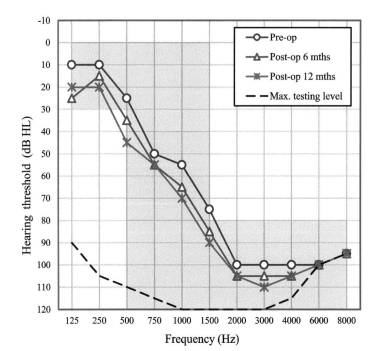

Figure 7.71.4 Pre- and postoperative hearing thresholds.

Hearing Preservation, Calculation in [%]			
Legend:		**Follow-up**	
S	**Hearing Preservation**	**6 months**	**12 months**
75 – 100%	Complete HP		
26 – 74%	Partial HP	**S = 85.7%**	**S = 80.6%**
1 – 25%	Minimal HP		
No detectable hearing	Loss of hearing		

Figure 7.71.5 Hearing preservation results.

72. Female, 64 years – cochlear implant

Bilateral gradually progressive hearing loss since the age of 50. Bilateral tinnitus. Intermittent mild vertigo. She has used hearing aids bilaterally since the age of 61 (Figures 7.72.1–7.72.5).

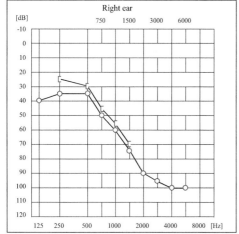 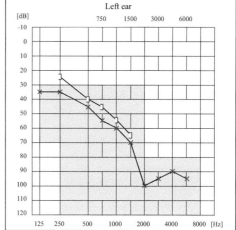

Figure 7.72.1 **Preoperative pure-tone audiometry.**

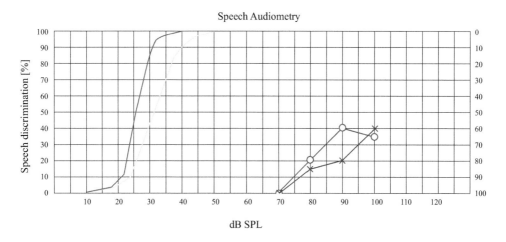

Figure 7.72.2 **Preoperative speech audiometry.**

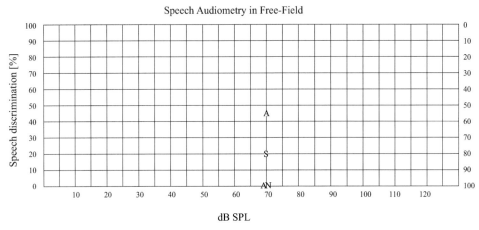

Speech Audiometry in Free-Field

LEGEND:
A – right ear in hearing aid, left ear in active masking
S – left ear in hearing aid, right ear in passive masking
AN – right ear in hearing aid, SNR + 10 dB, left ear in passive masking

Figure 7.72.3 **Preoperative speech audiometry in free-field.**

PDT-EAS, CI left ear, Cochlear™ Nucleus® CI422

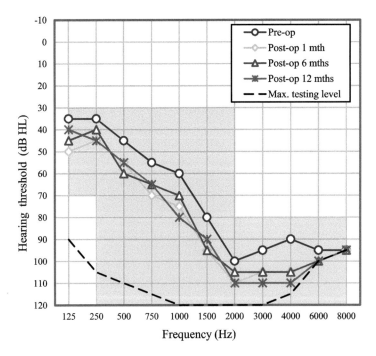

Figure 7.72.4 **Pre- and postoperative hearing thresholds.**

Hearing Preservation, Calculation in [%]				
Legend:		Follow-up		
S	Hearing Preservation	1 month	6 months	12 months
75 – 100%	Complete HP			
26 – 74%	Partial HP	S = 71.8%	S = 76.5%	S = 72.9%
1 – 25%	Minimal HP			
No detectable hearing	Loss of hearing			

Figure 7.72.5 Hearing preservation results.

73. Female, 64 years – bone conduction implant

Bilateral recurrent otitis media with effusion since the age of 18, more often in the left ear. Right-sided myringoplasty with tube placement at the age of 58 and attico-antro-mastoidectomy with the excision of middle-ear lesions. Left ear: double removal of cholesteatoma (in another clinic) and revision modified radical surgery at 57. After 1 year, second-look surgery – no recurrence of cholesteatoma. The left external ear canal posterior wall reconstruction with BonAlive® bioactive glass (at 62). Right-sided tinnitus. Periodic vertigo with the feeling of instability. She does not use hearing aids (Figures 7.73.1–7.73.4).

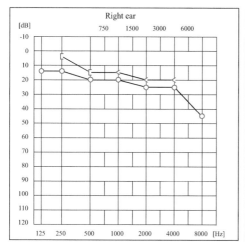
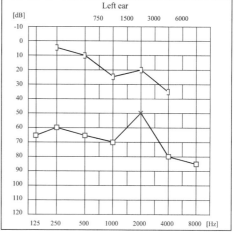

Figure 7.73.1 Preoperative pure-tone audiometry.

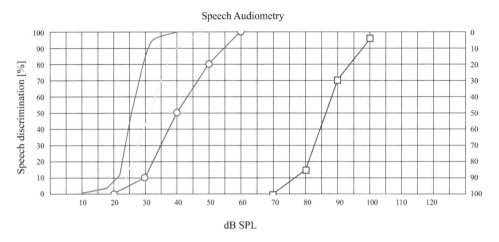

Figure 7.73.2 Preoperative speech audiometry.

Med-El Bonebridge (BB) BCI602, left ear

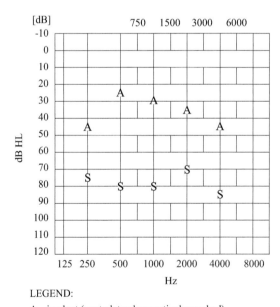

LEGEND:

A – implant (contralateral ear actively masked)

S – unaided (contralateral ear actively masked)

Figure 7.73.3 Pure-tone audiometry in a free-field for aided (A) and unaided (S) conditions after 3-month follow-up.

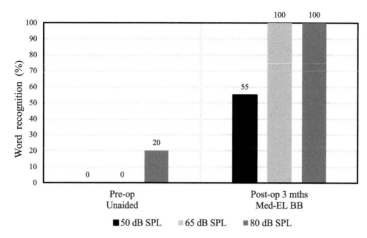

Figure 7.73.4 Word recognition score for unaided and aided conditions in quiet at 50, 65, and 80 dB SPL after 3-month follow-up. Non-implanted ear in active masking.

74. Female, 64 years – cochlear implant

Bilateral progressive hearing loss since childhood. Left-sided tinnitus since about 35 years of age. She had used hearing aids for about 6 months but stopped due to a lack of benefits. Head imaging: CT of the temporal bones and MRI – no pathologies (Figures 7.74.1–7.74.5).

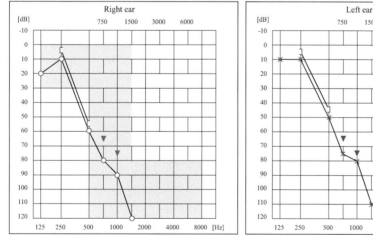
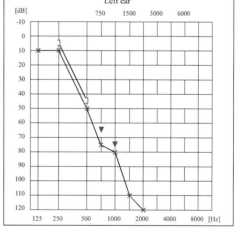

Figure 7.74.1 Preoperative pure-tone audiometry.

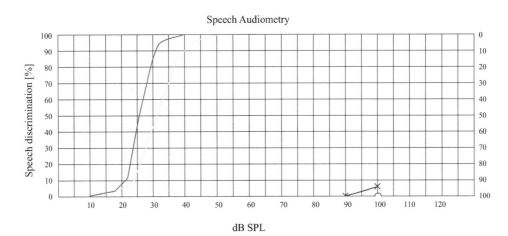

Figure 7.74.2 **Preoperative speech audiometry.**

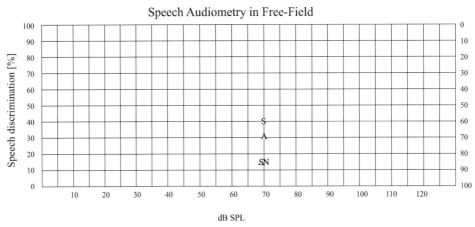

LEGEND:
A – right ear in hearing aid, left ear in passive masking
S – left ear in hearing aid, right ear in passive masking
AN – right ear in hearing aid, SNR + 10 dB, left ear in passive masking
SN – left ear in hearing aid, SNR + 10 dB, right ear in passive masking

Figure 7.74.3 **Preoperative speech audiometry in free-field.**

PDT-EC (from 250 Hz), CI right ear, Med-El SYNCHRONY FLEX28™

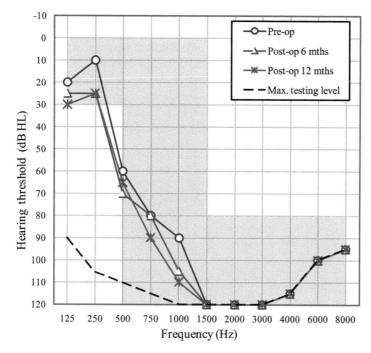

Figure 7.74.4 Pre- and postoperative hearing thresholds.

Hearing Preservation, Calculation in [%]			
Legend:		Follow-up	
S	Hearing Preservation	6 months	12 months
75 – 100%	Complete HP		
26 – 74%	Partial HP	S = 85.7%	S = 78.6%
1 – 25%	Minimal HP		
No detectable hearing	Loss of hearing		

Figure 7.74.5 Hearing preservation results.

75. Female, 65 years – bone conduction implant

In childhood, head trauma with left tympanic membrane perforation. In the past, some episodes of otitis media in the left ear. Radical surgery of the left ear at the age of 15. Reconstruction of the posterior wall of the left external ear canal using the Bon-Alive bioactive glass. There was an attempt of the hearing-aid fitting, but subjectively no benefits (Figures 7.75.1–7.75.4).

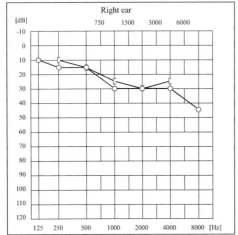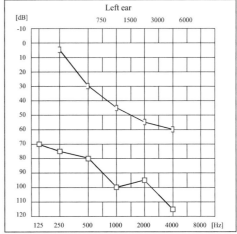

Figure 7.75.1 **Preoperative pure-tone audiometry.**

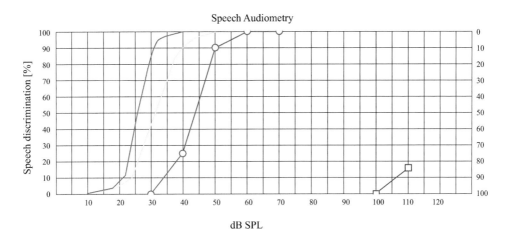

Figure 7.75.2 **Preoperative speech audiometry.**

Cochlear Baha Connect, left ear

Pure-Tone Audiometry in Free-Field

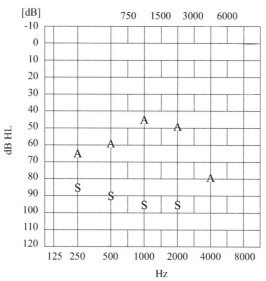

LEGEND:

A – implant (contralateral ear actively masked)

S – unaided (contralateral ear actively masked)

Figure 7.75.3 Pure-tone audiometry in a free-field for aided (A) and unaided (S) conditions after 12-month follow-up.

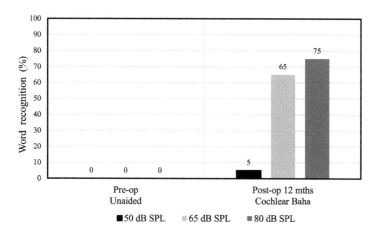

Figure 7.75.4 Word recognition score for unaided and aided conditions in quiet at 50, 65, and 80 dB SPL after 3-month follow-up. Non-implanted ear in active masking.

76. Male, 65 years – cochlear implant

Sudden left-ear hearing loss at the age of 48. The hearing loss in the right ear is gradually progressing for a few years. Bilateral tinnitus: more intense on the left side. Intermittent mild vertigo. He has used a hearing aid on the left ear since the age of 49. Head imaging: MRI – no pathologies (Figures 7.76.1–7.76.5).

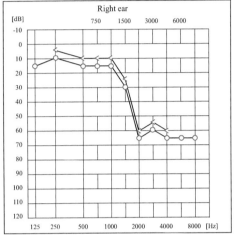 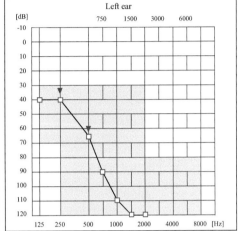

Figure 7.76.1 Preoperative pure-tone audiometry.

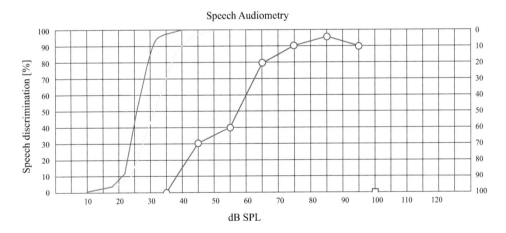

Figure 7.76.2 Preoperative speech audiometry.

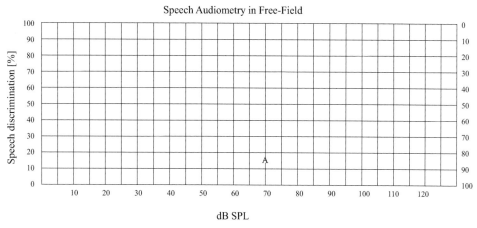

LEGEND:
A – left ear in hearing aid, right ear in active masking

Figure 7.76.3 Preoperative speech audiometry in free-field.

PDT-EAS, CI left ear, Oticon NEURO Zti EVO

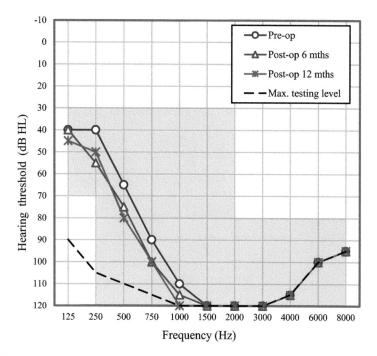

Figure 7.76.4 Pre- and postoperative hearing thresholds.

Hearing Preservation, Calculation in [%]			
Legend:		Follow-up	
S	Hearing Preservation	6 months	12 months
75 – 100%	Complete HP		
26 – 74%	Partial HP	S = 79.5%	S = 74.4%
1 – 25%	Minimal HP		
No detectable hearing	Loss of hearing		

Figure 7.76.5 Hearing preservation results.

77. Male, 65 years – cochlear implant

Bilateral gradually progressive hearing loss since the age of 45. Bilateral tinnitus. Vertigo since the age of 55. He had used hearing aids bilaterally since the age of 56 but stopped using them in the left year after 7 years due to the lack of hearing benefits. Head imaging: MRI – meningioma of 8 × 26 mm in front of the cerebral falx, numerous vascular lesions, no other lesions (Figures 7.77.1–7.77.5).

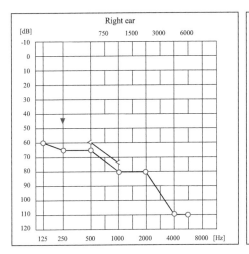
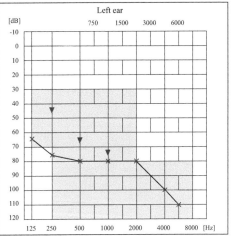

Figure 7.77.1 Preoperative pure-tone audiometry.

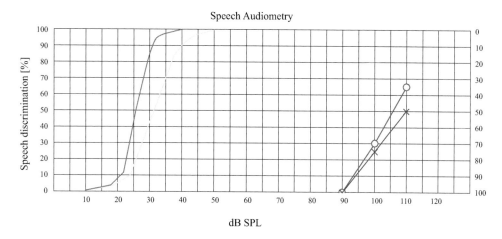

Figure 7.77.2 **Preoperative speech audiometry.**

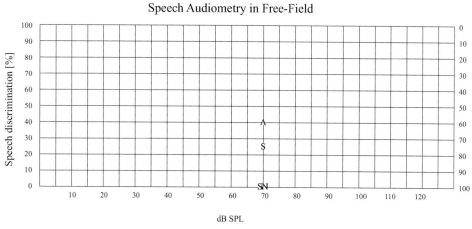

LEGEND:
A – right ear in hearing aid, left ear in passive masking
S – left ear in hearing aid, right ear in passive masking
AN – right ear unaided, left ear in passive masking
SN – left ear unaided, right ear in passive masking

Figure 7.77.3 **Preoperative speech audiometry in free-field.**

PDT-EAS, CI left ear, Advanced Bionics HiFocus™ SlimJ

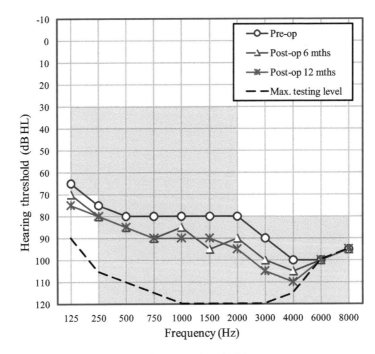

Figure 7.77.4 Pre- and postoperative hearing thresholds.

Hearing Preservation, Calculation in [%]			
Legend:		**Follow-up**	
S	Hearing Preservation	6 months	12 months
75 – 100%	Complete HP		
26 – 74%	Partial HP	S = 75.4%	S = 68.4%
1 – 25%	Minimal HP		
No detectable hearing	Loss of hearing		

Figure 7.77.5 Hearing preservation results.

78. Male, 65 years – cochlear implant

Bilateral gradually progressive hearing loss since the age of 40. For many years, he worked in noise without ear protectors. Subjectively worse hearing in the left ear. He has a hearing aid for the right ear but subjectively no hearing benefits (Figures 7.78.1–7.78.5).

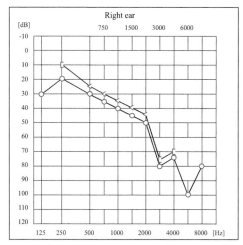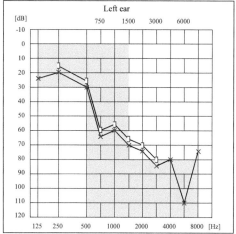

Figure 7.78.1 **Preoperative pure-tone audiometry.**

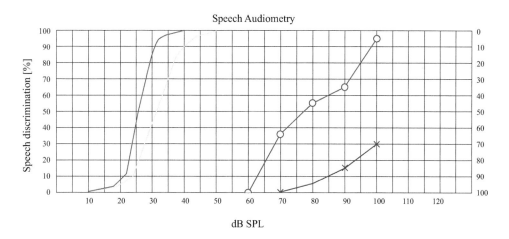

Figure 7.78.2 **Preoperative speech audiometry.**

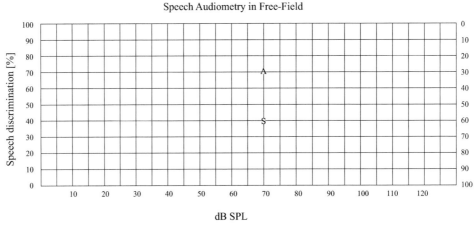

Figure 7.78.3 Preoperative speech audiometry in free-field.

PDT-EC (from 500 Hz), CI left ear, Med-El SYNCHRONY FLEX24™

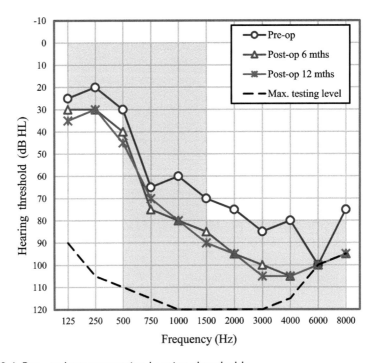

Figure 7.78.4 Pre- and postoperative hearing thresholds.

Hearing Preservation, Calculation in [%]			
Legend:		Follow-up	
S	Hearing Preservation	6 months	12 months
75 – 100%	Complete HP		
26 – 74%	Partial HP	S = 71.4%	S = 68.6%
1 – 25%	Minimal HP		
No detectable hearing	Loss of hearing		

Figure 7.78.5 Hearing preservation results.

79. Female, 59 years – middle-ear implant

Hearing problems of unknown etiology in both ears for about 10 years. In the patient's opinion, the hearing loss does not progress. Subjectively worse hearing in the left ear. No prior ear surgeries. Bilateral tinnitus, stronger on the left side. Positional vertigo when she tilts her head back. Hearing aids for both ears since 2013 with hearing benefits; currently, she cannot use them due to recurrent otitis (Figures 7.79.1–7.79.4).

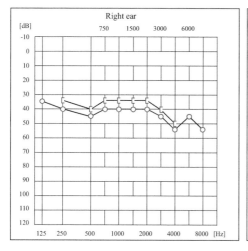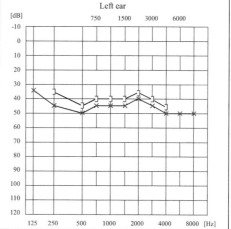

Figure 7.79.1 Preoperative pure-tone audiometry.

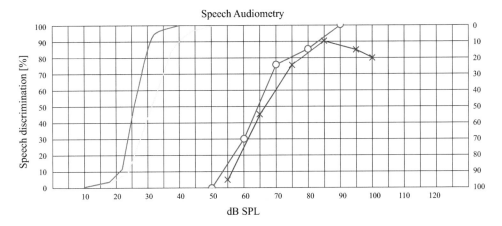

Figure 7.79.2 **Preoperative speech audiometry.**

Med-El Vibrant Soundbridge (VSB) left ear

Pure-Tone Audiometry in Free-Field

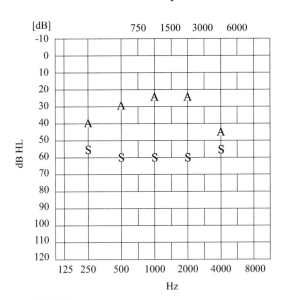

LEGEND:

A – implant (contralateral ear passively masked)

S – unaided (contralateral ear passively masked)

Figure 7.79.3 **Pure-tone audiometry in a free-field for aided (A) and unaided (S) conditions after 12-month follow-up.**

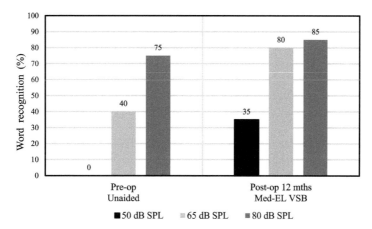

Figure 7.79.4 Word recognition score for unaided and aided conditions in quiet at 50, 65, and 80 dB SPL after 12-month follow-up. Non-implanted ear in passive masking.

80. Male, 66 years – cochlear implant

Bilateral gradually progressive hearing loss since about the age of 40. In the past, some episodes of otitis media with effusion. She has used a right-ear hearing aid since the age of 60 (Figures 7.80.1–7.80.5).

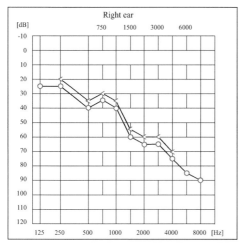

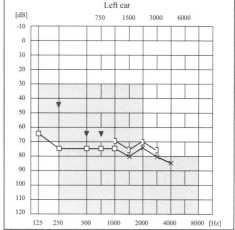

Figure 7.80.1 Preoperative pure-tone audiometry.

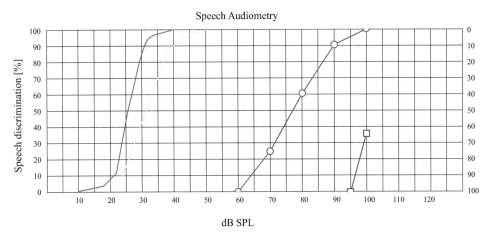

Figure 7.80.2 **Preoperative speech audiometry.**

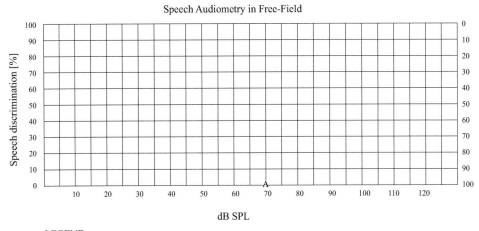

LEGEND:
A – left ear in hearing aid, right ear in active masking

Figure 7.80.3 **Preoperative speech audiometry in free-field.**

PDT-EAS, CI left ear, Advanced Bionics HiFocus™ SlimJ

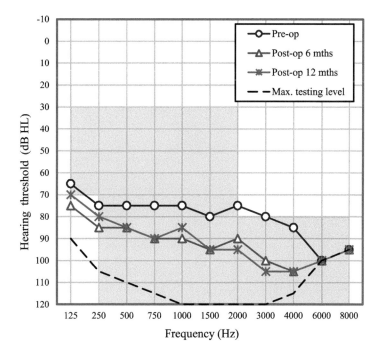

Figure 7.80.4 Pre- and postoperative hearing thresholds.

Hearing Preservation, Calculation in [%]			
Legend:		**Follow-up**	
S	Hearing Preservation	6 months	12 months
75 – 100%	Complete HP		
26 – 74%	Partial HP	S = 60.6%	S = 62.1%
1 – 25%	Minimal HP		
No detectable hearing	Loss of hearing		

Figure 7.80.5 Hearing preservation results.

81. Male, 66 years – cochlear implant

Bilateral gradually progressive hearing loss since the age of 55. He was treated with gentamicin in childhood. In the interview, he admitted that for many years he was exposed to impulse noise – he was often at the shooting range. There was an attempt of the hearing-aid fitting, but no benefits. HCV. Head imaging: MRI – no pathologies (Figures 7.81.1–7.81.5).

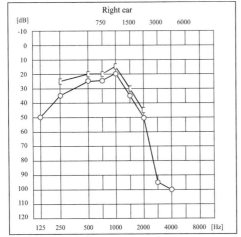 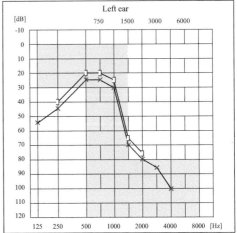

Figure 7.81.1 **Preoperative pure-tone audiometry.**

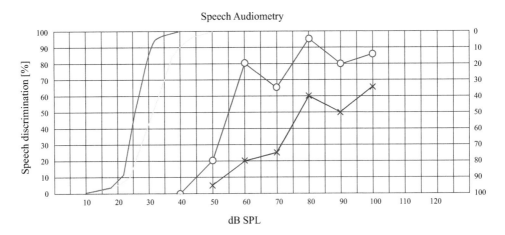

Figure 7.81.2 **Preoperative speech audiometry.**

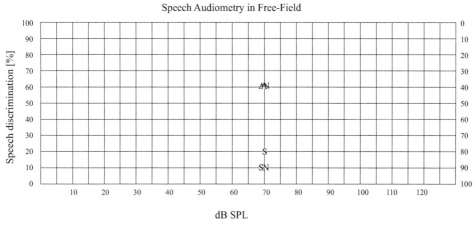

Figure 7.81.3 Preoperative speech audiometry in free-field.

PDT-EC (from 1000 Hz), CI left ear, Med-El SONATA FLEX20

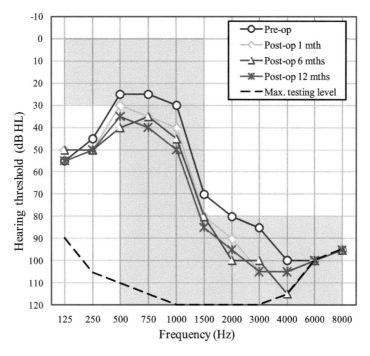

Figure 7.81.4 Pre- and postoperative hearing thresholds.

Hearing Preservation, Calculation in [%]					
Legend:		Follow-up			
S	Hearing Preservation	1 month	6 months	12 months	
75 – 100%	Complete HP				
26 – 74%	Partial HP	S = 86.0%	S = 80.0%	S = 79.0%	
1 – 25%	Minimal HP				
No detectable hearing	Loss of hearing				

Figure 7.81.5 Hearing preservation results.

82. Female, 67 years – cochlear implant

Sudden right-ear deafness accompanied by vertigo at the age of 40 – no hearing improvement after treatment. She was then diagnosed with Meniere's disease in the right
ear. Initially, episodes of vertigo occurred several times a month. Over the years, the
attacks became less frequent and severe. Hearing loss is gradually progressing. Sudden
left-ear deafness at the age of 65. Hearing improvement after treatment. Intermittent
left-ear tinnitus. She does not use hearing aids (Figures 7.82.1–7.82.5).

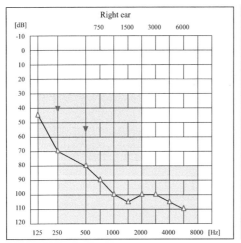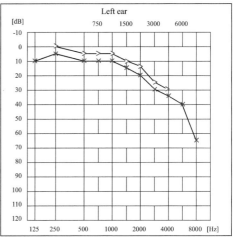

Figure 7.82.1 Preoperative pure-tone audiometry.

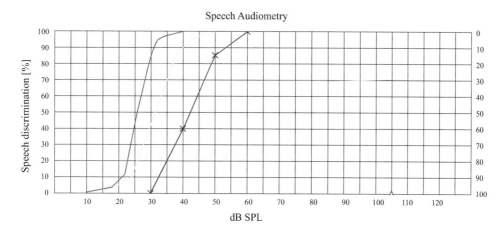

Figure 7.82.2 **Preoperative speech audiometry.**

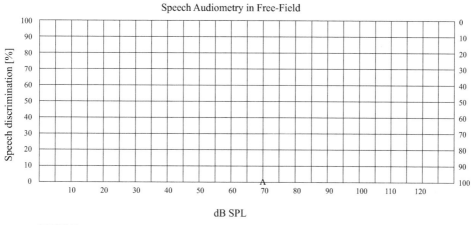

LEGEND:
A – right ear in hearing aid, left ear in active masking

Figure 7.82.3 **Preoperative speech audiometry in free-field.**

PDT-EAS, CI right ear, Oticon NEURO Zti EVO

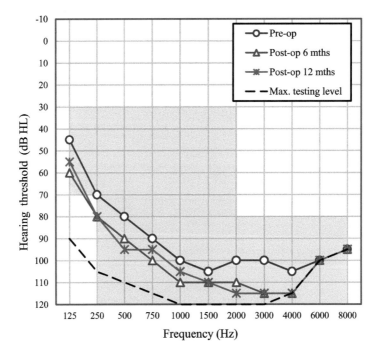

Figure 7.82.4 Pre- and postoperative hearing thresholds.

Hearing Preservation, Calculation in [%]			
Legend:		**Follow-up**	
S	**Hearing Preservation**	**6 months**	**12 months**
75 – 100%	Complete HP		
26 – 74%	Partial HP	**S = 56.8%**	**S = 59.1%**
1 – 25%	Minimal HP		
No detectable hearing	Loss of hearing		

Figure 7.82.5 Hearing preservation results.

83. Female, 67 years – cochlear implant

Bilateral gradually progressive hearing loss since the age of 58. Intermittent tinnitus. She has used hearing aids on both sides since the age of 59 but subjectively limited hearing benefits (Figures 7.83.1–7.83.5).

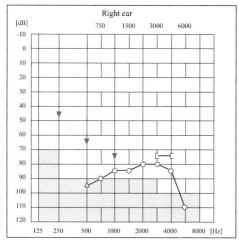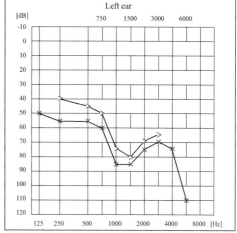

Figure 7.83.1 **Preoperative pure-tone audiometry.**

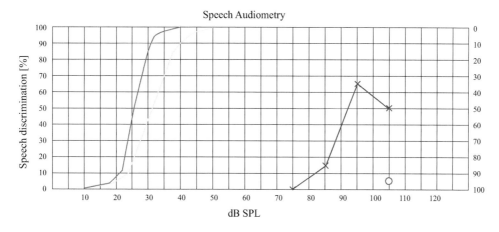

Figure 7.83.2 **Preoperative speech audiometry.**

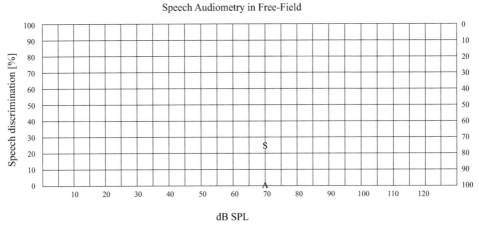

Figure 7.83.3 Preoperative speech audiometry in free-field.

PDT- ES, CI right ear, Advanced Bionics HiFocus™ SlimJ

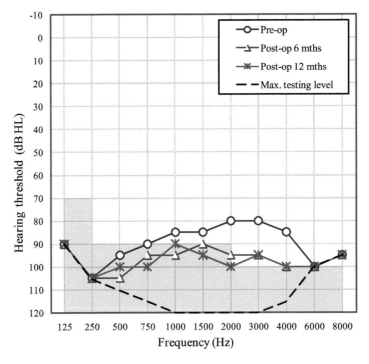

Figure 7.83.4 Pre- and postoperative hearing thresholds.

Hearing Preservation, Calculation in [%]			
Legend:		**Follow-up**	
S	**Hearing Preservation**	**6 months**	**12 months**
75 – 100%	Complete HP		
26 – 74%	Partial HP	S = 65.9%	S = 63.6%
1 – 100%	Minimal HP		
No detectable hearing	Loss of hearing		

Figure 7.83.5 Hearing preservation results.

84. Male, 67 years – cochlear implant

Bilateral gradually progressive hearing loss since about 45 years of age. Episodes of chronic otitis media with effusion. Two right-ear surgeries: exploratory tympanotomy with the removal of lesions and myringoossiculoplasty. No otitis media since then. Right-sided tinnitus for many years. No vertigo. He had used hearing aids on both sides, but he stopped due to a lack of hearing benefits after about a year (Figures 7.84.1–7.84.5).

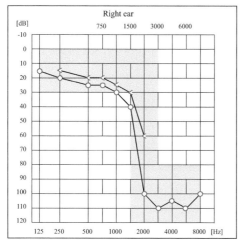
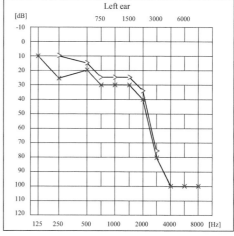

Figure 7.84.1 Preoperative pure-tone audiometry.

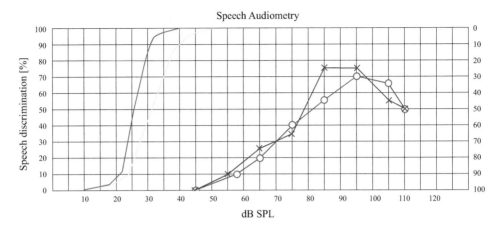

Figure 7.84.2 Preoperative speech audiometry.

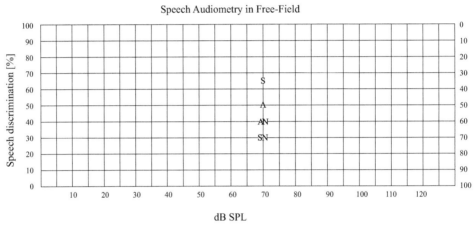

LEGEND:
A – right ear in hearing aid, left ear in passive masking
S – left ear in hearing aid, right ear in passive masking
AN – right ear in hearing aid, SNR + 10 dB, left ear in passive masking
SN – left ear in hearing aid, SNR + 10 dB, right ear in passive masking

Figure 7.84.3 Preoperative speech audiometry in free-field.

PDT-ENS, CI right ear, Med-El SONATA FLEX20

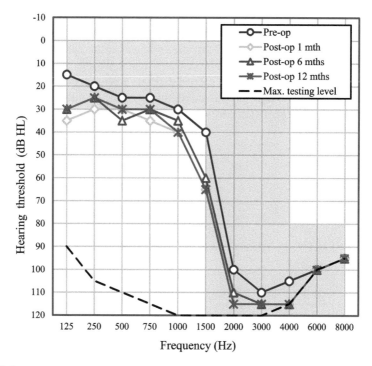

Figure 7.84.4 Pre- and postoperative hearing thresholds.

Hearing Preservation, Calculation in [%]				
Legend:		**Follow-up**		
S	**Hearing Preservation**	**1 month**	**6 months**	**12 months**
75 – 100%	Complete HP			
26 – 74%	Partial HP	S = 80.7%	S = 84.4%	S = 82.6%
1 – 25%	Minimal HP			
No detectable hearing	Loss of hearing			

Figure 7.84.5 Hearing preservation results.

85. Female, 69 years – cochlear implant

Chronic otitis media with effusion in the right ear since around 30 years of age. Surgery to remove post-inflammatory changes in the right ear at the age of 54. Left-ear rapidly progressive hearing loss since about 60 years of age. Episodes of vertigo and constant left-sided tinnitus – suspicion of Meniere's disease. Left-sided ventilation tube placement at the age of 67. Vertigo has subsided since then. She has used a hearing aid on the right ear for several years (Figures 7.85.1–7.85.5).

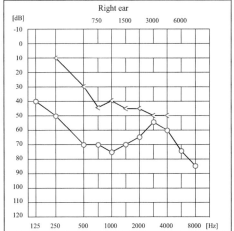
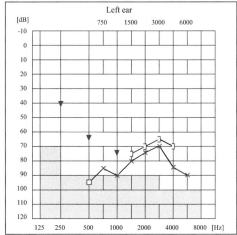

Figure 7.85.1 **Preoperative pure-tone audiometry.**

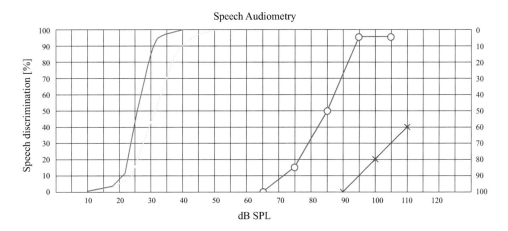

Figure 7.85.2 **Preoperative speech audiometry.**

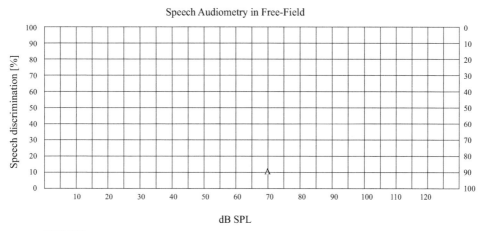

Speech Audiometry in Free-Field

LEGEND:
A – left ear in hearing aid, right ear in active masking

Figure 7.85.3 Preoperative speech audiometry in free-field.

PDT-ES, CI left ear, Advanced Bionics HiRes 90K™ Advantage

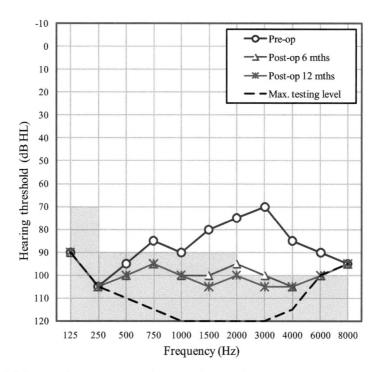

Figure 7.85.4 Pre- and postoperative hearing thresholds.

Hearing Preservation, Calculation in [%]			
Legend:		Follow-up	
S	Hearing Preservation	6 months	12 months
75 – 100%	Complete HP		
26 – 74%	Partial HP	S = 50.0%	S = 44.0%
1 – 25%	Minimal HP		
No detectable hearing	Loss of hearing		

Figure 7.85.5 Hearing preservation results.

86. Male, 69 years – cochlear implant

Bilateral gradually progressive hearing loss since around 60 years of age. At the age of 63, significant deterioration of hearing in the right ear during hospitalization in the intensive care unit (as a result of complications following kidney stone removal surgery). In the interview, he admitted he was exposed to noise at work for many years. Right-ear tinnitus. Intermitted, mild vertigo. He does not use hearing aids. Head imaging: MRI – no pathologies (Figures 7.86.1–7.86.5).

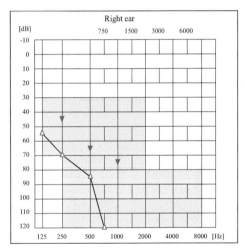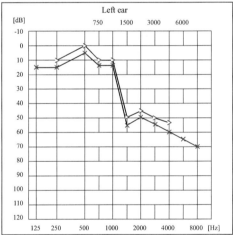

Figure 7.86.1 Preoperative pure-tone audiometry.

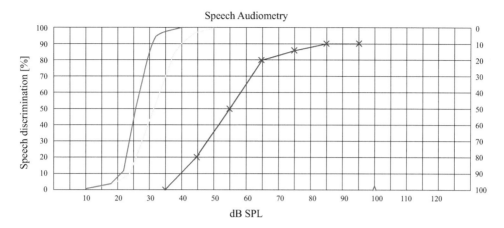

Figure 7.86.2 **Preoperative speech audiometry.**

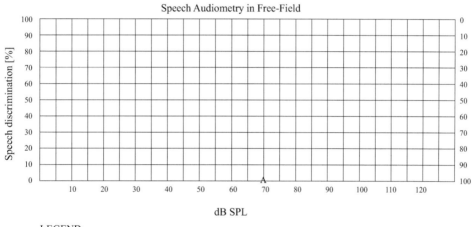

LEGEND:
A – right ear in hearing aid, left ear in active masking

Figure 7.86.3 **Preoperative speech audiometry in free-field.**

PDT-EAS, CI right ear, Oticon NEURO Zti EVO

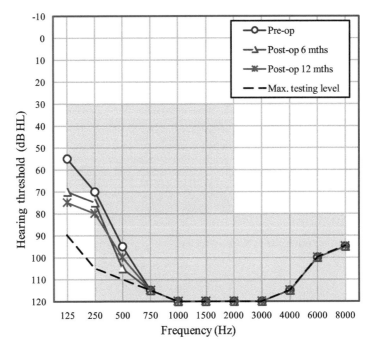

Figure 7.86.4 Pre- and postoperative hearing thresholds.

Hearing Preservation, Calculation in [%]			
Legend:		**Follow-up**	
S	**Hearing Preservation**	**6 months**	**12 months**
75 – 100%	Complete HP		
26 – 74%	Partial HP	**S = 64.7%**	**S = 58.8%**
1 – 25%	Minimal HP		
No detectable hearing	Loss of hearing		

Figure 7.86.5 Hearing preservation results.

87. Male, 69 years – cochlear implant

Bilateral gradually progressive hearing loss since the age of 50. There was an attempt of the hearing-aid fitting, but no benefits. Head imaging: MRI – no pathologies (Figures 7.87.1–7.87.5).

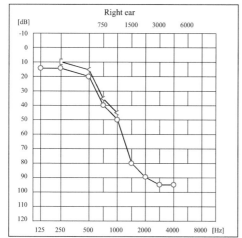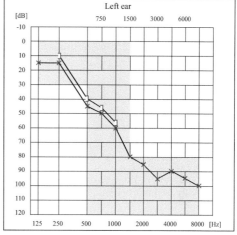

Figure 7.87.1 **Preoperative pure-tone audiometry.**

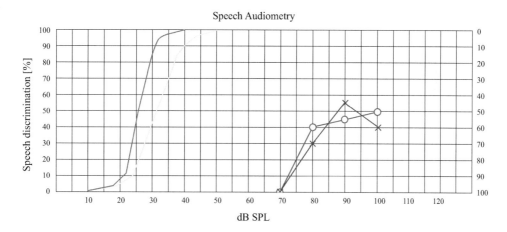

Figure 7.87.2 **Preoperative speech audiometry.**

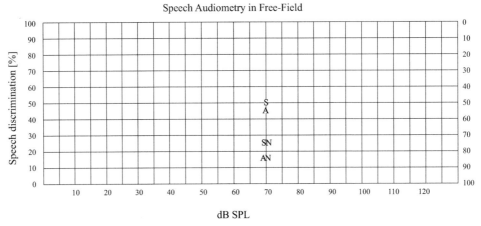

LEGEND:
A – right ear in hearing aid, left ear in passive masking
S – left ear in hearing aid, right ear in passive masking
AN – right ear in hearing aid, SNR + 10 dB, left ear in passive masking
SN – left ear in hearing aid, SNR + 10 dB, right ear in passive masking

Figure 7.87.3 Preoperative speech audiometry in free-field.

PDT-EC (from 250 Hz), CI left ear, Med-El SONATA Medium

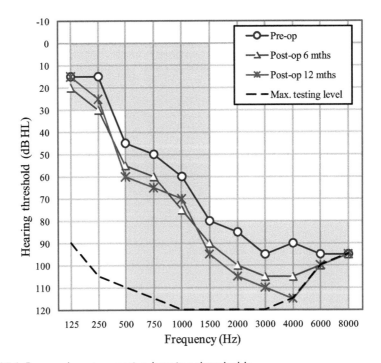

Figure 7.87.4 Pre- and postoperative hearing thresholds.

Hearing Preservation, Calculation in [%]			
Legend:		**Follow-up**	
S	**Hearing Preservation**	**6 months**	**12 months**
75 – 100%	Complete HP		
26 – 74%	Partial HP	S = 77.3%	S = 73.2%
1 – 25%	Minimal HP		
No detectable hearing	Loss of hearing		

Figure 7.87.5 Hearing preservation results.

D. ELDERLY PATIENTS

88. Female, 7I years – cochlear implant

Bilateral gradually progressing hearing loss since the age of 50. Tinnitus: none. Vertigo: transient. She has used a hearing aid in the left ear since the age of 60 and in the right ear since the age of 64 (Figures 7.88.1–7.88.5).

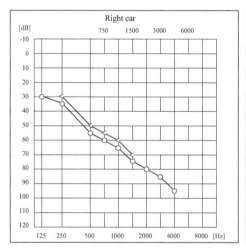
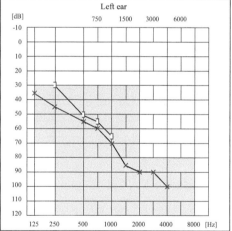

Figure 7.88.1 Preoperative pure-tone audiometry.

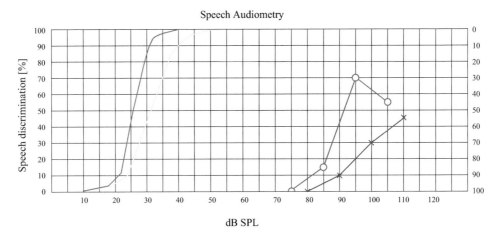

Figure 7.88.2 **Preoperative speech audiometry.**

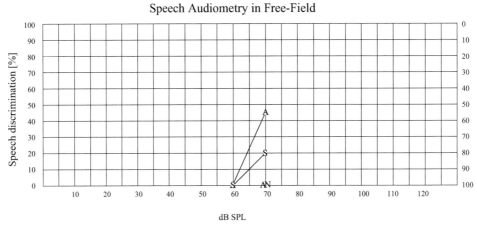

LEGEND:
A – right ear in hearing aid, left ear in passive masking
S – left ear in hearing aid, right ear in passive masking
AN – right ear in hearing aid, SNR + 10 dB, left ear in passive masking

Figure 7.88.3 **Preoperative speech audiometry in free-field.**

PDT-EAS, CI left ear, Med-El CONCERTO FLEX24™

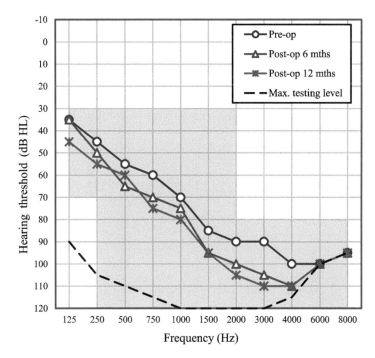

Figure 7.88.4 Pre- and postoperative hearing thresholds.

Hearing Preservation, Calculation in [%]			
Legend:		Follow-up	
S	Hearing Preservation	6 months	12 months
75 – 100%	Complete HP		
26 – 74%	Partial HP	S = 80.5%	S = 72.7%
1 – 25%	Minimal HP		
No detectable hearing	Loss of hearing		

Figure 7.88.5 Hearing preservation results.

89. Male, 73 years – cochlear implant

Bilateral gradually progressing hearing loss for many years, recurrent otitis media. Previous left-ear surgeries: epitympanotomy with myringoplasty (at 71), exploratory tympanotomy with lesion removal (at 72). Previous right-ear surgeries: cleaning and removing inflammatory lesions (in 70), attico-antro-mastoidectomy with middle-ear lesion removal, drain tubes, and myringoplasty (at 71). He has used a hearing aid in the left ear but with little hearing benefits in his subjective opinion. Right ear – no hearing aid (Figures 7.89.1–7.89.5).

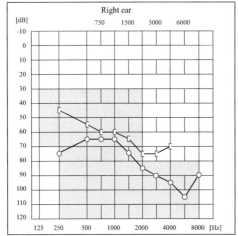 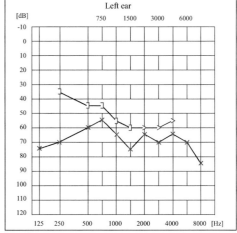

Figure 7.89.1 **Preoperative pure-tone audiometry.**

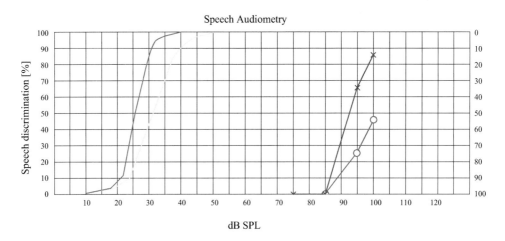

Figure 7.89.2 **Preoperative speech audiometry.**

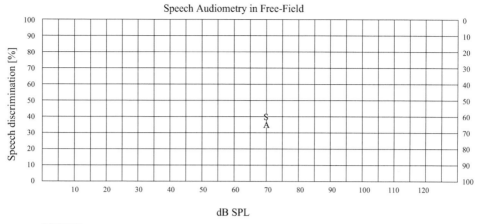

Figure 7.89.3 Preoperative speech audiometry in free-field.

PDT-EAS, CI right ear, Oticon Neuro Zti EVO

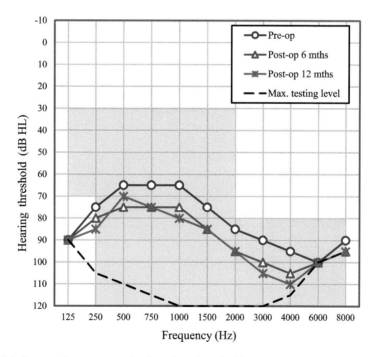

Figure 7.89.4 Pre- and postoperative hearing thresholds.

Hearing Preservation, Calculation in [%]			
Legend:		Follow-up	
S	Hearing Preservation	6 months	12 months
75 – 100%	Complete HP		
26 – 74%	Partial HP	S = 74.6%	S = 69.8%
1 – 25%	Minimal HP		
No detectable hearing	Loss of hearing		

Figure 7.89.5 Hearing preservation results.

90. Female, 74 years – cochlear implant

Bilateral gradually progressing hearing loss since the age of 36 due to bilateral otosclerosis. Bilateral stapedectomy: in the left ear at the age of 51, in the left ear at the age of 57. Bilateral tinnitus. Vertigo: periodic loss of balance related to head movements, with compensated damage to the labyrinth. She has used hearing aids on both ears since the age of 57 (Figures 7.90.1–7.90.5).

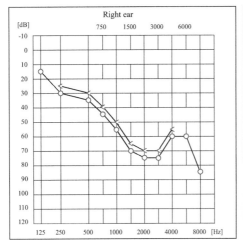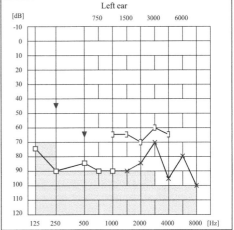

Figure 7.90.1 Preoperative pure-tone audiometry.

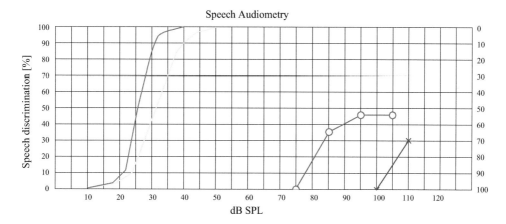

Figure 7.90.2 **Preoperative speech audiometry.**

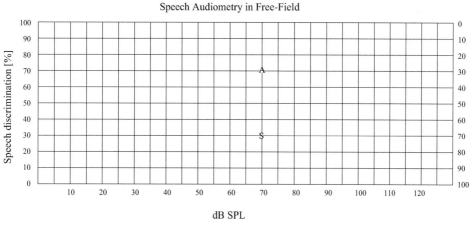

LEGEND:
A – right ear in hearing aid, left ear in passive masking
S – left ear in hearing aid, right ear in active masking

Figure 7.90.3 **Preoperative speech audiometry in free-field.**

PDT-ES, CI left ear, Oticon Neuro Zti EVO

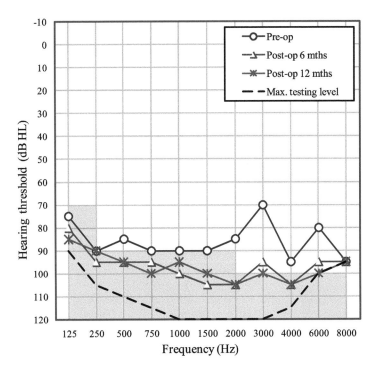

Figure 7.90.4 Pre- and postoperative hearing thresholds.

Hearing Preservation, Calculation in [%]			
Legend:		**Follow-up**	
S	**Hearing Preservation**	**6 months**	**12 months**
75 – 100%	Complete HP		
26 – 74%	Partial HP	**S = 54.7%**	**S = 52.8%**
1 – 25%	Minimal HP		
No detectable hearing	Loss of hearing		

Figure 7.90.5 Hearing preservation results.

91. Male, 76 years – cochlear implant

Bilateral progressive hearing loss since childhood. He has used a hearing aid in the right ear since the age of 66. Left ear: no hearing aid. Head imaging: CT and MRI – no pathologies (Figures 7.91.1–7.91.5).

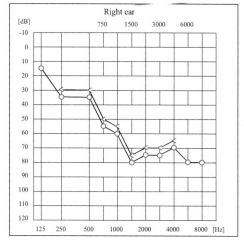 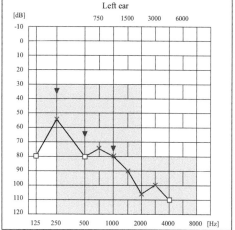

Figure 7.91.1 **Preoperative pure-tone audiometry.**

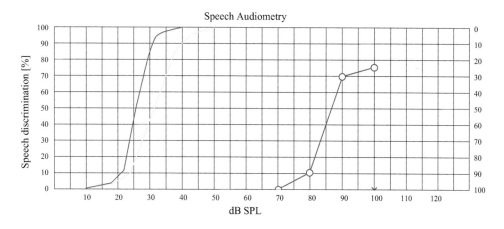

Figure 7.91.2 **Preoperative speech audiometry.**

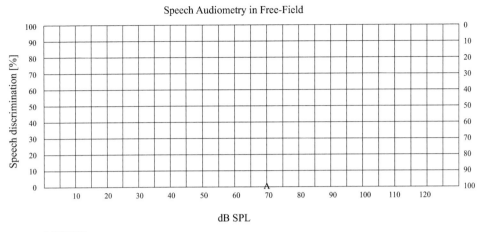

LEGEND:
A – left ear in hearing aid, right ear in active masking

Figure 7.91.3 Preoperative speech audiometry in free-field.

PDT-EAS, CI left ear, Advanced Bionics HiRes™ Ultra CI, HiFocus™ SlimJ

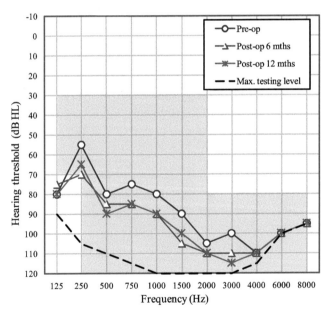

Figure 7.91.4 Pre- and postoperative hearing thresholds.

Hearing Preservation, Calculation in [%]			
Legend:		**Follow-up**	
S	**Hearing Preservation**	**6 months**	**12 months**
75 – 100%	Complete HP		
26 – 74%	Partial HP	S = 72.9%	S = 70.8%
1 – 25%	Minimal HP		
No detectable hearing	Loss of hearing		

Figure 7.91.5 Hearing preservation results.

92. Female, 77 years – cochlear implant

Bilateral gradually progressing hearing loss for many years. Bilateral, bothersome tinnitus. Occasional vertigo. She suffered from meningitis in childhood. She does not use hearing aids – there was an attempt of the hearing-aid fitting, but no benefits in the patient's subjective opinion (Figures 7.92.1–7.92.5).

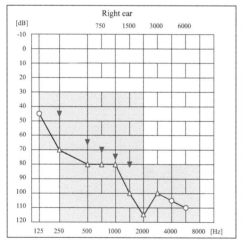
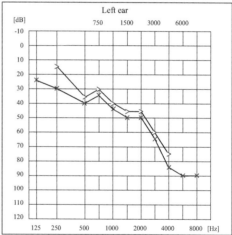

Figure 7.92.1 Preoperative pure-tone audiometry.

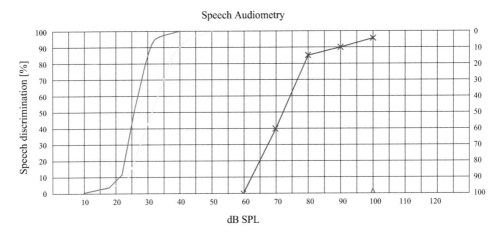

Figure 7.92.2 **Preoperative speech audiometry.**

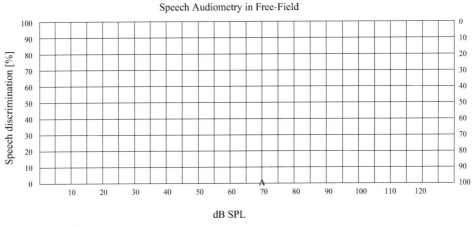

LEGEND:
A – right ear in hearing aid, left ear in active masking

Figure 7.92.3 **Preoperative speech audiometry in free-field.**

PDT-EAS, CI right ear, Oticon Neuro Zti EVO

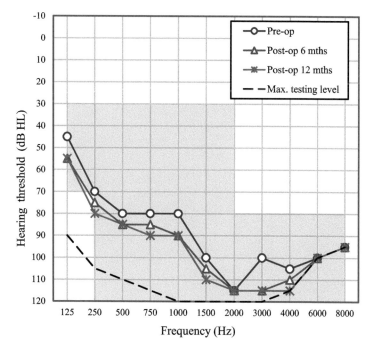

Figure 7.92.4 Pre- and postoperative hearing thresholds.

Hearing Preservation, Calculation in [%]			
Legend:		**Follow-up**	
S	**Hearing Preservation**	**6 months**	**12 months**
75 – 100%	Complete HP		
26 – 74%	Partial HP	S = 75.0%	S = 66.7%
1 – 25%	Minimal HP		
No detectable hearing	Loss of hearing		

Figure 7.92.5 Hearing preservation results.

93. Female, 77 years – cochlear implant

Bilateral gradually progressing hearing loss of unknown etiology since the age of 55. Bilateral tinnitus, more annoying on the left side. She has used hearing aids bilaterally since the age of 65 (Figures 7.93.1–7.93.5).

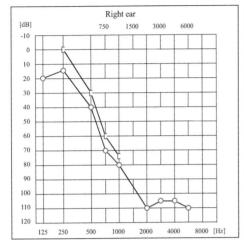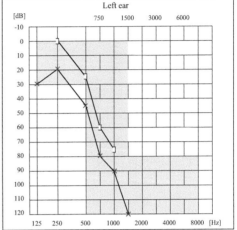

Figure 7.93.1 Preoperative pure-tone audiometry.

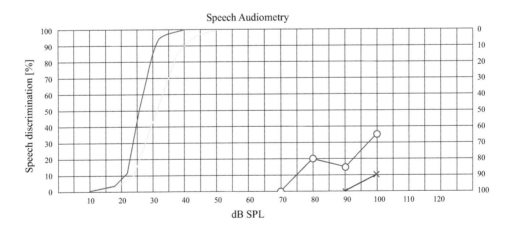

Figure 7.93.2 Preoperative speech audiometry.

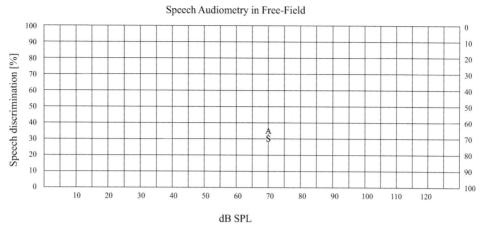

Speech Audiometry in Free-Field

LEGEND:
A – right ear in hearing aid, left ear in passive masking
S – left ear in hearing aid, right ear in passive masking

Figure 7.93.3 Preoperative speech audiometry in free-field.

PDT-EC (from 250 Hz), CI left ear, Med-El SONATA FLEX24™

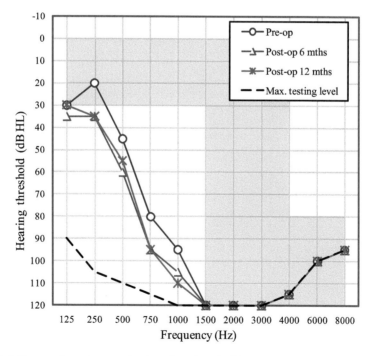

Figure 7.93.4 Pre- and postoperative hearing thresholds.

Hearing Preservation, Calculation in [%]			
Legend:		Follow-up	
S	Hearing Preservation	6 months	12 months
75 – 100%	Complete HP		
26 – 74%	Partial HP	S = 77.8%	S = 79.6%
1 – 25%	Minimal HP		
No detectable hearing	Loss of hearing		

Figure 7.93.5 Hearing preservation results.

94. Female, 79 years – cochlear implant

Bilateral chronic otitis media with effusion since childhood. Right-ear stapedotomy at the age of 57 and reoperation – without hearing improvement. Significant hearing deterioration in the right ear after the modified radical surgery (in another center). Left-ear tympanoplasty at the age of 65 (in another center). Sudden hearing deterioration in the left ear at the age of 73. Bilateral bothersome tinnitus. She has used a hearing aid in her left ear since the age of 89. Right ear: no hearing aid (Figures 7.94.1–7.94.5).

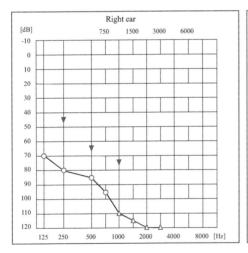 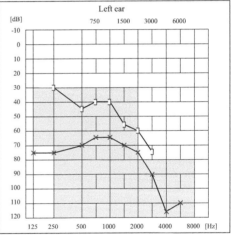

Figure 7.94.1 Preoperative pure-tone audiometry.

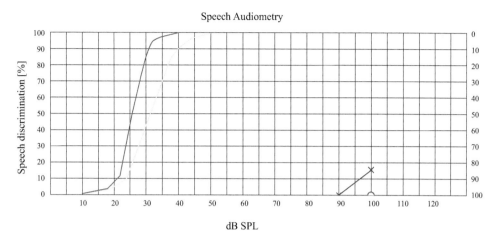

Figure 7.94.2 **Preoperative speech audiometry.**

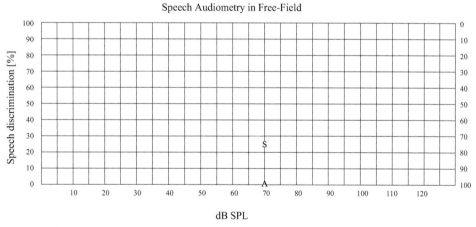

LEGEND:
A – right ear in hearing aid, left ear in passive masking
S – left ear in hearing aid, right ear in passive masking

Figure 7.94.3 **Preoperative speech audiometry in free-field.**

PDT-ES, CI right ear, Advanced Bionics HiRes™ 90K Advantage

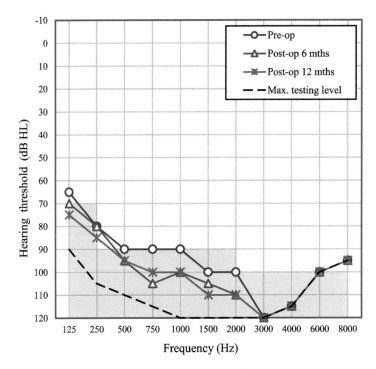

Figure 7.94.4 Pre- and postoperative hearing thresholds.

Hearing Preservation, Calculation in [%]			
Legend:		**Follow-up**	
S	**Hearing Preservation**	**6 months**	**12 months**
75 – 100%	Complete HP		
26 – 74%	Partial HP	**S = 69.7%**	**S = 63.6%**
1 – 25%	Minimal HP		
No detectable hearing	Loss of hearing		

Figure 7.94.5 Hearing preservation results.

95. Male, 79 years – cochlear implant

Bilateral gradually progressing hearing loss for several decades. At the age of 74, he had a traffic accident with a head injury (no fractures within the skull bone). A significant deterioration of hearing in the left ear after the accident. Bilateral tinnitus, more annoying on the left side. He does not use hearing aids. There was an attempt of the hearing-aid fitting, but no hearing benefits in the patient's subjective opinion. Head imaging: MRI of the head with contrast – no pathologies (Figures 7.95.1–7.95.5).

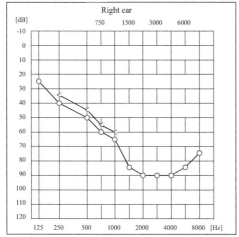
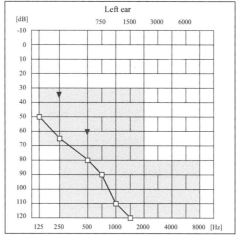

Figure 7.95.1 **Preoperative pure-tone audiometry.**

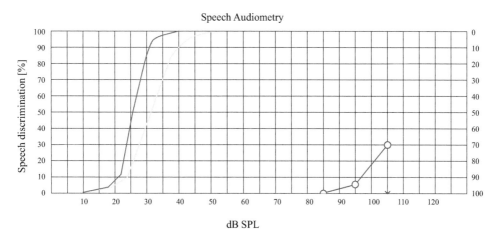

Figure 7.95.2 **Preoperative speech audiometry.**

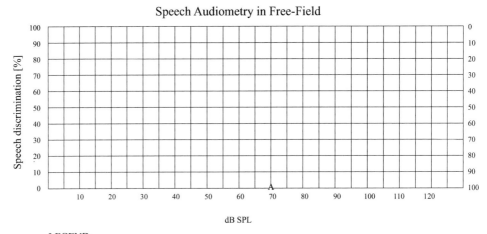

LEGEND:
A – left ear in hearing aid, left ear in active masking

Figure 7.95.3 Preoperative speech audiometry in free-field.

PDT-EAS, CI left ear, Advanced Bionics HiFocus™ SlimJ

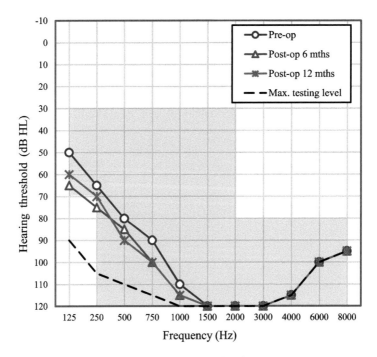

Figure 7.95.4 Pre- and postoperative hearing thresholds.

Hearing Preservation, Calculation in [%]			
Legend:		Follow-up	
S	Hearing Preservation	6months	12 months
75 – 100%	Complete HP		
26 – 74%	Partial HP	S = 69.0%	S =72.4%
1 – 25%	Minimal HP		
No detectable hearing	Loss of hearing		

Figure 7.95.5 Hearing preservation results.

96. Male, 82 years – cochlear implant

Bilateral gradually progressing hearing loss for several decades. Bilateral tinnitus. Hearing aids used bilaterally but inconsistently due to limited hearing benefits. Head imaging: MRI – no pathologies (Figures 7.96.1–7.96.5).

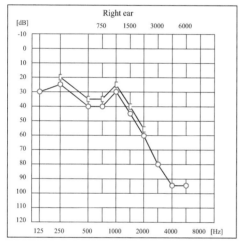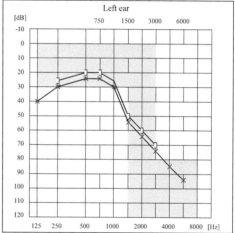

Figure 7.96.1 Preoperative pure-tone audiometry.

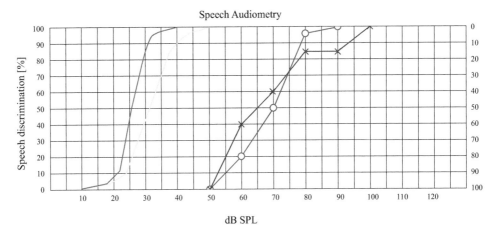

Figure 7.96.2 **Preoperative speech audiometry.**

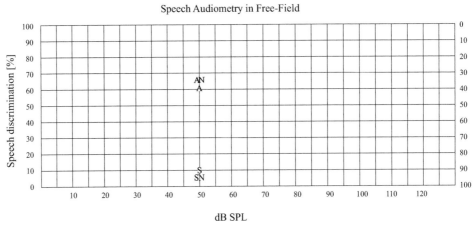

LEGEND:
A – left ear in hearing aid, rght ear in passive masking
S – left ear unaided, right ear in passive masking
AN – right ear in hearing aid, left ear in passive masking
SN – right ear unaided, left ear in passive masking

Figure 7.96.3 **Preoperative speech audiometry in free-field.**

PDT-ENS, CI left ear, Med-El SONATA FLEX20

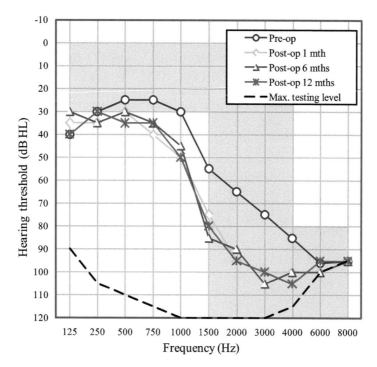

Figure 7.96.4 Pre- and postoperative hearing thresholds.

Hearing Preservation, Calculation in [%]				
Legend:		Follow-up		
S	Hearing Preservation	1 month	6 months	12 months
75–100%	Complete HP			
26–74%	Partial HP	S = 77.2%	S = 78.1%	S = 76.4%
1–25%	Minimal HP			
No detectable hearing	Loss of hearing			

Figure 7.96.5 Hearing preservation results.

97. Female, 84 years – cochlear implant

Bilateral rapidly progressing hearing loss since the age of 75. Left-sided tinnitus. She has used hearing aids bilaterally since the age of 77 – initially, there were hearing benefits. Head imaging: CT – no pathologies (Figures 7.97.1–7.97.5).

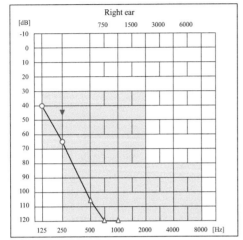
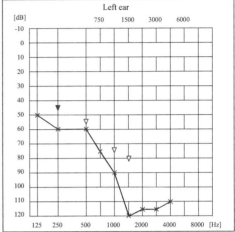

Figure 7.97.1 **Preoperative pure-tone audiometry.**

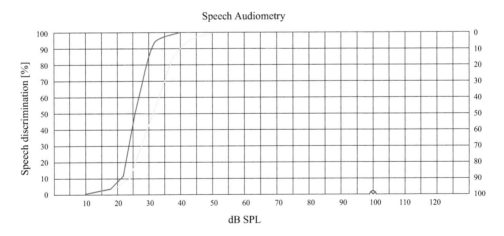

Figure 7.97.2 **Preoperative speech audiometry.**

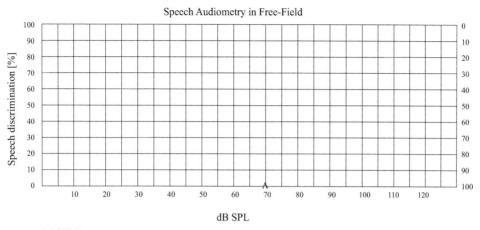

Speech Audiometry in Free-Field

LEGEND:
A – right ear in hearing aid, left ear in passive masking

Figure 7.97.3 Preoperative speech audiometry in free-field.

PDT-EAS, CI right ear, Med-El SONATA Medium

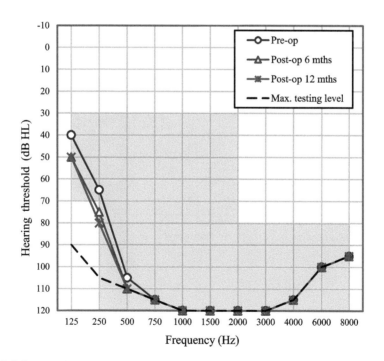

Figure 7.97.4 Pre- and postoperative hearing thresholds.

Hearing Preservation, Calculation in [%]			
Legend:		**Follow-up**	
S	**Hearing Preservation**	**6 months**	**12 months**
75 – 100%	Complete HP		
26 – 74%	Partial HP	**S = 73.7%**	**S = 68.4%**
1 – 25%	Minimal HP		
No detectable hearing	Loss of hearing		

Figure 7.97.5 Hearing preservation results.

98. Male, 85 years – cochlear implant

Sudden idiopathic deafness in the left ear at the age of 64. Since the age of 67, gradually progressing hearing loss in the left ear. He uses hearing aids bilaterally, but there is no hearing benefit on the left side in the patient's subjective opinion. Head imaging: MRI and CT – no pathologies (Figures 7.98.1–7.98.5).

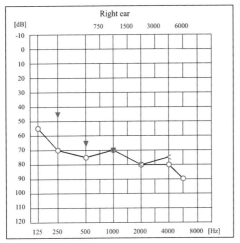
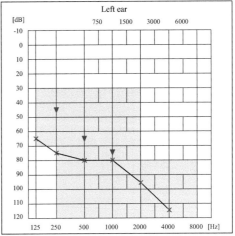

Figure 7.98.1 Preoperative pure-tone audiometry.

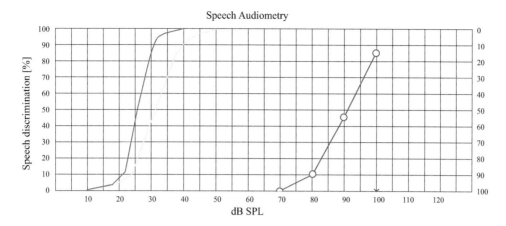

Figure 7.98.2 **Preoperative speech audiometry.**

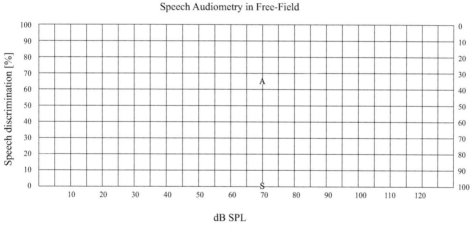

LEGEND:
A – right ear in hearing aid, left ear in passive masking
S – left ear in hearing aid, right ear in passive masking

Figure 7.98.3 **Preoperative speech audiometry in free-field.**

PDT-EAS, CI left ear, Oticon Neuro Zti EVO

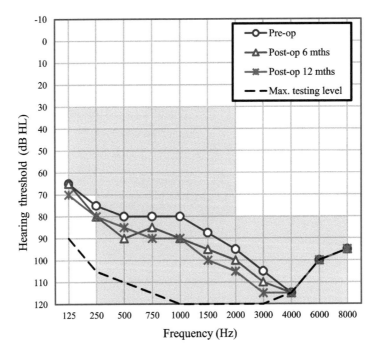

Figure 7.98.4 Pre- and postoperative hearing thresholds.

Hearing Preservation, Calculation in [%]			
Legend:		**Follow-up**	
S	**Hearing Preservation**	**6 months**	**12 months**
75 – 100%	Complete HP		
26 – 74%	Partial HP	S = 79.6%	S = 71.0%
1 – 25%	Minimal HP		
No detectable hearing	Loss of hearing		

Figure 7.98.5 Hearing preservation results.

Chapter 8

Role of the pharmacology (glucocorticoids) in hearing preservation in the partial deafness treatment (PDT)

Magdalena B. Skarżyńska
Institute of Sensory Organs

CONTENTS

INTRODUCTION

Preservation of hearing in patients undergoing cochlear implantation, crucial in patients with partial deafness, depends in the first place on surgical technique and selection of an appropriate electrode (Skarżyński et al. 2002, 2003, 2007b). An interesting research question is what other, not surgical, factors affect hearing preservation in patients with partial deafness. One of the factors under investigation is the effect of glucocorticoid administration in patients undergoing cochlear implantation (Sweeney et al. 2015, Rah et al. 2016).

Glucocorticoids play an important role in the pharmacological treatment of many otorhinolaryngological disorders, such as Meniere's disease, sudden sensorineural hearing loss (SSNHL), or tinnitus. They are used as a complementary treatment in the ENT surgery procedures such as cochlear implantation (Chrousos 2015, Alles et al. 2006). The effectiveness of pharmacotherapy in treating these disorders is sometimes hard to determine. It depends on many factors, such as the adverse effects of drugs, often causing the treatment to be discontinued, and possibly other therapies applied. Unfortunately, the adverse effects of glucocorticoid treatment may be severe, particularly in patients with additional risk factors, and often make it necessary to suspend the pharmacotherapy.

DOI: 10.1201/9781003164876-8

A widely discussed problem among the ENT clinical specialists and scientists studying pharmacokinetics is the optimal way of glucocorticoid administration (local or systemic) in otorhinolaryngological disorders. Complementary glucocorticoid treatment reduces the oxidative stress and inflammatory reactions and, in effect, may help inhibit the apoptosis of the hearing cells. The main challenge for the effective delivery of a drug to its action localization is the blood-labyrinth barrier (BLB) and the inner ear's anatomical inaccessibility.

PHARMACOLOGICAL CHARACTERISTICS, THE ROLE, PHARMACOLOGICAL ACTIVITY, AND ADVERSE EFFECTS OF GLUCOCORTICOIDS

According to the Anatomical Therapeutic Chemical (ATC) Classification System, glucocorticoids are classified as H02 AB. The human adrenal cortex synthesizes the following three types of steroids: corticosteroids produced in zona fasciculata, mineralocorticoids produced in zona glomerulosa, and androgens in zona reticularis. One of the main differences between corticosteroids and androgens is the number of carbon atoms in a molecule: 21 in corticosteroids and 19 in androgens. The main glucocorticoid in the human body is cortisol, while the main mineralocorticoid aldosterone (Brunton et al. 2017).

The glucocorticoid receptor is present in the cytoplasm in an inactive form until it binds with a glucocorticoid molecule. This reaction activates the receptor, and the resulting glucocorticoid-glucocorticoid receptor complex is translocated to a cell nucleus. There, it gets into interaction with the specific short DNA sequences called glucocorticoid-responsive elements (GREs), which enable gene transcription induction. It is a complex process due to the interaction with particular cofactors and proteins (Brunton et al. 2017). A negative response to a glucocorticoid is also possible. Webster and Cidlowski (1999) have reported identifying the genes that are negatively regulated by glucocorticoids. An example of a negative, so-called down-regulation is the inhibition of the expression of genes responsible for encoding cytokines or enzymes (e.g., collagenase), which both play an essential role in immune and inflammatory reactions. Down-regulation plays a crucial role in the immunosuppressive and anti-inflammatory effects of glucocorticoids.

Two glucocorticoids with the highest anti-inflammatory activity are dexamethasone and betamethasone. Prednisone, prednisolone, triamcinolone, and 6α-methylprednisolone have 4–5 times stronger anti-inflammatory activity than cortisol. Moreover, they all have a longer half-life than cortisol. Examples of glucocorticoids, their anti-inflammatory properties, and biological half-life are shown in Table 8.1.

Glucocorticoids are biologically and pharmacologically active compounds with two fundamental functions: anti-inflammatory and immunosuppressive. Glucocorticoids affect:

1. Lipid metabolism. One of the effects of corticosteroid treatment is the redistribution of fat tissue, medically known as Cushing's syndrome.
2. Carbohydrate and protein metabolism. Glucocorticoids stimulate the liver to form glucose in a biochemical reaction (gluconeogenesis) from amino acids and glycerol and stimulate the liver to release glucose from glycogen. Simultaneously,

Table 8.1 Properties and activity (anti-inflammatory activity and biological half-life) of corticosteroids (Brunton et al. 2017)

	Anti-inflammatory activity	Biological half-life $t_{1/2}$
Cortisol	1	Short: $t_{1/2}$ = 8–12 h
Cortisone	0.8	Short: $t_{1/2}$ = 8–12 h
Fludrocortisone	10	Intermediate: $t_{1/2}$ = 12–36 h
Prednisone	4	Intermediate: $t_{1/2}$ = 12–36 h
Prednisolone	4	Intermediate: $t_{1/2}$ = 12–36 h
6α-Methylprednisolone	5	Intermediate: $t_{1/2}$ = 12–36 h
Triamcinolone	5	Intermediate: $t_{1/2}$ = 12–36 h
Betamethasone	25	Long: $t_{1/2}$ = 36–72 h
Dexamethasone	25	Long: $t_{1/2}$ = 36–72 h

lipolysis reaction and protein breakdown increase, and consequently, blood glucose level increases. Patients with diabetes or other forms of hyperglycemia should be particularly strictly observed when treated with glucocorticoids. Glucocorticoids induce protein metabolism-increasing and procuring compounds, such as amino acids, for further reactions.

3. Water and electrolyte balance. Glucocorticoids have a negative impact on Ca^{2+} metabolism, reducing its absorption from the digestive system and increasing its elimination through kidneys. To prevent osteoporosis, Ca^{2+} supplementation and physical activity adequate to a patient's condition are necessary. Glucocorticoids also reduce osteoblast activity and stimulate osteoclast activity. Sometimes, glucocorticoid treatment may cause increased Na^+ retention and decreased K^+ concentration because of an interaction with the mineralocorticoid receptor. These changes in ion concentration may affect the cardiovascular system.

4. Immunosuppressive and anti-inflammatory effects. Glucocorticoids may suppress or prevent anti-inflammatory reactions in different ways. They reduce the diapedesis of granulocytes and proliferation of Th lymphocytes and inhibit/reduce the activation of macrophages, neutrophils, mast cells, and cytokines (interleukins 1, 2, 3, 4, 5, 6, 8), and tumor necrosis factor TNF-α. They reduce the COX-2 (cyclooxygenase 2) expression and reduce prostanoid concentration by lowering their production. They increase the activity of catecholamines and reduce the production of histamine (Munck et al. 1984, Brunton et al. 2017).

5. Impaired wound healing. Due to the reduced synthesis of collagen and glycosaminoglycans and fibroblast function disorders, as a result, wound healing may be impaired.

Glucocorticoid treatment in ENT disorders sometimes requires a high-dose application or extended time of treatment, which increases the risk of adverse effects.

The adverse effects of glucocorticoid therapy include:

1. Repression of infection or injury response,
2. Risk of opportunistic infections,
3. Risk of hyperglycemia,
4. Risk of muscular dystrophy,

5. Risk of Cushing's syndrome,
6. Risk of glaucoma (generally in genetically predisposed patients),
7. Risk of osteoporosis.

Sudden cessation of glucocorticoid treatment may cause adrenocortical insufficiency, especially if the therapy was long-lasting or high dose. The dose should be reduced slowly, not suddenly (Brunton et al. 2017).

PHARMACOKINETICS OF GLUCOCORTICOIDS AND REVIEW OF DIFFERENT ANIMAL MODEL STUDIES

Pharmacokinetics is affected by several factors that are summarily described by the acronym LADME:

1. L: liberation,
2. A: absorption,
3. D: distribution,
4. M: metabolism,
5. E: elimination.

The active substance liberation speed depends on the drug's form (tablet, capsule, syrup, injection, other) and the speed of transport of the drug from the application site. One of the primary factors affecting pharmacokinetics is the active substance's solubility, which depends on the environment's pH and size of the molecule. In the initial stages of the pharmacokinetic process, binding of drugs with proteins is crucial: larger protein means a more extended therapeutic activity of a drug because a drug bound to a protein is inactive, serving as a reserve of a drug in the organism. The absorption depends on the lipophilicity and solubility of drugs. According to the literature, only a few medications can be used in the ENT practice with any effects because of the difficulties related to achieving the sufficient concentration of the active substance in the inner ear (Salt & Plontke 2018). These are aminoglycosides (mainly gentamicin) used, for example, in Meniere's disease (Lange 1989) and corticosteroids (dexamethasone and triamcinolone) in the pharmacotherapy of the idiopathic sudden sensorineural hearing loss (ISSHL) or other cases of acute hearing loss (Hamid & Trune 2008). From the pharmacokinetics perspective, the inner ear is a multicompartment model with physiologically balanced inner ear fluids (perilymph and endolymph) due to the BLB (Liebau & Plontke 2015, Plontke et al. 2017). The process of transport of drug molecules also depends on many factors, such as the route and mode of administration (single or repeated administration), dose, drug's pH, or solution's osmolarity. The same factors also influence the clearance of the drug and its elimination from the organism.

Plontke et al. (2017) have published the results of an animal model study comparing the effects of dexamethasone and 0.9% saline solution delivered during implantation in a guinea pig. Both were administered intravenously 60 min before implantation. In conclusion, they had noted that dexamethasone could reduce the damage of cells when the electrode enters the cochlea's turns or the apical region. They did not observe any relationship between dexamethasone and the reduction of cochleostomy-related fibrosis.

The *in vitro* studies showed a positive correlation between the reduction of the auditory cell damage after applying a glucocorticoid administered in the form of a dexamethasone-releasing polymer electrode coating and the TNF-α expression. The animal model studies have shown that glucocorticoids, applied in the form of dexamethasone coating of the electrode, can significantly reduce the hearing cell damage (pharmacokinetic and morphological analyses) thanks to their anti-inflammatory and immunomodulating characteristics (Liu et al. 2016). However, another study report published by Honeder et al. (2016) did not confirm the positive impact of steroids on preserving residual hearing in a guinea pig. The discrepancy may be due to the different types of steroids used in both studies: dexamethasone in the former and triamcinolone in the latter.

Douchement et al. (2015) have studied the effects of the glucocorticoid on HP during cochlear implantation using a gerbil model. The animals were implanted bilaterally: an electrode with controlled dexamethasone delivery (1% or 10% concentration) on one side and a conventional electrode on the other side. The hearing was tested at 4–6 weeks after surgery and 1 year after. The results after 1 year showed much better results in high frequencies, while the results for the low frequencies were ambiguous and hard to interpret.

Other researchers studied the efficacy of preoperative and intraoperative models of steroid administration for HP. Preoperatively, 5 mg/mL of dexamethasone was administered systemically, then topically (off-label) during the cochlear implantation procedure. Pure-tone audiometry (PTA) was performed at four frequencies: 250, 500, 1000, and 2000 Hz. The statistically significant differences were observed between the study and the control group, confirming the beneficial effect of glucocorticoid administration (Cho et al. 2016).

TOPICAL AND SYSTEMIC ADMINISTRATION OF GLUCOCORTICOIDS

There are two possible ways of glucocorticoid administration in the treatment of otologic disorders. Topical administration (e.g., transtympanic injection) allows achieving a high glucocorticoid concentration in the middle ear, but due to anatomical conditions (Eustachian tube), some portion of the drug may leak out. Topical administration to the middle and inner ear eliminates the 'first-pass' effect that occurs when the drug is administered orally. The main advantages of local drug administration are:

1. Lower dosage,
2. A high concentration of the active substance in the administration site,
3. Possibly better effects of therapy, as the drug reaches its target location directly,
4. Reduced risk of adverse effects,
5. Bypassing the BLB that limits the penetration of exogenous substances into the inner ear structures.

The topical administration of the drug may involve intracochlear delivery (as stem cell or gene therapy) and extracochlear delivery (e.g., intratympanic injection). It is also possible to combine both delivery modes (Plontke et al. 2017). The systemic drug delivery in otorhinolaryngological disorders is classified as noninvasive, as it incurs no damage to the anatomical structures such as the tympanic membrane. The adverse effects related to systemic administration can lead to the discontinuation of treatment. The BLB in the inner ear is one of the obstacles in achieving a high concentration of a drug in the cochlea.

APPLICATION OF GLUCOCORTICOIDS IN THE COCHLEAR IMPLANT PROCEDURE IN PATIENTS WITH PARTIAL DEAFNESS IN THE WHC

The prospective study described in this section aimed to assess the glucocorticoid administration effects in patients with partial deafness undergoing a cochlear implantation procedure (Skarżyńska et al. 2018). It was the first study of this type carried out in the WHC. It is continued in different patient groups, with various cochlear implants and electrodes and different glucocorticoid administration algorithms.

The aim of this study was to assess two different regimens of glucocorticoids (dexamethasone and dexamethasone with prednisone) administration in patients with partial deafness undergoing cochlear implantation. According to the study protocol, the implant used in this study was the Med-El system with a 28 mm-long electrode (Flex28™). The effect of glucocorticoid treatment on hearing was determined at six intervals: preoperatively, at the time of speech processor activation, and 1, 6, 9, and 12 months after the activation.

The study group consisted of 46 patients who were divided randomly into three subgroups. Patients in the first group received steroids intravenously (Figure 8.1), following the protocol of 0.1 mg/kg body mass dexamethasone intravenously 30 min before the surgery and then the same doses intravenously every 12 h for the next 3 days.

In the second group, patients underwent a prolonged, combined treatment. Three days before surgery, a dose of 1 mg/kg body mass/day was administered orally. Then, 30 min before the surgery, a 0.1 mg/kg body mass dose of dexamethasone was injected intravenously. For the next 3 days, dexamethasone was administered intravenously every 12 h (similarly to the first group). Then for the next 3 days, a dose of 1 mg/kg body mass/day was administered orally. After this time, the dose of prednisone was reduced by 10 mg/day. The gradual reduction of the dose was introduced to prevent adverse effects. The scheme of glucocorticoid therapy in the second group of patients is shown in Figure 8.2. Dexamethasone under the brand name Dexaven® (solution for injection

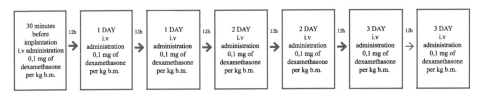

Figure 8.1 Scheme of steroid administration in the first subgroup of patients in the study of Skarżyńska et al. (2018).

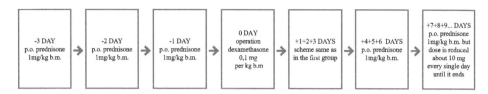

Figure 8.2 Scheme of administration of steroids in the second subgroup of patients in the study of Skarżyńska et al. (2018).

4 mg/mL) and prednisone under the brand name Encorton® (1, 5, 10, and 20 mg tablets) were administered according to the protocol of the study.

The third subgroup was a control group. Patients enrolled in this group underwent a standard cochlear implantation procedure without steroid treatment.

Pharmacokinetic of glucocorticoids used in the study

In the study, two different algorithms of the delivery of two different glucocorticoids were proposed. Both substances belong to the same pharmacological group (glucocorticoids ATC H02 AB) but have different pharmacokinetic and pharmacodynamic properties. Dexamethasone is a synthetic glucocorticoid (molecular weight: 392.46 g/mol) with immunomodulating and anti-inflammatory effects. In the ENT clinical practice, it is usually administered intravenously or in off-label use, such as in transtympanic injections. It is also used in the treatment of the nonbacterial otitis externa. After an intravenous injection of dexamethasone, the mean time to peak concentration (C_{max}) is 10–30 min, and the half-life ($t_{1/2}$) ranges from 2.2 to 3.8 h. The proteins responsible for transporting dexamethasone are also responsible for transporting the adrenal cortex hormones. Dexamethasone is chiefly metabolized in the liver and eliminated with bile. Only 2.6% of the chemically unchanged dose is eliminated by kidneys.

The second steroid used in this study, prednisone, is a synthetic glucocorticoid (a derivative of cortisone) classified in the ATC Classification System H02 AB 07. Prednisone is a prodrug that transforms into an active metabolite – prednisolone, which has a strong anti-inflammatory effect. The bioavailability of prednisone in oral administration ranges from 70% to 90%. The mean time to peak concentration (C_{max}) is from 1 to 2 h. Half-life ($t_{1/2}$) is 3.4–3.8 h in plasma and 18–36 h in tissue. Prednisone's binding with plasma proteins ranges from 70% to 73%, and the prednisolone binding to the plasma proteins is higher (90%–95%). Similarly, like dexamethasone, prednisone is metabolized mostly in the liver and eliminated with bile. Pharmacodynamic and pharmacokinetic data were based on the characteristics of medical products used in the study.

Methodology: outcome measures and qualification criteria

The primary measure used to assess the study outcomes was the PTA mean hearing threshold in 11 frequencies in the range 125–8,000 Hz, measured at six intervals (periods:

preoperative, at processor activation, and 1, 6, 9, and 12 months post-activation). The HP rate was calculated based on the HP classification proposed by Skarżyński et al. (2013) (Chapter 6).

The protocol of this study has the appropriate Bioethical Commission approval. Patients included in the study had severe to profound hearing loss and were divided according to Skarżyński's partial deafness treatment (PDT) classification (Chapter 1) into two groups: PDT-EC (partial deafness treatment – electric complement stimulation) and PDT-EAS (partial deafness treatment – electric-acoustic stimulation) (Skarżyński et al. 2013, 2015).

The inclusion criteria were:

- Hearing loss in the range of 65–120 dB at 250–1,000 Hz and 75–120 dB at 2,000–8,000 Hz;
- Cochlear duct length CDL = 3.65 × A − 3.63 (from the round window to helicotrema) in the CT imaging;
- Cochlea length equal to or more than 27.1 mm.

Patients with severe and advanced chronic diseases, whose condition could worsen after the extended or high-dose treatment with glucocorticoids, as well as patients taking medications that could interact with the drugs used in this study, were excluded from the study. Consequently, the exclusion criteria were:

1. Presence of symptoms or disorders that are a contraindication for using glucocorticoids, or where particular caution is indicated, such as advanced diabetes, advanced hypertension, neoplastic disease, osteoporosis, infections (bacterial, viral, or fungal).
2. Taking medications that diminish the effects of glucocorticoids or may have harmful interactions with glucocorticoids.
3. Taking medications that increase the effects of glucocorticoids.

Table 8.2 presents the study's clinical characteristics in the PICO framework (P – population, I – intervention, C – comparison, O – outcome).

Results and observations

Nonparametric statistical tests were used in the statistical analysis. Preoperatively, there were no statistically significant differences in hearing thresholds between patients in each of the three subgroups, including the control group, which means that all study participants had similar hearing levels in the preoperative period.

Deterioration of mean hearing thresholds in PTA was observed from the first follow-up interval, which is at the time of sound processor activation. Statistically significant differences were observed between the second subgroup (combined steroid treatment: prednisone + dexamethasone) and the control group: patients in the second study subgroup have obtained better PTA results in low frequencies than the control group. A similar observation was made in the measurements taken at 1, 6, 9, and 12 months after the activation of the sound processor – patients who underwent the

Table 8.2 PICO (P – population, I – intervention, C – comparison, O – outcome) according to the protocol of the Skarżyńska et al.'s (2018) study

P – Population	≥18 years cochlear duct length ≥27.1 mm (measured with CT imaging) hearing threshold 10–120 dB HL at 125–250 Hz hearing threshold 35–120 dB HL at 500–1,000 Hz hearing threshold 75–120 dB HL at 2,000–8,000 Hz
I – Intervention	Two schemes of glucocorticoid administration: 1. intravenous dexamethasone (0.1 mg/kg of body mass) 30 min before the cochlear implant surgery, then same dose every 12 h for three consecutive days (six doses); dexamethasone used in this study was supplied in ampoules of a 2 mL solution (4 mg/mL) 2. prednisone administered orally for 3 days before (1 mg/kg of body mass), then 30 min before the cochlear implant surgery; intravenous dexamethasone (0.1 mg/kg of body mass) similarly to the first group; for 3 days after surgery, prednisone administered orally (1 mg/kg of body mass); next, the dose was daily reduced by 10 mg until it reached zero
C – Comparison	No steroids administered
O – Outcome	The desired outcomes were the smallest deterioration in the average pure-tone audiometry (PTA) results during the five examined in the study periods compared to the preoperative period

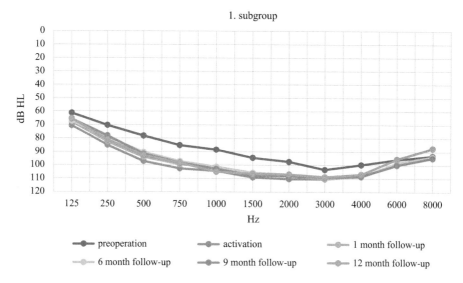

Figure 8.3 Average hearing thresholds in patients from the first subgroup with standard steroid treatment in the preoperative period, upon activation, at 1, 6, 9, and 12 months after CI (Skarżyńska et al. 2018).

combined (prolonged) glucocorticoid treatment had more stable hearing thresholds in all follow-up periods (Figures 8.3–8.6).

The rate of HP was calculated following the formula proposed by Skarżyński et al. (2013) and based on the PTA measurements taken 12 months after implant activation and preoperatively. The results were then divided into three groups according to the

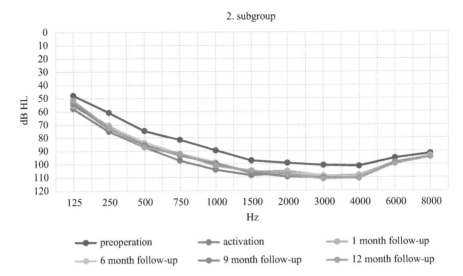

Figure 8.4 Average hearing thresholds in patients from the second subgroup with combined steroid treatment in the preoperative period, upon activation, at 1, 6, 9, and 12 months after CI (Skarżyńska et al. 2018).

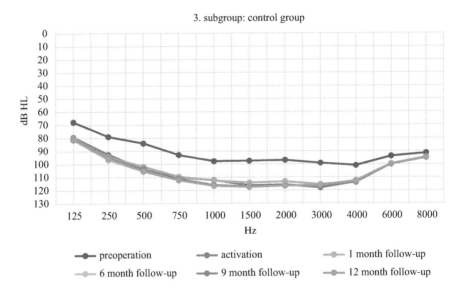

Figure 8.5 Average hearing thresholds in patients from the third subgroup (control) with standard steroid treatment in the preoperative period, upon activation, at 1, 6, 9, and 12 months after CI (Skarżyńska et al. 2018).

HP classification: minimal HP, partial HP, and complete HP (Table 8.3). The smallest variability of results and the highest overall HP rate (38%) were observed in the second subgroup. All patients from the second subgroup (prolonged steroid treatment) and almost 69% of patients from the first subgroup had partially or fully preserved hearing. The majority of the control group patients had minimal HP at 70.6% (see Table 8.3 and Figure 8.7).

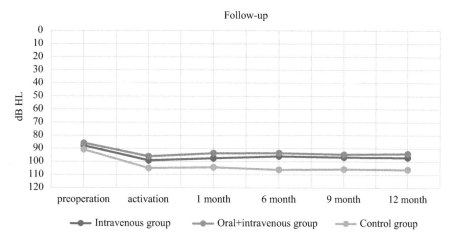

Figure 8.6 Average hearing thresholds in patients with standard steroid treatment (group 1), patients with prolonged steroid treatment (group 2), and control (group 3) in the preoperative period, upon activation, at 1, 6, 9, and 12 months after CI (Skarżyńska et al. 2018).

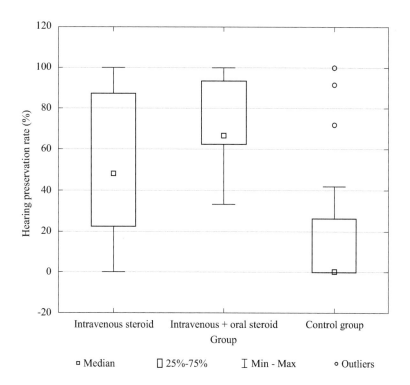

Figure 8.7 Hearing preservation (HP) rate in three subgroups (Skarżyńska et al. 2018).

Table 8.3 HP measured 12 months after implantation, in relation to the therapy applied –
the number and percent of patients (Skarżyńska et al. 2018)

	Minimal HP (0%–25%)	Partial HP (26%–75%)	Complete HP (≤ 75%)
Subgroup 1	5 (31.2%)	7 (43.8%)	4 (25.0%)
Subgroup 2	0 (0.0%)	8 (61.5%)	5 (38.5%)
Control group	12 (70.6%)	3 (17.6%)	2 (11.8%)

SUMMARY

This study was the first prospective analysis comparing two different glucocorticoid administration regimes in patients with partial deafness undergoing cochlear implantation. Its results confirm that the complementary glucocorticoid treatment helps stabilize hearing thresholds and preserve hearing in adults. According to the literature and the study results presented in this chapter, the combination treatment of intravenous dexamethasone and oral prednisone is the most effective treatment scheme.

Presently, researchers, clinicians, and commercial companies are looking to develop a new CI electrode capable of delivering glucocorticoids in a controlled way. The results of this study confirm that the administration of glucocorticoids aids in HP and stabilization of hearing thresholds in patients undergoing cochlear implantation. Other research reports support these findings, for example, Sweeney et al. (2015) and Cho et al. (2016). This report complements the earlier ones by reporting so far the longest follow-up period of 12 months from implant activation.

Summarizing, it should be underlined that pharmacotherapy (glucocorticoid treatment) combined with surgical skills and type of medical device (electrode) is useful as the complementary management in patients with partial deafness undergoing cochlear implantation, because it helps stabilize hearing thresholds and promotes HP.

Chapter 9

Otoneurological aspects of cochlear implantation in partial and total deafness

Magdalena Sosna-Duranowska
Institute of Physiology and Pathology of Hearing

CONTENTS

INTRODUCTION

The influence of cochlear implantation on vestibular function and balance is a complex issue. Cochlear implant (CI) provides deaf patients with audiological input providing them with a better orientation in the surrounding world. Consequently, the patients are more willing to participate in social life; their life quality gets better, and they are more physically active. Additionally, CI influences the rehabilitation process's effectiveness in patients suffering from any preoperative vestibular damage or other ailments impacting balance (Abramides et al. 2015, Parietti-Winkler et al. 2015). The possibility of eliciting vestibular evoked myogenic potentials by electric stimulation of the implanted electrode has also been described in the literature (eVEMP) (Parkes et al. 2017). The importance of this phenomenon is not fully known and demands further research. The negative aspects of cochlear implantation involve the risk of traumatizing the vestibular organ.

DOI: 10.1201/9781003164876-9

As specialists broaden the indications and qualification criteria for cochlear implantation, vestibular functionality preservation is gaining importance. Three situations require our particular attention:

1. Implantation of older people. In case of any vestibular damage, the central nervous compensation mechanism may be less effective due to the aging process and comorbidities.
2. Bilateral implantations, which are more and more frequent. The bilateral implantation may generate bilateral vestibular hypofunction, which is a challenging condition for specialists. Thus, the vestibular rehabilitation may not be entirely successful when the vestibular input is reduced or absent bilaterally (Gillespie & Minor 1999, McCall & Yates 2011). Other therapy options are minimal: somatosensory vibratory waist bell, vestibular prostheses/implants (not in common clinical use) (Della Santina et al. 2010, Phillips et al. 2015).
3. Partial deafness treatment (PDT) method introduced by H. Skarżyński has added new groups of CI candidates (Skarżyński et al. 2003, 2006, 2015). Patients with residual hearing at low frequencies (partial deafness) are today the massive part of all CI recipients. Our prospective cross-sectional study, conducted in the WHC, showed that these patients achieve better preoperative results of vestibular tests measured as cVEMP (cervical vestibular evoked myogenic potential), oVEMP (ocular vestibular evoked potential), caloric test, vHIT (video head impulse test), than those with total deafness (Sosna et al. 2019). Figure 9.1 presents an overview of the vestibular condition tests in patients with partial deafness before CI. It should be noted that better residual hearing at low frequencies means better vestibular organ's condition. It means that implanting persons with low-frequency residual hearing involves surgical ingerence into a normally functioning vestibulum more often than in patients with total deafness. During the cochlear implantation in partial deafness cases, the surgeon should do his best to protect the cochlear and the vestibular function.

IMPAIRMENT OF VESTIBULAR FUNCTION AFTER COCHLEAR IMPLANTATION – POSSIBLE MECHANISMS

Although the CI procedure does not directly interfere with vestibular structures, both the vestibulum and the cochlea share the same inner ear fluid space. This fluid may be responsible for transferring possibly damaging forces from one to the other. There are multiple factors involved, and the reasons why cochlear implantation influences the function of the vestibular organ is still a matter for further research. The most plausible factors causing postoperative organ dysfunctions are:

• Labyrinthine irritation and inflammation from foreign bodies (such as blood, bone dust, or electrode in the external ear), a reaction called serous labyrinthitis (Fina et al. 2003, Kubo et al. 2001);
• Intraoperative perilymph loss (Mangham 1987);
• Trauma caused by electrode's insertion into the tympanic duct may cause hair cells' damage or necrosis if endolymph and perilymph become mixed due to basilar membrane rupture (O'Leary et al. 1991, Tien & Linthicum 2002, Eshragi et al. 2015);

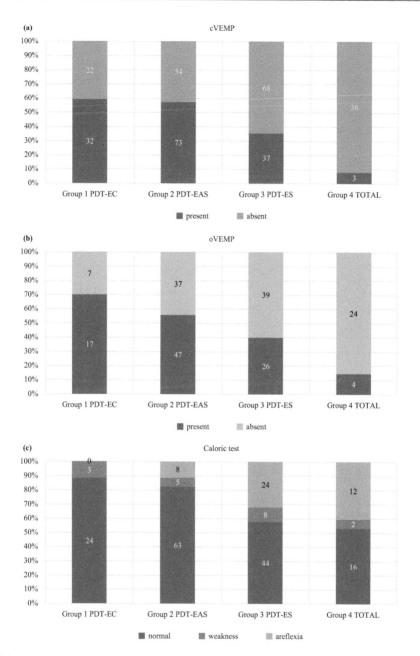

Figure 9.1 **Preoperative results of vestibular tests in patients with partial deafness: (a) cVEMP, (b) oVEMP, (c) caloric test (Sosna et al. 2019).**

- Misinsertion of an electrode into the vestibule;
- Otoconia dislodgement caused by intraoperative drilling, the spread of electric current during CI activation, or the ampullary cupula's irritation by bone dust mixed into the inner ear fluid may cause the benign paroxysmal positional vertigo (BPPV) (Viccaro et al. 2007).

Balance dysfunction may also appear later after cochlear implantation, related to other vestibular pathologies:

- Fibrosis and obliteration of the inner ear (Tien & Linthicum 2002);
- Endolymphatic hydrops resulting from disturbance of inner ear fluid homeostasis (Tien & Linthicum 2002);
- Perilymphatic fistula (Kusuma et al. 2005);
- Electric co-stimulation of vestibular nerve fibers (Coordes et al. 2012).

HEARING PRESERVATION TECHNIQUES AND PROTECTION OF THE VESTIBULAR ORGAN

There are some aspects connected with surgical procedures used to preserve low- and mid-frequency hearing during cochlear implantation that, we believe, can also protect the peripheral vestibular system:

- Insertion of an electrode through the round window lowers the risk of misinsertion into the vestibule since the round window is a good landmark that projects directly into scala tympani (Skarżyński et al. 2007b, 2014b);
- Use of soft electrodes reduces electrode insertion trauma;
- Reducing the insertion angle makes it less likely that any cochlear structure will be damaged since the cochlea is thicker in its basal region (Avci et al. 2014, Biedron et al. 2010);
- A micropuncture of the round window membrane with a surgical needle decreases intraoperative perilymph loss, and resignation from drilling in the cochlea lowers the risk of otoconia loss;
- Perioperative steroid administration is helpful because they have an anti-inflammatory effect, reduce reaction to foreign bodies, and prevent the endolymphatic hydrops risk (Skarżyńska et al. 2018).

VESTIBULAR SYMPTOMS AFTER COCHLEAR IMPLANTATION AND SPECIFICITY OF VESTIBULAR DISORDERS IN CI RECIPIENTS

Around half of CI recipients may have some vestibular symptoms that may appear preoperatively or in the postoperative period as early and delayed symptoms after implantation, either transient, paroxysmal, or persistent (Ito 1998, Zawawi et al. 2014). Figure 9.2 presents the recommended management algorithm for patients with postoperative vestibular symptoms.

There are some specific aspects of vestibular disorders among CI recipients:

1. The BPPV appears in patients with CIs twice as often as in the general population (Limb et al. 2005).
2. Epidemiology of BPPV localization after cochlear implantation is similar to the general population. Most often, the posterior semicircular canal is affected, then lateral and anterior. In sporadic cases, BPPV appears in a non-implanted ear.

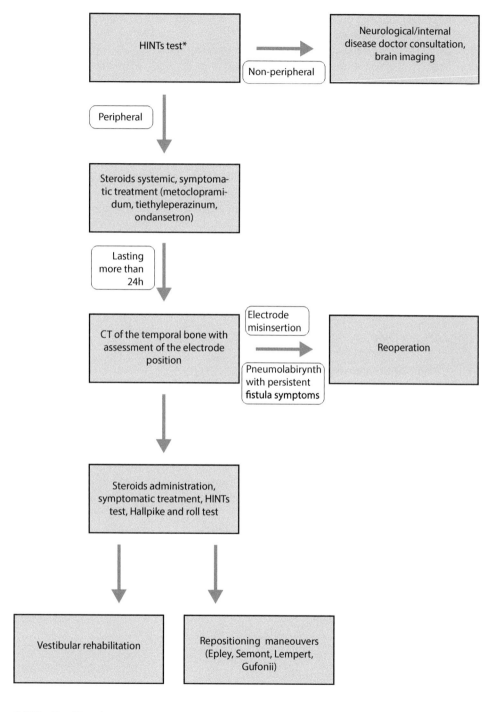

*HINTs – Head Impulse Test, Nystagmus, Skew Deviation Test

Figure 9.2 Vestibular symptoms after cochlear implantation in the early postoperative period and recommended management.

3. The significant part of CI recipients suffers from vestibular disorders (uni- or bilaterally) before cochlear implantation as the etiological factor of deafness often destroys the vestibular hair cells as well.

4. In deaf ears, delayed endolymphatic hydrops (DEH), also known as delayed Meniere's disease, may appear years, or even decades, after the onset of hearing loss, causing Meniere-like symptoms. There is no evidence that cochlear implantation procedure influences that process. The treatment is the same as in Meniere's disease (dietary restrictions, betahistine, diuretic treatment, intratympanic steroid injections, ventilation tube insertion, systemic steroid therapy, gentamycin intratympanic injections, endolymphatic sac surgery, or vestibular neurectomy) (Schuknecht 1978).

5. In CI patients, determination of the side affected by (delayed) Meniere's disease is difficult because there are no hearing fluctuations.

6. The main risk of cochlear implantation is paroxysmal vestibular system damage (partial or total). The central nervous compensation mechanism enables the disappearance of vestibular symptoms if unilateral vestibular damage occurs. Additional neurological, psychiatric, orthopedic, or rheumatoid comorbidities may limit the effectiveness of the central compensation mechanism (Whitney et al. 2020).

PREOPERATIVE OTONEUROLOGICAL TESTING

The battery of otoneurological tests that are currently in clinical use enables us to assess each part of the vestibulum separately (Jacobson et al. 2011):

- Sacculus with cVEMP that measures vestibulocollic reflex (Colebatch & Halmagyi 1992);
- Utricle – with oVEMP that measures vestibulo-ocular reflex (Todd et al. 2007);
- Lateral semicircular canal – with the caloric test for low-frequency stimuli and with a rotatory chair or vHIT for high-frequency stimuli;
- Superior and posterior semicircular canals with vHIT (MacDougall et al. 2009).

Till now, there is no consensus regarding the necessity of vestibular evaluation during the cochlear implantation procedure.

Each of these tests has its pros and cons, contraindications, and its tricky aspects. None is the 'gold standard' in the vestibular assessment. It should be recommended that as many tests as possible are made in each particular case to gain all the necessary information about the patient's vestibular status.

cVEMP, oVEMP

Advantages

- Quick and comfortable for patients, do not provoke vertigo nor vegetative symptoms;

- Assess the organs that are the most fragile to be damaged during electrode insertion due to anatomical proximity.

Disadvantages

- Dependable on many factors (neck muscle stiffness, false negatives by a conductive hearing loss if elicited by air-conducted stimuli, central nervous pathologies that include the arch of the vestibulospinal reflex cVEMP or vestibulo-ocular reflex oVEMP; false positives by 'third window syndrome');
- Strictly connected with the age; the amplitude and frequency of elicited responses decrease with age (Piker et al. 2015);
- VEMP responses are often absent before cochlear implantation, so they are useless in monitoring vestibular functions;
- No universal norms regarding latencies and amplitudes. There is no consensus on how to stimulate (tone burst vs. click, 500 Hz vs. 750 Hz vs. 1,000 Hz, stimulus parameters 2:2:2 or 2:1:2), and how to generate the constant contraction of sternocleidomastoideus muscle in cVEMPs (45° head rotation away from the stimulated ear vs. head elevation);
- Bone-conducted stimuli may be used to stimulate patients with conductive hearing loss. The specificity of this method in the case of cVEMP is doubtful, as it may generate the response both from the sacculus and from the utricle (both of them have ipsilateral projections to the sternocleidomastoideus muscle). cVEMP elicited by bone stimuli may be the alternative, not the replacement for cVEMP by air-conducted stimuli;
- In the case of oVEMPs, bone-conducted stimuli are a well-established way to assess the utricle function. It is indicated to stimulate with lower frequencies (100–125 Hz) that enable applying the 20–30 dB nHL lower stimuli. An accessory transducer (e.g., Radioear B81) should then be provided.

Caloric test

Advantages

- Old, well-established, reliable test in otoneurology; its role was never entirely replaced by the newer tests;
- Shows the present and past (once the damage has appeared, it will be detected by the caloric test regardless of the compensation level).

Disadvantages

- Limited application in patients presenting weak bilateral responses (then the differentiation between physiologically weak responses and bilateral hypofunction is needed by adding vHIT or rotatory chair test);
- May provoke vertigo and vegetative symptoms;
- Assesses only the lateral semicircular canal function (the population of neurons type II that respond to low frequencies 0.004–0.008 Hz stimuli);
- The way of heat transmission strongly influences the final result. There are some restrictions to use the caloric test: tympanoplasty with canal wall-down technique,

eardrum perforation, or inner ear malformations. The effect of the electrode in the cochlea on heat absorption is not well known either.

vHIT

Advantages

- The only test in common clinical use that assesses all semicircular canals;
- Quite comfortable for patients, as the head movements do not exceed $10°–20°$;
- Stimulates semicircular canals (neuron type II) with high-frequency stimuli 1–6 Hz that are more physiological for cupulas; more prominent correlation between the outcome and everyday functioning;
- Gives the absolute result concerning the particular vestibulum without the necessity to compare it with the opposite side.

Disadvantages

- Demands experience to achieve reliable results (head velocity must be >150°/s, which is quite tricky in left anterior, right posterior (LARP), right anterior left posterior (RALP) plane; the googles slipping off during the abrupt head motion);
- Test's sensitivity is questionable; the proportion between the detection of vestibular damage by caloric test and vHIT varies (Bell et al. 2015). It cannot replace the caloric test but should be used as a complementary test;
- It is, partially, a compensation test – if velocity applied to the patient's head is too small (<150°/s), the result may be falsely negative;
- Utmost care should be exercised while performing this test in patients with advanced cervical spine degenerative changes.

INCIDENCE OF VESTIBULAR DAMAGE AFTER PARTIAL DEAFNESS TREATMENT

The reduced or lost responses in cVEMP, oVEMP, caloric tests, or vHIT after cochlear implantation are reported in many papers. The incidence of vestibular damage after cochlear implantation (cochleostomy technique) is shown in Table 9.1.

The study conducted in the Otorhinolaryngosurgery Clinic of the Institute of Physiology and Pathology of Hearing included 107 CI patients (59 females, 48 males, age 10–80, mean 43.32 ± 18.44). Thirteen patients were already CI users and received a second implant on the opposite ear. Apart from five cases implanted with perimodiolar electrode, all patients were implanted with soft lateral wall electrodes.

Exclusion criteria were reimplantation, superior semicircular canal dehiscence syndrome, inner ear malformations, including the large vestibular aqueduct syndrome (LVAS) and total vestibular damage before CI confirmed by absent cVEMPs and oVEMPs, caloric test areflexia measured as the slow-component nystagmus velocity (SCV) <12°, and corrective saccades in all semicircular canals in the vHIT.

All patients were implanted with the round window surgical approach and hearing preservation techniques. The cVEMP, oVEMP, and caloric tests were performed before implantation and then at 1–3 months (cVEMP, oVEMP) and 4–6 months (caloric

Table 9.1 Incidence of vestibular damage after cochlear implantation in cochleostomy (literature review)

	cVEMP loss	Reduction of response in the caloric test	Gain reduction in all semicircular canals in vHIT	Time between cochlear implantation surgery and test
Krause et al. (2009)	–	32.00% (12/38)[a]	–	4 weeks
Krause et al. (2010)	43.00% (6/14) 43.00% (6/14)[b]	50.00% (8/16)[a]	–	2 months
Migliaccio et al. (2005)	–	–	9.00% (1/11)	4–6 weeks
Todt et al. (2008)	50.00% (8/16)	42.90% (9/30)[a]	–	–
Buchmann et al. (2004)	–	29.00% (8/28)[c]	–	4 months
Melvin et al. (2009)	31.25% (5/16)[d]	6.25% (1/16)[c]	3.60% (1/28)	1–2 months

[a] Change from a normal response to UW (unilateral weakened response) or from UW to areflexia.
[b] Decrease in VEMP amplitude by more than 50%.
[c] Decrease in SPV (slow-phase velocity).
[d] Loss of response or elevation of response threshold VEMP ≥ 10 dB nHL

tests) after CI. Loss of cVEMP responses was observed in 14 out of 73 (19.2%) and oVEMP in 8 out of 46 (17.4%) patients who registered responses preoperatively. In the case of the caloric test, the postoperative change of UW (unilateral weakness) >25% towards the implanted ear was reported in 6 out of 43 (13.95%) cases.

CONCLUSIONS

The surgical technique with the round window electrode insertion used in PDT preserves the vestibule's function better than traditional cochleostomy. Cochlear implantation may result in partial or total vestibular damage despite using the hearing preservation surgical techniques. We want to emphasize that the risk of vestibular damage can be decreased but never eliminated, even when hearing preservation techniques are applied (Sosna et al. 2019). Every patient should be informed about the possibility of vestibular damage and possible vestibular disorders before signing the operation's consent. Special care should be taken where the possibility of bilateral hypofunction of vestibule after cochlear implantation exists. Preoperative assessment of vestibular function should be performed especially in those patients:

- The candidates for bilateral cochlear implantation,
- With a history of vertigo/dizziness attacks,
- When there is an increased risk of implanting the better/only vestibule (e.g., cholesteatoma, otosclerosis/status post stapedotomy in the opposite ear),
- Patients without clear audiological and anatomical indications of which side should be implanted.

Chapter 10

The utility of the functional magnetic resonance imaging for assessment of brain functions in patients with partial deafness

Tomasz Wolak and Katarzyna Cieśla
Institute of Physiology and Pathology of Hearing

CONTENTS

INTRODUCTION – PROGRESS IN THE FIELD OF FMRI STUDIES

The functional magnetic resonance imaging (fMRI) technique is regarded as the most precise noninvasive method to evaluate brain networks performing certain cognitive functions. It is used increasingly more frequently in brain research. It is also becoming increasingly popular in clinical work, for example, locating speech processing centers in the brain before surgery. Each year, we witness giant steps forward in the development of magnetic resonance technology. MR scanners become smaller, lighter, and less demanding in maintaining the system of liquid-helium cooling of the magnet. At the same time, data acquisition becomes faster, more precise, and thus more affordable. Increasingly more popular are MR scanners with the 3 T magnetic field induction (for comparison, the Earth's magnetic field $\approx 30–60$ µT). Already, the first 7 T scanners have been introduced into research and clinical work. New imaging sequences enable obtaining perfect quality images in significantly less time than before. Today, a whole-head functional (fMRI, c.f. anatomical, MRI) scan of the brain can be acquired in less than 1 s. Registration of anatomical images of the entire head with 1mm spatial resolution may take about 1–2 min. There are also ongoing studies on counteracting the limitations of the MR technique. One of the recently developed techniques involves the so-called quiet sequences that eliminate excessive noise generated by the device during image acquisition.

DOI: 10.1201/9781003164876-10

Presently, it is also possible for people with implanted nonmagnetic metallic objects in their body to undergo an MR scan. Metal artifacts (image distortions caused by a metal object) are less extensive, which allows for radiological assessment of adjacent areas. Manufacturers of cochlear implants and middle ear implants use technologies that allow performing an MR test in a 3 T scanner without removing magnetic elements of the implant placed under the patient's skin. Unfortunately, during an MR study, the implant has to be switched off, and its outer parts must remain outside of the MR testing room. Therefore, as of today, it is still impossible to perform a functional brain study (to assess functional networks in the brain and not its anatomy) with an active implant. It is possible, however, to record structural images necessary for diagnosing and monitoring the progress of brain disease.

Figure 10.1 shows a 3 T magnetic resonance image of a head phantom with an example cochlear implant 'placed in the right ear.' The image was taken at the Bioimaging

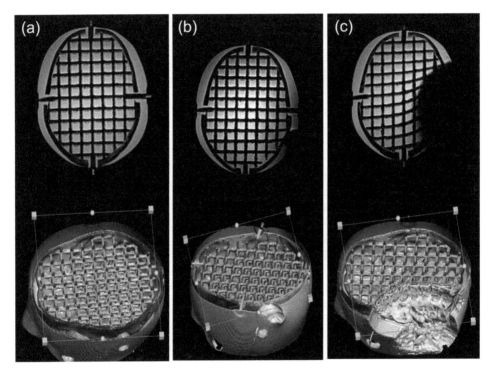

Figure 10.1 (a) Reference image of a head phantom, (b) an image of a head phantom with the internal part of an example cochlear implant with the magnet removed, (c) and an image of a head phantom with an example cochlear implant with the magnet remaining in place. The magnet in the external part of the implant (a coil connected via cable to the speech processor) holds to the external part of the implant under the skin, which also has a magnet. Both magnets enable the inductive transfer of power and information between coils. In some modern cochlear implants, self-rotating capsule magnets change their alignment according to the powerful magnetic field of an MR scanner, preventing the patient from feeling any pain related to the magnet's movement under the skin. (Source: own research.)

Research Centre of the Institute of Physiology and Pathology of Hearing in Kajetany. It demonstrates that an MR image obtained without removing the internal part of an implant misses only a few percent of the information, allowing the assessment of the larger part of the brain.

Technical progress in magnetic resonance imaging makes it possible today to obtain images of quality comparable to brain cross-sectional photography. The development of the parallel imaging technique, including the so-called multichannel coils, makes it possible to increase imaging speed and quality considerably. Simultaneously, techniques are being developed that can eliminate the previous problems of fMRI imaging, such as image distortions or low resolution. There are techniques today that enable recording functional brain images with a 1mm resolution. New brain activity scanning techniques such as the blood oxygenation-sensitive steady-state (BOSS) fMRI increase test sensitivity. Another novelty is the dynamic magnetic resonance spectroscopy that will enable observing biochemical reactions (changes in metabolite concentration) in the brain in response to tasks, similar to fMRI. Increasingly more often, imaging is based on other elements than hydrogen, such as helium, carbon, phosphorus, or xenon. The fMRI technique is also combined with other techniques such as event-related potentials (ERP), electroencephalography (EEG), transcranial magnetic stimulation (TMS), or functional near-infrared spectroscopy (fNIRS). The fusion of fMRI with other techniques increases the temporal resolution of the acquired data and provides combined information about the direct electric neuronal activity blood perfusion in brain regions engaged in the task. Magnetic resonance also enables fiber tracking, i.e., measuring the integrity of white matter tracks connecting brain regions.

Among the numerous fMRI applications in studying the brain's functional organization, many apply to sensory functions, particularly hearing. This chapter presents the fMRI technique basics and the possibilities of brain regions' imaging functions involved in processing auditory information. Bioimaging Research Center opened at the Institute of Physiology and Pathology of Hearing in 2009, is equipped with a state-of-the-art 3 T MR scanner and multiple devices for providing sensory/cognitive stimuli. We specialize in studies of the auditory system, particularly in people with hearing impairments. The last part of this chapter will focus on fMRI studies of the tonotopic organization (sound frequency-related) of the auditory cortex, including patients with partial deafness (PD).

DESCRIPTION OF THE FMRI TECHNIQUE

Thirty years ago, the first functional imaging tests using the fMRI technique had been conducted, revolutionizing our knowledge of the human brain functioning (first studies on rats were performed by Seiji Ogawa in 1990).

The assessment of brain functions using the fMRI technique is made indirectly by assessing brain oxygenation dynamics. Initially, registration of perfusion in individual brain areas had been possible only after intravenous administration of a contrast agent. Deoxyhemoglobin, the part of hemoglobin in the blood flow without oxygen, is strongly magnetic, in contrast to the oxygen-carrying oxyhemoglobin. Its level in blood changes following neuronal activity, as demonstrated by Ogawa (1990). Thanks to that discovery, it is possible to assess the brain's functional status using

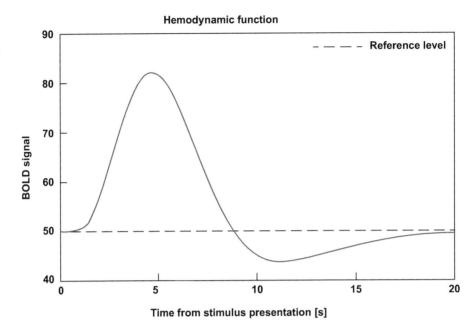

Figure 10.2 Hemodynamic response function (HRF) time series in BOLD fMRI.

magnetic resonance by observing a specific blood-oxygenation-level-dependent (BOLD) signal.

In a typical fMRI study, a person performs a task after being presented a specific stimulus, e.g., auditory. The reaction time of neurons to stimuli is relatively short (a hundred or so milliseconds), while a hemodynamic response function (HRF) is delayed (Figure 10.2). In typical cases, the BOLD signal delay from the start of stimulation is about 2 s. The time to the plateau is about 6 s. The exact HRF parameters depend on the region of the brain engaged in analyzing a stimulus. After the stimulation period, the BOLD signal drops within a few seconds below the baseline and stabilizes only after at least 20 s from stimulus presentation.

One should also remember that the change of a BOLD signal represents a summary activity of a population of neurons, which means that the same change of the BOLD signal may be due to a large activity of a small number of neurons or a small activity of a large number of neurons. There is indisputable theoretical and experimental evidence that the BOLD signal is strictly correlated with nervous tissue activity in the central nervous system.

Functional brain imaging provides information about the level of hemodynamic activity in the nervous system, reflecting the involvement of different brain structures in a specific task. The main advantages of that technique are complete noninvasiveness and high spatial resolution of the acquired data. The examination is painless and does not require the administration of any potentially harmful contrast.

A typical fMRI study (Figure 10.3) comprises several blocks of providing stimuli and control resting periods, during which a series of brain images is collected

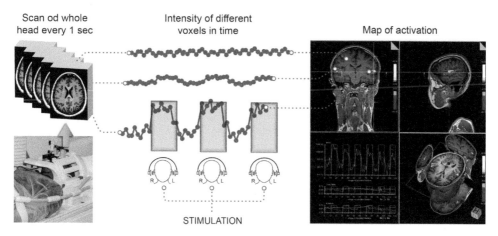

Scan od whole head every 1 sec

Intensity of different voxels in time

Map of activation

STIMULATION

Figure 10.3 fMRI examination diagram: study participant wearing headphones and goggles for sensory/cognitive stimulation placed inside the MR scanner bore. In a study, thousands of brain section images are registered during repeated stimulation. The detailed analysis of images combined with information about the type and time of stimuli allows pinpointing the active regions in the brain.

(performed using the echo-planar technique, EPI). The analysis involves following the whole time course of the experiment for each voxel (a single volume unit of the imaged tissue) individually to see any significant correlation between the signal change and the stimulation periods. The signal should get stronger during stimulation.

In functional brain studies, it is necessary to use devices for presenting stimuli during the task, such as special earphones and/or goggles. It is also essential to use adequate MR imaging sequences that are particularly sensitive to changes of the so-called T2 time, i.e., local changes of the magnetic field homogeneity.

Functional brain studies can be divided into individual studies (data collected in only one person) and group studies (of a larger population to obtain averaged group functional brain maps). In group studies, the typical voxel size is $2 \times 2 \times 2$ mm. In individual studies, the aim is to achieve a 1 mm or better resolution of the images, which is an indication for using MR scanners with at least 3 T magnetic field.

APPLICATION OF THE FUNCTIONAL MAGNETIC RESONANCE IN THE AUDITORY PATHWAY STUDIES

Technical solutions

An advantage of fMRI in auditory research is the relatively high sensitivity and specificity of this method in detecting task-related brain activity. Also, as there are no adverse effects related to this method, even small children can participate. It is also possible to perform multiple assessments of dynamic processes in the brain, such as the effects of auditory rehabilitation and training (Hall 2014, Hall et al. 2014).

Researchers are looking to identify markers in the specific brain activity patterns that could help predict a patient's progress after a specific medical intervention, such as cochlear implantation (Giraud et al. 2001b, Lazard et al. 2013). As mentioned, due to the interaction between the magnetic field and the implant's system, it is impossible to use the fMRI method to assess the processing of auditory information delivered through the implant. In these patients, the recommended brain imaging methods are PET or EEG.

A primary difficulty in the fMRI studies of auditory processing is the noise produced by the MR scanner during image acquisition, which may reach even 100 dB. The primary source of noise predominant in the 0.5–2 kHz range is the fast switching of current in the gradient coils – the electrodynamic forces cause mechanical vibrations that produce the mentioned noise (Talavage et al. 2004, Seifritz et al. 2006, Ravicz et al. 2000). The other sources of noise present during the whole fMRI test sequence are the air conditioning system and the compressor for cooling helium in the scanner's magnet. These devices generate noise at the level of about 70 decibels (Woods & Alain 2009). So-called silent sequences, available since 2012, reduce MR scanner noise by about 95%, but they can only be applied to acquire structural images. The first sequence of that type designed for functional imaging/echo-planar imaging (EPI) is presently in the testing phase and not commercially available.

Presently used sound stimulation methods require a specialized headphone system that works in the strong magnetic field. Four types of MR-compatible headphones are commercially available: pneumatic, piezoelectric, electrodynamic, and electrostatic. Pneumatic headphones have a narrow bandwidth up to 6–8 kHz and can only serve for communicating with the participant or presenting simple language tasks. The sound quality provided by other types of headphones is excellent, and they can be used in studies of more sophisticated auditory processing.

In studies of the auditory system, especially in studies of the tonotopic organization (frequency-related) of the cortex, precise calibration of the presented sounds is essential. The digitally generated stimuli are played through an integrated or dedicated soundcard. The quality of the soundcard (amplifiers and power outputs) affects the fidelity of the delivered sound. The soundcard transforms a digital signal into an analog one. The signal is again transformed into a digital form and sent through an optical fiber to the MR scanner. Then, the signal is again converted from digital into analog and sent to the headphones. Usually, headphones used in MR studies have an analog input. This entire track of transmission of the sound stimuli creates a constant delay and some distortions. This is not fundamentally relevant for studies of the auditory cortex's tonotopic organization, but each pipeline part's parameters should be as good as possible. Particularly important in these studies is the linearity of sound intensity in relation to its frequency (frequency characteristics).

fMRI studies of the auditory cortex often employ a *sparse* sequence, where brain images are collected at specific intervals, as short as possible, when the MR scanner is silent. This way, the scanner noise does not affect brain responses. The repetition time (TR, which is the length of time between consecutive acquisitions of the same image slice/volume) in the *sparse* sequence is a few seconds (4–18 s). For example, if the TR = 10 s and the studied area is divided into 40 slices, one slice is collected each 62.5 ms, which gives 2.5 s to collect the signal from all slices and 7.5 s waiting time to start another acquisition. When there is no noise from gradient coils, it is possible to stimulate the auditory cortex using lower sound intensity than if the images were collected continuously. If the TR is longer, then the effect of cortex stimulation by the scanner noise is smaller (lesser masking of the auditory stimuli). The stimulation protocol is planned so that at the moment of image acquisition, the hemodynamic response amplitude is as high as possible. If we assume, as above, the following values of an imaging sequence: TR = 10 s, TA = 2.5 s (TA – real time needed to collect all slices of the studied volume – head) and 40 slices, then the signal from central slices of the head will be recorded about 1–1.5 s after the start of acquisition. If stimulation happens about 5 s before the start of acquisition, then, assuming a 6 s delay from the start of stimulation to a maximum of the hemodynamic response, this provides optimal signal acquisition parameters. To obtain additional information about the shape and the temporal course of the HRF, which often is valuable information, we can apply an additional *jitter* (random delay) of the distribution of stimuli in time. As a result, the HRF is sampled at different points in its time course. The sparse model of acquisition requires collecting more data volumes (which increases the sequence duration) to obtain sufficient statistical power (number of averages) for each sample of the HRF (Figure 10.1). *Sparse* acquisition random delays allow determining the rate of the signal change and the individual shape of the HRF in a specific region for each person. It is handy for regional analysis of the brain data, i.e., focused on selected brain areas and not the whole brain. The disadvantage of *sparse* is, as mentioned, that it takes longer than continuous data acquisition, so participation in an examination may cause weariness and growing attention loss. Moreover, the risk of movement artifacts increases. A solution could be dividing the imaging sequence into several shorter sessions.

The organization of the hearing pathway

An overview of applications of fMRI techniques in studies of the auditory system can be found in the following review publications: King et al. (2018), Talavage et al. (2014), Wong (2010), Hall et al. (2014), Price (2012). As discussed in them, the fMRI technique can be used to assess many aspects of auditory information processing in the central nervous system. Examples include tonotopic (related to sound frequency) cortex organization, analysis of acoustic stimuli of various levels of complexity, processing of different aspects of language (phonology, syntax, semantics), production of speech, auditory memory and imagination, and reading. At the Institute of Physiology and Pathology of Hearing, we conduct fMRI research on all these sensory and cognitive processes; however, in the present paper, we focus on assessing the tonotopic organization of the human cortex.

The brain processes information hierarchically. The majority of sensory information is transferred from the receptors through the thalamus to the primary cortex centers. Each sense has a corresponding area in the brain, which maps information from receptors preserving the topology. For example, auditory receptors are tonotopic, which means that sounds of a given frequency are preferentially encoded in a specific region in the cochlea. The cochlea's tonotopic organization is preserved at all levels of the auditory pathway, from cochlear nuclei, olivary nuclei, inferior colliculi, medial geniculate nuclei to the primary auditory cortex (PAC) in the region of Heschl's gyri in bilateral temporal lobes in the brain. Similarly, the sense of sight: receptors – rod and cone cells in the retina – are represented in the visual cortex, preserving their spatial organization called retinotopy. Sensory centers in one cerebral hemisphere receive sensory information from the contralateral side of the body; that is, the auditory cortex in the left hemisphere receives most information from the right-side cochlea (about 70%), and the remaining 30% comes from the ipsilateral cochlea.

Information reaching primary cortical centers is further processed in the secondary and tertiary centers, also called associative centers/cortices. The secondary centers are mostly unimodal (related to one sense) and specialize in finding the distinctive features of incoming information (e.g., the Wernicke area specializes in detecting the speech sounds – phonemes – in auditory information). These centers throughout human life are to learning and narrow their specialization. The tertiary, associative centers combine information from many senses and enable recording or reproducing their meaning from memory. Learning means coding in memory the distinctive patterns of information provided by senses. Cognitive processes, including attention, motivation, emotions, and the context, in which information was presented, play an essential role in learning and memory (Hickok & Poeppel 2007). The nervous system's, including the auditory system, ability to undergo functional and structural changes under the influence of experience is called neuroplasticity. Generation of an auditory sensation requires, therefore, not only an efficient sensory organ (outer, middle, and inner ear) and the pathway through which the information reaches the brain, but also efficient processing of that information in the brain.

OWN STUDIES OF THE AUDITORY CORTEX RESPONSES IN NORMAL HEARING

Evaluation of tonotopic organization of the auditory cortex

fMRI studies of the tonotopic organization of the auditory cortex and the relationship between the location and intensity of signal change in the auditory cortex and sound frequency/intensity have been conducted in several neuroimaging centers around the world (e.g., Talavage et al. 2004, Langers et al. 2007, Woods & Alain 2009, Woods et al. 2009, Humphries et al. 2010, Da Costa et al. 2011, Striem-Amit et al. 2011).

The most recent fMRI studies confirm that there is one area on the lateral plane of the Heschl's gyrus representing low frequencies and two high-frequency areas in the polar pole and temporal pole of the temporal plane. Some researchers interpret that stable functional configuration as a high-low-high frequencies gradient alongside the Heschl's gyrus (two collinear gradients) (Woods et al. 2009, Hertz and Amedi 2010). Other researchers, and it's a prevalent opinion, claim that frequencies are represented in the auditory cortex as a V-shape, where the low-frequency area connects two high-frequency areas that cross the Heschl's gyrus obliquely/transversely (Langers & van Dijk 2012, Humphries et a. 2010, Striem-Amit et al. 2011, Da Costa et al. 2011, Moerel et al. 2012, Herdener et al. 2013). Different interpretations result probably from a different spatial resolution of the collected imaging data across studies. Presumably, low-field MR scanners (1.5 T) used in the earlier studies had been unable to differentiate the two high-frequency areas, especially that, in some people, they are very close to one another (Langers & van Dijk, 2012).

At the Institute of Physiology and Pathology of Hearing, we have developed a method of imaging the auditory cortex's tonotopic organization in a 3T MR scanner

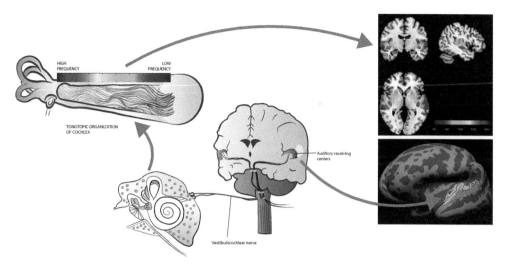

Figure 10.4 Tonotopic organization of a cochlea reflects the tonotopic organization of the primary auditory cortex in temporal lobes.

by applying a sparse sequence. The examination involves three sessions, each 8 min long. Within these 8 min, image acquisition takes 2 s (scanner noise is then at the level of 90–100 dB), and auditory stimulation is presented during the remaining 6 s. In a series of our studies, images of the auditory cortex's tonotopic organization were obtained using complex tones with various central frequencies, from low to high: 400, 800, 1600, 3200, and 6400 Hz. Each central frequency tone was played during an examination run 24 times. Sounds were presented at 80 dB through electrostatic headphones. Additionally, quiet periods were introduced to obtain a baseline level of BOLD signal change, also 24 times. The proposed study paradigm allows obtaining robust maps of frequencies in the auditory cortex showing the expected V-shaped frequency gradients in the Heschl's gyrus area in both temporal lobes (Figure 10.4).

Assessment of the relationship between sound intensity and the auditory cortex activation

In the subsequent studies in healthy subjects, we have used the same set of complex sounds with the following central frequencies: 400, 800, 1600, 3200, and 6400 Hz. This time, sounds were calibrated to three different levels: 40, 60, and 80 dB (Wolak et al. 2017a). Our goal was to investigate the relationship between the level of sound intensity and the activated area's location and size in the auditory cortex. As shown in Figure 10.5, the area of activation in the PAC was found to enlarge almost linearly with an increase of sound intensity. At the same time, however, the location of the center of activation for a given central frequency level remained the same.

We searched to explain the obtained results, showing larger based on mechanisms occurring in the inner ear. When quiet sounds are presented, for example, at 40 dB,

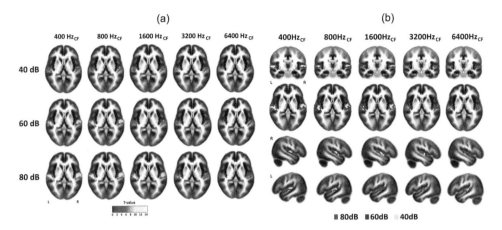

Figure 10.5 (a) The pattern of activation of the auditory cortex in response to complex sounds with subsequent central frequencies (0.4–6.4 kHz) and different intensity levels: 40, 60, and 80 dB, (b) location of active areas for different stimulus intensities (Wolak et al. 2017b).

displacement (vibration) of the basilar membrane in the cochlea is relatively small, so only a limited part of the cochlea is stimulated, and thus, a small number of the auditory nerve endings sends impulses to upper auditory structures. An increase in sound intensity induces an increase of the basilar membrane's activation area, also engaging a larger number of neurons. When sound intensity is very high, basilar membrane vibrations involve practically the whole cochlea, gradually recruiting all neurons adjacent to the maximum displacement region. In addition, there are two kinds of neurons in the auditory nerve. If low-intensity sounds (below 40 dB) are presented, only the so-called low-threshold neurons respond. At the level of 40–60 dB, these neurons become saturated, and, gradually, the sound coding process also engages high-threshold neurons. For sound levels of 90–100 dB, these neurons also become saturated (Wolak et al. 2016, 2017a).

An additional effect registered in our fMRI study was the broader area of excitation accompanying sounds with lower, compared to higher, central frequencies at the same intensity level. That effect can also be explained by physiological mechanisms at the level of the organ of Corti in the inner ear. A soundwave entering the cochlea passes first the basilar membrane areas representing high frequencies, then mid- and then low frequencies (this is related to the membrane's mechanical features, the passive mechanism). When the sound is loud after stimulation with low frequency, neurons located at the basal and central part of the cochlea are stimulated (those responsible for high and mid-frequencies). Therefore, areas representing low-frequency ranges in the auditory cortex are larger than those representing high-frequency ranges. The higher the sound intensity, the effect is more pronounced.

Our fMRI studies show that if the applied sound intensity exceeds 60 dB in people with normal hearing, statistically significant group results can be obtained in a reasonable time (about 30 min). Conversely, in a group of 12 persons, with stimulation at 40 dB, we failed to obtain a group effect for 6,400 Hz frequency, which is a high frequency and thus induces smaller cortical activations than lower frequencies. Another significant outcome of that study was the conclusion that for the sounds of increased intensity (>60 dB), the maximum activation is located in the same area of the auditory cortex for lower-intensity sounds. This crucial fact enables using sounds of higher intensity in the fMRI studies of the PAC's tonotopic organization, although they produce less precise results.

Own studies in patients with partial deafness

For many years, it has been believed that the functional organization of the auditory system structures is stable throughout life. Today, studies taking advantage of the advanced electrophysiological and neuroimaging methods, such as fMRI, provide evidence of neuroplastic changes in all structures of auditory pathways related to the increased or reduced auditory stimulation, even in adulthood (Skarżyński P.H. et al. 2013, Illing and Rosskothen-Kuhl 2008, Kral & Tillein 2006). The term 'neuroplasticity' means the ability of the nervous system to adapt to changing conditions. In humans, functional reorganization of auditory pathways results from:

- Musical training (e.g., Herholz & Zatorre 2012, Pantev et al. 1998, Baumann et al. 2008);
- Auditory fatigue (e.g., Skarżyński P.H. 2012, Skarżyński P.H. et al. 2013);
- A period of hearing deprivation (e.g., Langers et al. 2007, Thai-Van et al. 2010, Lazard et al. 2010, 2013, Sharma et al. 2015, Wolak et al. 2019);
- Tinnitus (e.g., Langers et al. 2012, Roberts et al. 2012, Pantev et al. 2012);
- Hearing rehabilitation with cochlear implants (e.g., Seghier et al. 2005, Guiraud et al. 2007, Giraud et al. 2001a; Sharma et al. 2015, Thai-Van et al. 2010, Gordon et al. 2006).

The Institute of Physiology and Pathology of Hearing, in the years 2010–2011, had started the first in the world program of fMRI studies involving patients – candidates for cochlear implantation (Skarżyński et al. 2012c). A series of studies focused on patients with various types of PD, as proposed by Skarżyński et al. (2010). This classification differentiates patients with PD according to their audiogram type prior to cochlear implantation: PDT-AS (acoustic stimulation), PDT-EC (electric complementation), PDT-EAS (electric-acoustic stimulation), and PDT-ES (electric stimulation).

Our first fMRI study used two chirp-type sounds (one sweeping frequencies from 50 to 950 Hz and the other representing a frequency range from 3 to 5 kHz, rising in 1 s time) for auditory stimulation. We aimed to investigate how the sounds passing through the basilar membrane in the inner ear are reflected in the auditory cortex. We observed activations in the auditory cortex in both hemispheres. In the PDT-EC group (candidates for cochlear implantation to electrically complement their residual normal low-frequency hearing), the activations were more extensive compared to the other tested group and involved areas corresponding to low- and mid-range frequency sounds. These patients were unable to hear high-frequency sounds, and thus, there were no corresponding responses visible in the brain. In the PDT-EAS group (candidates for acoustic amplification via a hearing aid of the preserved residual hearing in low frequencies and electric stimulation, i.e., a cochlear implant, to provide hearing in the remaining frequency ranges), activations in the PAC were limited to the areas responsible for low-frequency hearing. Although the results may seem obvious, they were the first in the world objective visualization of the location and size of regions responsible for the sensation of hearing in people with a specific hearing impairment such as PD.

The second series of tests was an fMRI study of the auditory cortex's tonotopic organization in patients with sensorineural hearing loss. Patients in the study group had symmetrical, sloping hearing loss (more severe in higher-frequency range); the control group included persons with normal hearing matching the study group in terms of age and sex. The study used complex tones with the following central frequencies: 400, 800, 1600, 3200–6400 Hz (Wolak et al. 2016, 2017b).

As shown in Figures 10.6–10.8, the first result of the study was that in people with normal hearing, neuronal activation areas in response to the presented stimuli were seen bilaterally in the auditory cortex for all frequency ranges. In patients, no neuronal responses were observed for 3,200 Hz and 6,400 Hz sounds – these sounds were presented in the MR scanner at a higher hearing threshold than the group average. The study patient group's neuronal activation areas were observed for stimuli 400 Hz_{f0}, 800 Hz_{f0}, and 1,600 Hz_{f0} in both cerebral hemispheres, precisely in the same regions of the auditory cortex as in the control group (f0 is the central frequency).

We also observed that for low-frequency sounds (central frequency = 400 Hz), in patients, the active area covered more than 90% of the PAC volume calculated based on the Juelich probabilistic atlas. In people with normal hearing, it was 85% (Figure 10.6b) (Morosan et al. 2001). For all other frequencies, the activation area was much larger in people with normal hearing than in the patient group. We saw even more interesting results when we replaced the Juelich atlas mask with an area calculated as a sum of active regions for all applied frequencies in the study (Figure 10.6a). The latter area was larger than the one in the atlas. In that area, the difference in activation size for 400 Hz was 12% points (72% in the control group, 84% in the study group). In all other frequency ranges, we observed more extensive activation in people with normal hearing. We suspect that the activated areas' size in the auditory cortex reflects the pathophysiological effects characteristic for the cochlear hearing loss. In people who perceive mostly/more strongly low-frequency sounds, the tonotopic organization of the auditory cortex might change due to neuroplasticity. The effect was more pronounced in people who had not been able to hear high-frequency sounds from birth or in whom PD had appeared before the language acquisition period (age 3–7 years).

In the further analysis of the results, we should keep in mind that in sensorineural hearing impairments, the outer hair cells become damaged in the first place. These cells play a crucial role in hearing, as they amplify the basilar membrane motions, especially those caused by low-frequency sounds (the active mechanism). That mechanism enables us to hear sounds below 50 dB HL. More severe hearing loss also involves gradual damage to the inner hair cells.

More precisely, in the group of patients with hearing loss <55 dB HL in low-frequency ranges, we assume there was damage to the outer hair cells of various degree, inducing broadening of auditory filters and slight loudness recruitment (increased perceived loudness disproportionate to the increase in the signal intensity level). Simultaneously, the inner hair cells were relatively preserved, so the entirety of auditory information is transmitted to the higher structures of the auditory system. In effect, the

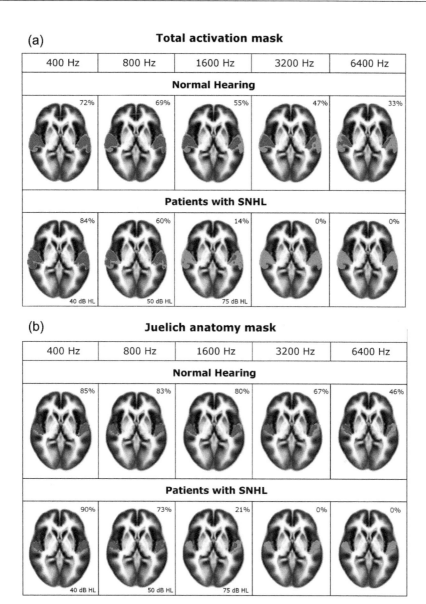

Figure 10.6 (a) Activation maps corresponding to sounds representing successive octaves/central frequencies (red) in relation to the complete activation mask (green) – mean results in the patient and the control group; numbers indicate the hearing threshold and percentage area of activation for each tone in relation to the area calculated as the sum of activations revealed for all tones; *p* < 0.05 FWE (family-wise error correction), (b) activation maps corresponding to sounds representing successive octaves (red) in relation to the TE1.0, TE1.1, and TE1.2 regions of the primary auditory cortex according to Juelich's atlas (green) obtained for the control group (upper row) and the study group of patients with sensorineural hearing loss (lower line); numbers indicate the hearing threshold and percentage area of activation for each tone in relation to the area of the primary auditory cortex; *p* < 0.05 FWE.

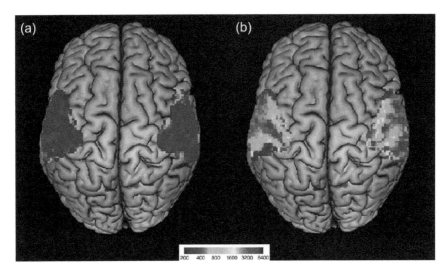

Figure 10.7 Mean tonotopic maps (*maximum intensity projection*): (a) a map calculated as a mean of 32 persons with normal hearing, (b) mean maps of 24 persons with partial deafness in high frequencies; each color represents frequencies presented on a scale below. (Source: own research.)

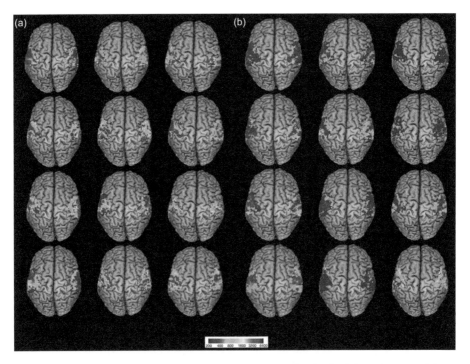

Figure 10.8 Examples of tonotopic maps obtained in individuals: (a) with normal hearing and (b) with partial deafness. (Source: own research.)

fMRI findings revealed larger representations of sound in the auditory cortex in this group with sensorineural hearing loss than in persons with normal hearing. A hearing loss more severe than 55 dB HL entails significant damage to the outer hair cells, broadening of auditory filters, significant and progressing loudness recruitment, and various degrees of damage to the inner hair cells. When the inner hair cells do not code sound, it is not transmitted to higher auditory structures, including the brain. For this group of patients, depending on whether the broadening of filters/loudness recruitment or limited bottom-up transmission of information is dominant, fMRI maps will show an enlarged or diminished representation of sounds in the auditory cortex (Moore 1995).

In the presented study, we also measured responses to the same sounds in the auditory cortex in patients with tinnitus and hearing loss. We failed to detect any specific patterns of the tonotopic organization in this group of patients. Thus, we have confirmed the reports published in the literature (Burton et al. 2012, Langers et al. 2012).

Figures 10.7 and 10.8 show group mean maps of the tonotopic organization of the auditory cortex. In this instance, they have been calculated using the 'the winner takes it all' approach. Considering that cortical activation for supra-threshold sounds is not fully selective in the cochlea nor the cortex, we present here the area that was the most active for a given frequency range (but not exclusively). The maps obtained in people with sensorineural hearing loss reflect the dominance of low- and mid-range frequencies related to high-frequency sensorineural hearing loss.

In sum, the outcomes of the presented series of fMRI studies confirm that the observed activation patterns in the auditory cortex reflect in the first place the peripheral phenomena occurring in the inner ear, including the passive and active mechanisms of the basilar membrane. However, we suggest that the tonotopic organization of the auditory cortex in patients with sensorineural hearing loss may be subject to slight reorganization – representation in cortical areas of the most potent perceived stimuli (most representative frequencies transmitted from the inner ear) may be enlarged. We speculate that central mechanisms may also be involved in the observed neuroplasticity effects. We demonstrated that the functional magnetic resonance technique is an objective measure of processes occurring along the auditory pathway.

Structural studies of the auditory cortex

One of our ongoing research projects involves combining the functional data with structural images of the auditory cortex. Disregarding individual differences in terms of location, shape, and size of the PAC may lead to erroneous assessments in group functional studies (see, e.g., Figure 10.11).

Rademacher, who was the author of the first studies in that area, published probability maps of the location of the PAC in the brain in the so-called Talairach space (Rademacher et al. 2001) that is a standardized coordinate system of the brain enabling comparisons of brains across individuals in one reference frame. Rademacher's maps have demonstrated differences in auditory cortex structures between individuals and between the right and the left hemisphere of an individual.

The study published by Morosan et al. (2001) presented a postmortem analysis of 27 brains (14 female, 13 male, aged 37–85, 90% right-handed). Nine of them, besides a cytoarchitecture study (the study of the organization of various types of cells), also had magnetic resonance images taken. Based on the cytoarchitecture study, which was the largest so far with respect to the auditory cortex, the authors prepared detailed topographical models of the PAC area. They set the three main goals for the study. The first one was to determine the range/anatomical variation of shape, size, and reach of the PAC area in the temporal lobes. The second was the analysis of the relationship between the Heschl's gyri and the PAC's borders. The study's third aim was a 3D reconstruction and overlaying these areas on a standard brain to compare the results with previous anatomical and functional studies. Morosan and colleagues observed significant differences between individuals concerning the PAC's location, especially in the coronal and sagittal plane of the brain (displacement by about 5–7 mm). Additionally, they found significant differences between cerebral hemispheres in individual brains in the location of the center of the PAC area in the frontal/coronal plane. The maximum individual asymmetry (i.e., the difference between hemispheres) was from 9 mm in the sagittal and axial planes to 13 mm in the frontal plane. An important question was how much the probability map of the PAC location agrees with PAC's location based on the Heschl's gyri location. The PAC area's average location was found in this study to differ in all dimensions from the PAC location determined in relation to Heschl's gyri in previous studies (Talairach & Tournoux 1988, Penhune et al. 1996). These results suggest that in calculating a mean brain image from a group of individuals, important information may be lost regarding individual differences in the anatomy. It is an essential conclusion in the context of the auditory fMRI studies, as group comparisons require referring all patients to a common set of coordinates (for example, a Talairach space or the MNI (Montreal Neurological Institute) coordinate system).

Figures 10.9 and 10.10 present examples of brain images of people with normal hearing, obtained using our study paradigm. As we can see, there are several variants

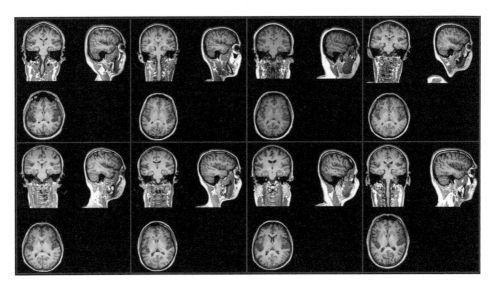

Figure 10.9 Examples of Heschl's gyrus segmentation in people with normal hearing (different variants found in own studies): red – first gyri/first branch of the Heschl's gyrus, blue – the second gyrus/branch of the Heschl's gyrus.

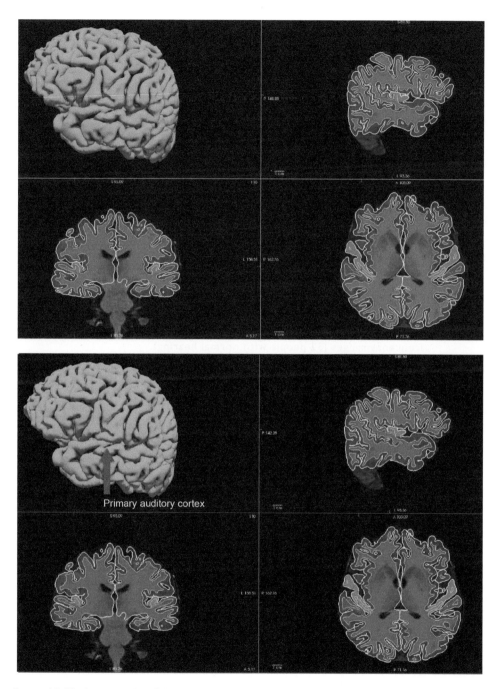

Figure 10.10 **An example of the cerebral cortex segmentation and Heschl's gyri – a variant with two gyri in both cerebral hemispheres. (Source: own research.)**

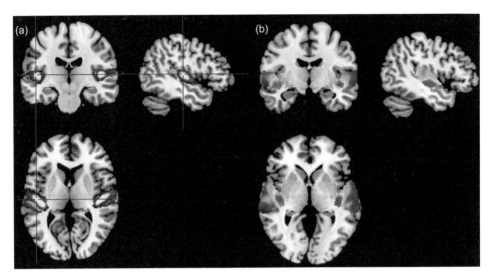

Figure 10.11 (a) A statistical map presenting the probable locations of different variants of the Heschl's gyrus (yellow-red for the first Heschl's gyrus and green for the second), (b) a tonotopic map of the primary auditory cortex calculated based on the mean representation of active areas in response to different frequency ranges (32 people with normal hearing).

of Heschl's gyrus across brains and hemispheres: with one gyrus (I-shaped), incomplete double gyri (Y-shaped), full double gyri (II), incomplete triple gyri (IY), and full triple gyri (III). The first variant is the most prevalent; the last one is the rarest. We should note that Heschl's gyri's variants do not have to be symmetrical in both hemispheres; for example, the left hemisphere may have a double gyri variant (bifurcation) while the right a single gyrus variant.

Figure 10.11 shows the location of Heschl's gyri and the tonotopic map with the gradient of frequencies represented in the auditory cortex, both obtained in the same study group (a group mean map). The gradient is clearly visible along the anterior margin (anteromedial direction) of the Heschl's gyrus. A similar gradient is also present in some people on the posterior margin (posteromedial direction) of the second Heschl's gyrus, but it is not visible on the map. This is because the frontal margin is present in a large majority of people exactly in the same place, but the number of gyri and their variants differ across individuals, and thus, the posterior gradient is somewhat 'blurred' (locations in different people do not overlap).

An alternative to the classical structural MR assessment is the technique measuring myelination (amount of the myelin sheath) in gray matter, which can also be used for segmentation of the Heschl's gyri. This technique helps to determine the location and size of the PAC area. Myelin is a sheath formed by oligodendrocytes covering nerve fibers in the central nervous system. Its amount is measured using T1- and T2-dependent MR images (Glasser & Van Essen 2011). Figure 10.12 shows a map of myelin content in the gray matter (top) and cross-sections of the gray matter in the area of Heschl's gyri. Areas with higher myelin content are visible in the cerebral cortex in the

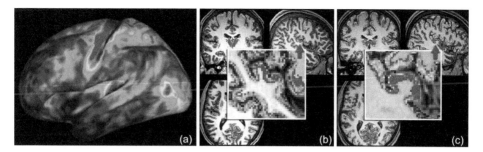

Figure 10.12 Images of myelin distribution in gray matter calculated based on high-resolution MR images; red color represents increased myelination, green low–myelination.

locations corresponding to the primary cortex for different senses. More myelinated areas in the Heschl's gyrus allow verifying its location and size. That additional measure is essential, particularly in cases when the results of Heschl's gyrus segmentation method and functional assessment (fMRI) are ambiguous.

SUMMARY

This review presents possible applications of the fMRI technique for auditory system studies. The fMRI study design should allow for the strengths and limitations of that technique, such as noise during the examination and an always-present strong magnetic field. Multiple studies conducted at the Institute of Physiology and Pathology of Hearing, described in this chapter, demonstrate the extent of possible applications of the fMRI technique in assessing brain functions in patients with hearing impairments such as PD. Today, modern magnetic resonance scanners enable combining the assessment of brain functions and structures as well as the degree of myelination of neuronal connections. The MR technique is applied to assess auditory processing the higher-than-cochlea levels of the auditory pathway, whose integrity is crucial in adapting to the altered sound signals in hearing impairments. In the future, we may expect that this method will be used for predicting, based on brain findings, the benefits of cochlear implantation (there have been such attempts made already) and that it will be possible to study brain functions in patients equipped with hearing devices, including cochlear implants. Assessment of neuroplastic processes in different populations of patients, including various types of PD, would provide additional information to develop optimized rehabilitation approaches for patients.

Chapter 11

Audiological rehabilitation in the partial deafness treatment program strategy – eliminating participation limitations

Małgorzata Zgoda, Agnieszka Pankowska and Joanna Ćwiklińska
Institute of Physiology and Pathology of Hearing

CONTENTS

INTRODUCTION

The primary model of disability in rehabilitation studies is the functional model adopted from sociological sciences (Nagi 1991). According to that model, we can look at the loss of listening skills as a dynamic process comprising four interconnected subprocesses. These subprocesses include (1) pathological process at the molecular level in auditory receptors, (2) damage manifesting as the sensory deficit, (3) functional limitations (inability to perform specific tasks, such as understanding spoken communications), and (4) difficulties encountered in the social sphere (that is, difficulties in complying with social expectations) (Brandt & Pope 1997, Nagi 1991). Audiological rehabilitation is a problem-solving exercise aimed at limiting the adverse effects of hearing loss by creating conditions conducive to activity and restoring full participation in life situations (Stephens & Hétu 1991, Chisolm at al. 2007, Sweetow & Palmer 2005). The basis of audiological intervention is providing an adequate hearing prosthesis to compensate for the loss of auditory functions caused by hearing impairment. Audiological rehabilitation also requires other strategies of help aimed at neutralizing activity and participation limitations. These strategies include perception training, support, and education (Boothroyd 2007, Dillon 2001). Partial deafness (PD) appearing at different ages brings consequences for the patient's functioning. The model of audiological rehabilitation for patients with PD after cochlear implantation adopted in the Institute of Physiology and Pathology of Hearing is concurrent with the functional model of disability based on the International classification of functioning, disability and health (ICF) (Lorens 2014).

DOI: 10.1201/9781003164876-11

PATIENTS WITH PARTIAL DEAFNESS – THEIR SPECIFIC DIFFICULTIES AND NEEDS IN HEARING, LANGUAGE, AND COMMUNICATION PERSPECTIVE

PD is diagnosed when the patient's hearing sensitivity in low frequencies is normal or slightly lowered, and there is no reception in high frequencies (Skarżyński et al. 2007b). These patients are often disinclined to use classic hearing aids because they do not improve their speech understanding. Medicine could not offer them any other solution until 2002, when the first cochlear implantation with preservation of the existing natural hearing in a person with that type of hearing loss has changed their prospects for the better. According to the newest concept of partial deafness treatment (PDT) presented in Chapter 1, it is possible to treat patients with PD and various degrees of hearing loss (Skarżyński et al. 2014b).

The greatest challenge for patients with PD is understanding spoken communications (Obrycka et al. 2012). The specific problems of these persons should not be considered only in the sphere of hearing possibilities and skills, but also in the sphere of language and communication.

The degree and type of hearing loss affect patients' communication skills, speech and language development levels, and social functioning. For example, among patients after PDT, several groups are using acoustic stimulation in different configurations: acoustic stimulation with hearing aids or middle ear implants (PDT-AS), electro-natural stimulation (PDT-ENS), electric complementation (PDT-EC), or electric-acoustic stimulation (PDT-EAS). Before cochlear implantation, problems most often observed in these patients are limited ability to receive, differentiate, and recognize environmental sounds (in silence as well as with interfering sounds), reception of speech with visual support (watching interlocutor's face, lipreading), limitations in following and understanding spoken communications in difficult acoustic conditions, significant limitations in differentiating and recognizing similarly sounding words, and disruption of prosody and articulation. Simultaneously, their ability to communicate verbally using multiword, grammatically correct expressions is preserved (Skarżyński et al. 2014a, Pankowska et al. 2014). Disorders and abnormalities noted in the diagnostic process affect patients' daily functioning. Limited access to many sounds, including speech, may affect their participation in the social life, determine their use of media, be responsible for the feeling of otherness, and be conducive to deterioration of the overall mental condition. Patients strongly stress the lack of support from their social environment, which, misled by their 'normal' speech communication, cannot understand their information reception limitations. They avoid meeting in a larger group with family or friends. They draw attention to the fact that when they reveal their problem, other people focus on short-term help that mostly involves speaking louder, which directly translates as failing to comprehend the patient's specific needs. Proportionally to the degree of hearing loss, these persons are anxious to pick up the phone and talk without visual support. When this situation continues, patients become more isolated, stop seeking new contacts, are afraid of ridicule, and significantly underrate their worth. Studies conducted in that group of patients confirm these problems and limitations (Obrycka et al. 2012).

In children and youths, we observe limitations in the reception of signals and speech, limited awareness of the phonological dimension of language, problems with applying grammatical rules organizing their statements, and widely defined school difficulties. These problems stem from the fact that speech perception is a complex process that combines physiological and phonemic hearing, auditory memory, and the ability to associate the acoustic patterns of words with concepts. These components are closely interconnected; each next has a more complex function and is dependent on the previous one. The physiological hearing provides a base for developing phonemic hearing. If – because of damaged hearing organ – audibility in some frequency band-width is worse, it will lead to inaccurate reception of speech sounds from that band-width. It disturbs the ability to distinguish, identify, and differentiate speech sounds (phonemic hearing). Disordered phonemic hearing, based on the auditory analysis and synthesis, leads to difficulties in learning to read and write. Difficulties in speech perception are also related to problems with auditory memory (that is, the ability to remember auditory patters such as the number and order of syllables in the word, the number of phonemes in a syllable, the sequence of words connected logically and grammatically, and the ability to associate sounds with ideas (lack of the correct au-ditory patterns).

Without a cochlear implant (CI), lack of hearing sensitivity, particularly in high frequencies, significantly limits the ability to understand communications transmitted through hearing. Simultaneously, the extant ability to hear and react to low-frequency sounds may mask the problems in the first years of a child's life. A child, perceived and treated by people around it like a person with normal hearing, grows up in an environ-ment where using speech and receiving communications through hearing is a natural method of building contact with family and environment. Difficulties and limitations in understanding communication's content affect the development of bonds and rela-tionships with family and friends and establishing the position in a group (Putkiewicz et al. 2011).

Patients from the PDT-ES group usually have such limitations in access to sounds and speech that any communication may only happen in a visual-auditory way or even only visual (lipreading, manual codes); sometimes, its range is minimal. It is observed mostly in persons with prelingual hearing impairment. Their auditory development is usually a result of planned auditory training. Provision with hearing aids usually gives these patients access to some perception clues, but there is no chance to differentiate or identify speech sounds. The degree and character of hearing loss also affect patients' language competencies that vary widely between individuals. During preoperative di-agnostics, disorders are observed in three dimensions: phonological (sounds and pros-ody), syntactic (grammar), and lexical (vocabulary). Moreover, there is a relationship between rehabilitation method, education, and influence of the closest environment before cochlear implantation and patient's ability, motivation, and willingness to com-municate, participate actively in a dialog, express and describe thoughts, states, emo-tions, and needs. Pedagogical and psychological influences also play an essential role.

Persons with postlingual hearing loss possess acoustic and acoustic-motor models of speech. They had participated actively in communication and developed language naturally in line with their age. For them, the loss of the ability to perceive acoustic stimuli is primarily a limitation in a social sphere. It is connected to the feeling of help-lessness, rejection, with a loss of a previous life.

A rehabilitation program developed for each patient individually should account for all the above factors. Patients can be divided into two groups: adults, and children and youths. That division refers to patients' age at the time of the diagnosis and determines differences of needs and difficulties caused by the limited access to sounds.

THE GOALS OF HEARING REHABILITATION

Activation of a CI system and subsequent changes of the electric stimulation parameters give the patient the ability to detect acoustic stimuli and receive sounds in the whole frequency range. A well-designed auditory rehabilitation process will build or re-build a patient's ability to perceive signals and speech. Best results can be achieved with the help of a multidisciplinary team of experts comprising an otolaryngologist, clinical engineer, speech and language therapist, pedagogue, and psychologist. Cooperation and exchange of information between these specialists aid in determining long- and short-term goals, monitoring the effects, selecting the parameters of electric stimulation, and making full use of the restored acoustic perception in the course of hearing therapy.

In working with youths and adults, the most important goals are adequate auditory training (particularly in the first two years after CI activation) and social activity stimulation. Auditory training stages include reaction to the signal, discrimination, identification, and speech understanding. The basic-level exercises include reaction to the signal (conditioning to the stimulus) and discrimination (differentiation). The typical conversation level involves training in the identification (recognition) of sounds, particularly speech, in closed set exercises. The speech understanding level involves open-set exercises aimed at developing the ability to conduct casual conversations (Skarżyński et al. 2004b). The building of auditory skills in subsequent levels allows patients to improve signal perception and hearing and communication skills. Duration of exercises on each level should be different in patients with prelingual and postlingual hearing loss. In patients with prelingual hearing loss, detection, discrimination, and identification of sounds must give them a basis for building a stock of auditory impressions and learning to compare and order them according to specific features. They will be their reference base for analogies to speech sounds. Training with lexical material should start from exercises with sentences, then words, and in the end with single speech sounds. The training should utilize first visual-auditory way, then auditory-visual, and finally auditory. It should be noted that not all persons with prelingual hearing loss are going to be able to develop the ability of auditory-only speech reception.

In patients with postlingual hearing loss, the training follows the same scheme, but it can refer to the patient's past auditory experiences. The auditory training is in the first stage conducted in favorable acoustic conditions, while later also with interfering sounds. The work with the patient aims to create opportunities to acquire auditory skills useful in daily social situations.

CHARACTERISTICS OF WORKING WITH
DIFFERENT GROUPS OF PATIENTS

In the group of patients using acoustic stimulation (PDT-AS) through the middle ear implant system, the auditory training goals are set after the implant activation, based on audiological tests, including speech audiometry and sentence tests, phonemic hearing tests, or tests of auditory differentiation of phonemes. The rehabilitation program should involve training in hearing through the middle ear implant and recognizing and understanding speech in different acoustic conditions. It should be noted that these patients quickly adapt to speech perception with middle ear implants, and the process of rehabilitation is faster than, for example, in the PDT-ES group. A vital element of the rehabilitation process is encouraging patients' participation in different social situations that demand making practical use of newly acquired auditory speech perception ability. Observing and defining audiogenic and psychologically conditioned communication limitations is crucial in this group of patients. Based on these observations, it is possible to invite specialists from the relevant fields to join the rehabilitation program.

Patients from the PDT-ENS, PDT-EC, and PDT-EAS groups with CIs can successfully combine the natural and the 'electric' hearing. After implantation, they gain the ability to perceive sounds in the whole frequency range. Nevertheless, adequately organized auditory training is necessary to teach them how to integrate acoustic sensations perceived through a natural hearing with sensations delivered through a CI. The program of auditory rehabilitation after cochlear implantation in these patients is based on methods also used in the rehabilitation of profoundly or totally deaf CI users, with modified sound and lexical materials (Solnica & Pankowska 2013). Rehabilitation work should include auditory exercises with environmental sounds (mainly middle and high frequency) and word material such as sentences in closed sets, half-open and open, pairs of similar words (with different consonants), multi- and one-syllable words, syllables. Material presented to patients should include in the first place high-frequency speech sounds that are the hardest or impossible to perceive, differentiate, and recognize for persons with PD before cochlear implantation (Stelmachowicz et al. 2004).

The PDT-ES group includes patients with the most severe degrees of hearing loss and nonfunctional, if any, residual hearing. This was the first group of CI candidates at the start of the program in Poland in 1992. It is still the most numerous and diverse in hearing, language, and communication benefits group of CI candidates.

The post-implantation rehabilitation program should account for the following factors:

- At what age did the hearing loss occur?
- When was it diagnosed?
- When did rehabilitation, early comprehensive specialist care commence?
- What is the degree and type of hearing loss?
- Does the patient use hearing prostheses systematically?
- How well does the auditory prosthesis compensate the auditory functions?
- What is the etiology of hearing loss or deafness?
- Is the hearing impairment the only developmental deficit?
- What are the patient's intellectual abilities and level of emotional maturity?

Patient's status and competencies before implantation determine the primary goals of rehabilitation after CI system activation.

PEDIATRIC POPULATION – ADDITIONAL REMARKS

In the rehabilitation of hearing in the youngest group of patients, most work focuses on auditory education and principles, methods, and strategies of the auditory-verbal method, with significant involvement of parents and child's closest environment. They all should cooperate to build and develop a child's ability of auditory signals, and speech reception. Auditory education comprises activities directed at acquiring and developing auditory skills before the speech acquisition period. In effect, children with profound hearing impairment obtain a collection of auditory experiences analogous to hearing persons. A CI is a tool that provides such an opportunity. A continuation of that work is appropriate auditory training, a set of exercises ordered according to increasing difficulty level. It aims to perfect the acquired auditory skills and use them in practice together with vocabulary training. This approach is in line with the auditory-verbal therapy (AVT) method. The AVT method's foundation is the diagnosis at the earliest possible time, provision with the latest available device, and immediate commencement of therapy with significant involvement of parents supported at all times by authorized specialists.

It is necessary to precisely define at this stage two terms that are integral in the AVT method: hearing and listening. Hearing is a passive process dependent on the status of a hearing organ. On the other hand, listening is an active process involving the ability to perceive sounds and derive information from them consciously. Provision with a CI prepares patients to hear sounds. Hearing rehabilitation introduces the patient to the process of listening and consequently to acquiring language intentionally as well as incidentally. This way, the patient can acquire the 'common' language, with a rich vocabulary, correct grammatically, and rich in elements expressing feelings and emotions.

Experience of working with the youngest CI users confirms that therapy organized according to the auditory-verbal method brings about the desired effects (Estabrooks et al. 2020, Pankowska et al. 2013). According to the philosophy of the auditory-verbal method, all therapy participants are partners. It means that all can present their rations, feelings, impressions, emotions; create and co-develop strategy; and use and modify techniques. It should be noted that there is a risk of conflict if the rules are presented unclearly and not fully understood. Based on observations of various rehabilitation processes, we can infer that the dominant tradition of rehabilitation care in Poland consists in the leading role of the therapist, with the child and parents being the more or less active observers and recipients of ideas and suggestions. The AVT rules firmly order us to change this picture. A therapist should be an instructor and guide, a parent should lead the process, and a child, engaged continuously in cooperation with parents, should be not a recipient but a partner in the act of communication. Parents' active participation enables them to learn the presented techniques and create roles on their own. Parents should cooperate with the therapist to adjust the forms of play and activity to the child's interests and abilities. The foundation of the language is its development through natural interactions in matters that are important and interesting for the child. Only parents have enough determination to pursue rehabilitation goals consistently (Estabrooks et al. 2020).

If parents and therapists agree that due to a child's individual predispositions and needs, it is necessary to resign from the auditory-only stimulation, then the CI obliges us to combine auditory sensations with visual, but always in that order. Only with this assumption, that child will be able to experience hearing and learn to listen.

SUMMARY

Adults and children with PD experience difficulties in the sphere of speech perception (receiving, identifying, and understanding). Incomplete speech information they receive is enough to recognize the start and the end of communication and cope better or worse with recognizing a sentence's content. Their problems start when they have to differentiate two similarly sounding words relying only on hearing (Pankowska et al. 2012).

Limited perception of sounds, particularly in the range of middle and high frequencies, affects the quality and legibility of speech. In spite of a limited stock of acoustic sensations, patients with PD can acquire a vocabulary base enabling verbal communication. In communication situations, they aid themselves with lipreading – visual canal provides essential support for following and understanding a communication content (Solnica et al. 2012). Limited access to the full range of sound frequencies impacts their functioning in the professional and social environments. Combined with limitations in using the media and participating in social events and meetings, it sets up a feeling of being different and in many cases is conducive to worsening of the overall mental condition (Putkiewicz et al. 2011).

Rehabilitation starts at the time of diagnosis and qualification of the degree and type of hearing loss. After cochlear implantation, it is continued in the form of comprehensive, multispecialty aid for patients within the framework of uniform, comprehensive care allowing for each group's specific needs and abilities. Tasks planned and implemented should restore patients' ability to perceive, compare, and recognize acoustic stimuli. Systematic training makes it possible to build or restore the ability to communicate verbally that is misdeveloped because of the hearing impairment.

Hearing, like all other senses, enables gathering and completing information about the surrounding world. Losing it, or being born without it, means losing access to some part of that information and, therefore, deprivation of knowledge about the surrounding world. Rehabilitation after cochlear implantation should be conducted in such a way that it can prepare patients to function first in favorable acoustic conditions such as a single sound source, and then in increasingly more challenging conditions such as with interfering noise, in a group conversation, and so on. This way, patients can achieve the best possible measure of activity and functioning in their social environments.

Chapter 12

Auditory development and speech perception in children after partial deafness cochlear implantation

Anita Obrycka and Artur Lorens
Institute of Physiology and Pathology of Hearing

CONTENTS

INTRODUCTION

Consequences of profound hearing loss have been studied extensively, but the effects of partial deafness (PD) (profound hearing loss limited to the high-frequency range) on auditory development and speech perception, particularly in young children, are less known. Nevertheless, there is ample evidence that these negative consequences exist, even though the speech of children with PD is usually intelligible. Elfenbein et al. (1994) report that fricatives and affricates' misarticulation is common in children with PD. Other studies report the findings of significant delays in vocabulary development, verbal abilities, reasoning skills, and increased errors in noun and verb morphology (e.g., cat vs. cats, keep vs. keeps) (Davis et al. 1986, Norbury et al. 2001). These performance deficits have been attributed to the inability to hear high-frequency sounds (Stelmachowicz et al. 2004).

Often, hearing deficits in children with PD remain beyond the scope of effective remediation with hearing aids (HAs). Limited audibility of high-frequency sounds in children with PD, even those fitted with HA, may cause phonological delays. An alternative solution for these children is cochlear implantation (CI). There are reasons, however, to proceed with caution in this regard. Studies' results suggest that the limited input of high-frequency sounds in children with PD fitted with HA may

DOI: 10.1201/9781003164876-12

contribute to phonological delays. However, the concern and fear exist that monaural implantation without hearing preservation and use of a HA on the opposite ear would be in the final reckoning less beneficial than binaural HAs. It is not clear that improved high-frequency audibility is more critical in this group of children than binaural processing with similar inputs. Therefore, there is a need for hearing preservation during cochlear implantation to facilitate binaural processing with equal input, at least in low frequencies (and in some cases in mid-frequencies). The decisive factor is the possibility to preserve the preoperative low-to-mid-frequency hearing during cochlear implantation.

This chapter presents an overview of pediatric auditory development from neurophysiological and psychoacoustical perspectives, focusing on children with PD and cochlear implants (CIs). We discuss the outcomes of hearing preservation that is the prerequisite of superior CI outcomes. We also present the published and unpublished studies on auditory development and speech perception in partial deafness treatment (PDT) with CI.

AUDITORY DEVELOPMENT

The progress of the research in anatomy, neurophysiology, and psychoacoustics in the last decades, has brought about remarkable advances in our understanding of human auditory development. We know that it is an extended process encompassing roughly the first 20 years of life and that it is hierarchical with a peripheral to a cortical gradient. It can be considered in three aspects: structural, functional, and behavioral. Considering these development aspects' milestones, Eggermont and Moore (2012) have distinguished two maturation process stages. They are related to two primary auditory processes: discrimination and identification.

The first stage begins in the third trimester of pregnancy when cochlear structures are already essentially developed, and lasts until about 6 months postnatal. Although the maturation process of outer and middle ear structures will continue after birth up to adolescence, they are ready to carry out their work. This period is also a time of rapid maturation of the auditory nerve, brain stem, and cortical layer I. Progressing myelination of axons in these structures increases the speed of neural conduction and improves the information transfer. Even though the auditory pathway's neural structures are still immature, functional and behavioral studies suggest that auditory processing abilities manifest early. Children younger than 6 months respond to environmental sounds and can accurately distinguish different acoustic stimuli. Development of perception skills mostly involves improving detection thresholds, spectral resolution, and high-frequency discrimination (Tharpe & Ashmead 2001, Olsho et al. 1988, Trehub et al. 1988, Eggermont 1991, Eggermont et al. 1996, Abdala & Sininger 1996). Therefore, this stage was labeled the discrimination stage.

The second stage of auditory development starts at the age of about 6 months. It manifests as the ability to use the extracted sound features to identify auditory objects. This ability is related to the onset of maturation of the deep cortical layers. At the beginning of that period, the ability to identify sounds starts to develop, and children begin to derive meaning from sounds. Between the age of 2 and 5 years, we observe the rapid development of perceptual language. Later childhood is the steady progress of speech perception in noisy or reverberant acoustic environments and sound localization ability. Those capabilities are not mature until the age of 15 years (Eggermont & Moore 2012).

Unquestionably, the auditory input drives auditory development. Appropriate auditory stimulation is the essential factor of survival and strengthening of synaptic connections, leading to improved auditory processing. In this way, age-related development of the auditory skills is strongly related to the auditory pathway's structural and functional maturation, particularly to the development of subsequent neural processing stages. The effects of profound hearing loss on auditory system maturation have been extensively studied (Kral et al. 2017, Kral & O'Donoghue 2010, Sharma et al. 2005, 2007). In children with congenital deafness, auditory input deprivation results in a lack of neuronal activity in the auditory pathway, which affects its further development. Simultaneously, the lack of appropriate neural activity leads to weakening or even losing synaptic connections (Kral et al. 2000). These effects have been observed and studied in people with profound hearing loss. However, less is known about the progress of the auditory system maturation in people with PD. The magnetoencephalographic study of humans with PD (steep-sloping audiograms) has provided evidence of an expanded representation of lesion-edge frequencies analogous to that found in animal studies (Dietrich et al. 2001).

AUDITORY DEVELOPMENT IN CI CHILDREN

In children with prelingual deafness, a CI was recognized as an effective way to deliver auditory input to the auditory system. Numerous studies confirm that cochlear implantation promotes auditory skills, including a child's ability to understand speech (Waltzman et al. 1994, Skarżyński et al. 2007a, Niparko et al. 2010, Kral & O'Donoghue 2010). Electrophysiological studies have been conducted to ascertain the optimal time of introducing the auditory input, the most effective from the point of view of supporting the auditory development of a prelingually deaf child (Sharma et al. 2002, 2007, Sharma & Dorman 2006). These studies have used cortical auditory evoked potentials (CAEPs) to analyze the first positive peak (P1) latency in the CAEP waveform. This latency represents the sum of all synaptic delays occurring in peripheral and central segments of the auditory pathway and is age-dependent. Therefore, it is considered to be a biomarker of maturation of the auditory system. The results confirm the existence of a critical period in auditory development. For example, Sharma et al. (2002) have found that in prelingually deaf children who received CIs before the age of 3.5, P1 latencies' development follows a typical trajectory.

On the other hand, in children implanted after seven years old, the P1 latencies were significantly longer than the norm. Therefore, we can conclude that experience with sounds in the period of the most intensive auditory pathway changes is crucial for its development. These electrophysiological findings are in agreement with behavioral studies showing faster speech and language development in children who received implants before 2 years old (Dettman et al. 2007, Holt & Svirsky 2008, Kral & O'Donoghue 2010, Niparko et al. 2010, Waltzman et al. 1994).

ASSESSMENT OF EARLY AUDITORY DEVELOPMENT OF CI CHILDREN

Auditory development should be evaluated and monitored based on age-appropriate tools. Out of three categories of tools, namely, questionnaires, closed- and open-set auditory assessment tests, the best choice for the assessment of early auditory development are questionnaires.

Questionnaires typically used in studies assessing the auditory development in children with HAs or CIs are IT-MAIS (Infant-Toddler Meaningful Auditory Integration Scale) (Zimmerman-Phillips et al. 1997), ASC (Auditory Skills Checklist) (Meinzen-Derr et al. 2007), PEACH (Parent's Evaluation of Aural/Oral Performance of Children) (Ching & Hill 2007), FAPI (Functional Auditory Performance Indicators) (Stredler-Brown & Johnson 2001), and LEAQ (LittlEARS Auditory Questionnaire) (Weichbold et al. 2005).

The quality and validity of assessment tools are crucial to ensure that it is possible to make inferences based on the obtained scores (American Educational Research Association; American Psychological Association; National Council on Measurement in Education, 2014; International Test Commission, 2000). Other traits of high-quality outcome measures include ease of administration, scoring, and interpretation (Andresen 2000). When assessing early auditory development, it is imperative to compare the results obtained after cochlear implantation with normative values to confirm the intervention's effectiveness. Of all tools mentioned above, LEAQ has the most considerable amount of evidence for its validity and fulfills all requirements of a high-quality diagnostic tool (Lorens et al. 2020).

LEAQ was designed to evaluate auditory development in children up to 2 years of age (Weichbold et al. 2005). It was validated for use in normal-hearing children as well as in a group of children with CIs (Weichbold et al. 2005, Obrycka et al. 2009, Coninx et al. 2009, Bagatto et al. 2011, Geal-Dor et al. 2011, Wang et al. 2013, García Negro et al. 2016, Obrycka et al. 2017).

Questions are arranged in the order of difficulty reflecting the most critical milestones of auditory development. The first questions focus on detecting and discriminating sounds, evaluated mainly based on a child's responses to human voices, music, environmental sounds, or sound-producing toys. Sound identification ability is tested based on a child's ability to recognize their name, link a name with an object, and identify a statement's emotional content. Final questions test comprehension in understanding spoken commands. The results of LEAQ can be evaluated based on the age-normative curve developed for this questionnaire. The normative values can be used to calculate the delay in auditory development. The idea of calculating the delay of auditory development with the LEAQ is illustrated in Figure 12.1.

To clarify the concept, let's consider an example. A 20-month-old CI child has scored 18 points in LEAQ (point A in Figure 12.1). Normally hearing children typically score 18 points at 12 months of age (point B in Figure 12.1). Therefore, the delay of auditory development of this child is eight months.

Moreover, long-term observation with LEAQ makes it possible to calculate the rate of auditory development understood as the average gain of LEAQ score in the time interval during which the child was observed. For example, if a child scores 4 points at CI activation and 22 points after the 6 months of CI use, we can calculate the individual rate of auditory development in terms of LEAQ scores. It is a quotient of

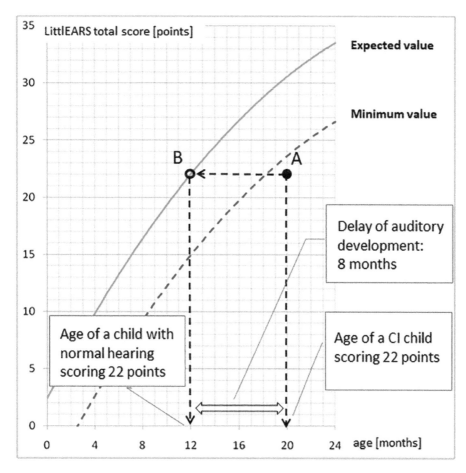

Figure 12.1 The model of calculating the delay of auditory development using the LEAQ age-related normative curve. Point A indicates the hypothetical result of a 20-month-old CI child; point B indicates the hearing age of a normally hearing child with the same score.

the difference between total scores for analyzed intervals and the number of months between intervals (here: $(22 - 4)/6 = 3$; the child developed at the rate of 3 points per month).

PARTIAL DEAFNESS

Total deafness and profound hearing loss are characterized by a nearly complete lack of inner hair cells. For this reason, these patients cannot gain any benefit from HAs, and in these cases, cochlear implantation is the treatment of choice. Pediatric cochlear implantation aims to provide critical stimulation to the child's auditory system and brain, thus allowing auditory development and, in this way, improving as far as possible its chances of developing spoken language.

A much more frequently occurring type of hearing impairment involves only a partial loss of inner hair cells, limited to some areas. In PD, it is the basal part of the cochlea responsible for the reception of high-frequency sounds. Therefore, high-frequency sounds, even amplified by HAs, are not audible or are perceived as severely distorted. The consequence of damaged or missing inner hair cells is the absence of the crucial connections from the ear to the brain, as 95% of the afferent auditory nerve fibers are from inner hair cells. If the degree of hearing loss is 60–80 dBHL or greater, inner hair cells are considered as being nonfunctional, as confirmed by the results of the animal studies (e.g., Liberman & Dodds 1984, Santi et al. 1982). In these cases, the use of a HA may not improve intelligibility (Turner 2006). Therefore, the term 'partial deafness' (PD), proposed by Skarżyński et al. (2003), distinguishes the high-frequency hearing loss, where only outer hair cells are damaged, and acoustic information can still be transmitted to the brain with the help of amplification. The authors of that study have observed that although HAs are insufficient to provide effective amplification for PD, CIs had not been recommended because implantation methods prevailing at that time could endanger the functioning part of the cochlea. They have introduced a new PD treatment method based on preserving existing low-frequency hearing during cochlear implantation. This method entails providing electric stimulation through a CI to complement the extant natural acoustic low-frequency hearing – the so-called electric complementation (PDT-EC). The first cases of partial deafness cochlear implantation (PDCI) in adults had produced outstanding results, which encouraged prof. H. Skarżyński to start performing PDCI in children (Skarżyński et al. 2007a). Since then, the term 'partial deafness' has commonly been used in the context of the cochlear implantation aimed at hearing preservation and electric-acoustic stimulation (PDT-EAS) (Prentis et al. 2010, Wilson 2012, Skarżyński & Lorens 2010a) or PDT-EC (Skarżyński et al. 2006, 2010). The PD concept has been gradually expanded to embrace normal hearing and mild, moderate, and even severe hearing loss in low frequencies accompanied by a profound hearing loss in high frequencies. As a way of ordering patients into more homogenous groups, Skarżyński proposed a classification based on the level of low-frequency thresholds (Skarżyński et al. 2010, 2015).

The term 'partial deafness' had been used in the literature earlier, but usually without an accurate description or definition. In 1950, Fowler observed that 'sudden partial deafness may be and often is, reversible if caused by impedance lesions, and when it occurs with Menieriform attacks' (Fowler 1950). In 1978, Sellars and Beighton, in the article titled 'The Aetiology of Partial Deafness in Childhood,' have described a child with PD as the one not suffering from profound sensorineural hearing loss but whose hearing loss is sufficiently handicapping to require special education (Sellars & Beighton 1978).

COCHLEAR IMPLANTATION WITHOUT AIMING FOR HEARING PRESERVATION IN CHILDREN WITH PD

Generally accepted practice is that children who have little potential for speech understanding may be offered CI. Cochlear implantation in these cases is motivated by the fact that acoustic stimulation with a HA, even exceptionally well fitted, produces limited benefits.

We should note that our understanding of what constitutes a 'limited benefit' has evolved over the last 30 years. Initially, only children who had very little residual hearing and did not show any sound awareness using HAs could be candidates for cochlear implantation. Gradually, pediatric cochlear implantation criteria have encompassed cases with better and better residual hearing.

This expansion can be illustrated by referring to the classification of HA users proposed by Osberger, Maso, and Sam (1993). They have divided children with sensorineural hearing loss into groups ranged from 'good' to 'poor' HA users based on the unaided and aided hearing thresholds. 'Bronze' HA users have an unaided pure-tone average (PTA) threshold greater than 110 dBHL, 'silver' from 100 to 110 dBHL, and 'gold' from 90 to 100 dBHL. More recently, a 'platinum' HA user group was defined for PTA between 60 and 90 dBHL (Eisenberg et al. 1998). Initially, pediatric CI's candidacy requirements included PTA of 100 dBHL or more ('silver' and 'bronze' HA users). Now, implantation criteria include 'silver' and 'gold' HA users. This widening of qualification criteria was motivated by studies demonstrating that implanted children in all three classes perform better than their HA-using peers with comparable hearing loss (Dowell et al. 2002; Eisenberg et al. 2004; Gantz & Davidson 2006, Leigh et al. 2011). Even in the 'platinum' group, children were shown to have a better hearing with a CI than with a HA.

Several studies report that children with at least some degree of residual hearing before cochlear implantation achieve better speech perception skills than those with poorer hearing, even if that residual hearing is lost or not used after implantation (Fitzpatrick et al. 2006, Mondain et al. 2002, Dettman et al. 2004, Rubinstein et al. 2000, Cullen et al. 2004). It shows that residual hearing in a CI candidate can be conducive to more successful implantation.

PRESERVATION OF HEARING AFTER COCHLEAR IMPLANTATION

Recently, many authors subscribe to the opinion that a CI surgery must aim to preserve residual hearing regardless of its level (Gantz et al. 2004, Gstöttner et al. 2004). This notion is related to the relaxation of the CI qualification criteria and the increasing numbers of children with residual hearing who receive implants.

There aren't many published reports of hearing preservation in children, although it has been widely reported in adults (Kiefer et al. 2004, Gantz et al. 2005, Fraysse et al. 2006, Skarżyński et al. 2003, 2007b, 2009). Skarżyński et al. (2002) have reported that in the group of 7 children and 19 adults implanted with the Combi 40 + system, only 19% of patients lost all measurable hearing after cochlear implantation. They investigated the influence of variables such as age and duration of deafness on preserving residual hearing and have found no correlation. In contrast, Kiefer et al. (1998) found that residual hearing preservation is more likely in children than in adults. Willingham and Manolidis (2004) have reported a comparison of steady-state auditory responses' (ASSR) thresholds before and after cochlear implantation in a group of 12 children implanted with MED-EL Combi 40+. They found no statistically significant differences in the implanted ear at 250, 500, 1k, 2k, 4k, and 8k Hz. These results confirm that the preservation of residual hearing in children is attainable at a level at least similar to adult patients.

It is clear that electric-acoustic stimulation (EAS), a combination of acoustic and electric hearing in one ear, requires an adequate residual hearing level. However, it is still unclear just how much residual hearing should remain to achieve effective EAS. Reports on EAS in adults published by James et al. (2005, 2006) and Fraysse et al. (2006) propose that an adult CI criterion for EAS should be a postoperative threshold of no more than 80 dB at 125 and 250 Hz, and 90 dB at 500 Hz. In such a configuration, a high-power HA can be used to take advantage of the residual hearing. If we carry over these criteria to children, we can assume that the platinum HA users with preserved hearing can be EAS benefiters, as they usually possess a sufficient residual hearing level.

COCHLEAR IMPLANTATION WITH HEARING PRESERVATION IN CHILDREN WITH PD

The first cochlear implantation in a child with PD was performed by H. Skarżyński (2007a). Despite the increasing numbers of pediatric PDCI patients, literature review yields scarce reports of studies on PD children with CI. In large part, published studies focus on surgical methods for preserving the residual hearing (Skarżyński et al. 2010, Brown et al. 2010) rather than patients' functional outcomes. Nevertheless, there is a growing amount of evidence that CIs are conducive to better auditory and speech development in children with PD than in those with HAs (Gratacap et al. 2015).

EARLY AUDITORY DEVELOPMENT AFTER COCHLEAR IMPLANTATION IN CHILDREN WITH PD

There is clinical evidence that the auditory development after cochlear implantation is different in children with PD than in children whose hearing loss is total or profound. In a clinical study conducted using the LEAQ, Obrycka et al. (2017) have examined 122 children implanted at the age of 6–22 months. Sixty-three children from the study group were described as having 'wide audibility' in HAs before implantation (free-field responses observed for at least 250, 500, and 1,000 Hz). Fifty-nine children had 'minimal audibility' in HAs before implantation; that is, they showed no responses in the free-field test, or only up to 500 Hz. It is difficult to measure audiometric thresholds in infants and toddlers precisely, so we can assume that 'wide audibility' corresponds to PD and 'minimal audibility' to profound hearing loss or deafness. The LEAQ scores in a period of up to 6 months of CI use were significantly higher in a group of children with PD compared to those with profound hearing loss or deafness (Figure 12.2b) despite the fact that children with profound hearing loss or deafness developed faster after cochlear implantation (Figure 12.2a). This is because children with PD have a smaller delay of auditory development before implantation compared to profoundly deaf children (they have higher LEAQ scores to start with). Therefore even with a slower developmental rate, they reach higher scores after 6 months.

Further analysis of the results revealed that in children implanted between 12 and 22 months of age, the average delay of auditory development in children with PD at the time of operation was significantly shorter than in children with profound

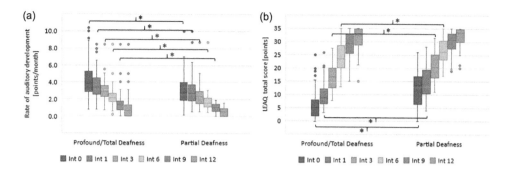

Figure 12.2 Early auditory development in children with partial deafness and profound hearing loss/deafness: (a) in terms of the auditory development rate, (b) in terms of LEAQ total score. Lines in the boxes indicate the medians, boxes – interquartile range, whiskers – range, dots – outliers, and asterisks – significant differences.

hearing loss or deafness. That delay decreased over time in both groups; nevertheless, the difference in the delay remains significant even after 12 months of CI use (Figure 12.3).

The evidence collected in this study suggests that even partial auditory input (as in congenital PD) promotes a measure of early auditory development before implantation. That is why PD children implanted after 12 months of age can effectively close the developmental gap between them and normally hearing children.

Before the age of 12 months, cochlear implantation seems to be the best chance for children with profound or total hearing loss to reach the same level of early auditory development as normally hearing children. Typically, their auditory development matches the normal curve within one year of CI use. In children with PD, it is not that crucial to implant them before 12 months of age. As mentioned, partial auditory input allows for developing the primary auditory skills: sound detection and discrimination. For this reason, the delay of auditory development in children with PD is lesser than in children with profound hearing loss or deafness.

SPEECH DISCRIMINATION IN CHILDREN WITH PD

Children with PD miss the essential information in high-frequency sounds crucial for speech discrimination (Stelmachowicz et al. 2004). Investigating the consequences of PD, we should keep in mind that the acoustic features of speech can be roughly divided into three major categories; each of them requires that cochlea transmits a different kind of information to the brain. These speech features are voicing, place of articulation, and manner.

The voicing is the presence of vocal-fold vibration in a speech sound, for example, voiceless /s/ versus voiced /z/. If a sound is voiced, periodic energy is increased across the entire spectrum of speech, particularly in lower frequencies. Voicing is the most resistant to the PD from all speech features because inner hair cells in the cochlea's apex can transmit voicing information.

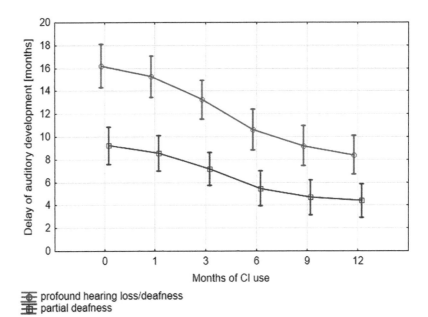

Figure 12.3 Delay of auditory development in children with partial deafness and children with profound hearing loss or deafness implanted between 12 and 24 months. Points indicate the mean values, and whiskers – confidence intervals.

The articulation place is the spectral information that signals where the sound is produced in the vocal tract, for example, at lips like /p/ or at the alveolar ridge, like /t/. That spectral information is located primarily in the higher-frequency regions of speech (Miller and Nicely 1955). It is most likely transmitted by frequency-place coding in the basal part of the cochlea. Thus, this speech feature is the most susceptible to PD, which consists in the damage or lack of inner hair cells in the cochlea's basal turn.

The manner is the distinction between types of consonants such as fricatives like /s/ or /z/ or stop consonants such as /k/ or /g/. In terms of acoustic and cochlear requirements, this speech feature lies in the middle between the voicing and the place of articulation.

PD involving severe to profound hearing loss in higher-frequency regions affects the ability to recognize even amplified speech. Available information about the physiology of hearing loss suggests that missing inner hair cells in the cochlea's basal areas will disrupt the perception of the spectral cues of speech. In such cases, electric stimulation with a CI can bypass that limitation and permit these spectral cues to be transmitted to the brain.

SPEECH DISCRIMINATION AFTER CI IN CHILDREN WITH PD

Speech discrimination after PDCI, especially in children, is a little-studied subject. Skarżyński and Lorens (2010a) have published a report on 25 children with PD implanted using the minimally invasive surgical technique where the electrode is inserted into the cochlea through the round window. This technique has been developed specially to increase the probability of hearing preservation. The children were divided into two groups according to their low-frequency hearing level: normal or close to normal and moderate to severe (platinum HA user group). In the observation period of 12 months, monosyllabic word recognition increased in the platinum group from 31% to 60% in quiet and from 1% to 19% in noise. In the group with normal or close to normal low-frequency hearing, the increase in quiet was from 34% to 67% and in noise from 7% to 47%.

The increase in performance in quiet conditions was comparable in both groups, but the benefit in noisy conditions was significantly larger in the group with better low-frequency hearing. This finding demonstrates that fair low-frequency hearing is a prerequisite of achieving large benefits in hearing in noise. In both groups, improvement of speech discrimination in noise exceeds that usually observed in profoundly deaf children who rely on only one CI (Dowell et al. 2002).

The rate and speed of improvement of auditory capacity suggest that the performance gain was due to CI intervention rather than any progress that would have occurred in rehabilitation with conventional HAs.

SUMMARY

This chapter presents an overview of pediatric auditory development from neurophysiological and psychoacoustical perspectives, focusing on children with a particular type of hearing loss named partial deafness. In PDCI, first described by Skarżyński, residual hearing at low frequencies can be relatively good or even intact. Thanks to hearing preservation round window surgical technique, PDCI has been shown to provide clinically significant auditory development gains for children with PD.

In PD children implanted between ages 1 and 2, a much more favorable auditory development pattern is observed than in deaf children implanted at the same age. The PDCI pattern of auditory development is, in fact, similar to the pattern observed in deaf children implanted very early (before the age of 1 year). This indicates that even partial auditory input (as in congenital PD) promotes some early auditory development before implantation. That is why PD children implanted after 12 months of age can effectively close the developmental gap between them and normal-hearing children. Therefore, speaking about early implantation, children with profound hearing loss should be implanted earlier than children with PD, preferably before the age of 1.

There is ample evidence in the literature of a reciprocal relationship between early auditory development and language skills development. As short-term gains in auditory development translate into a medium-term gain in the communication competency achieved with a CI, the appropriate assessment instruments are required, such as questionnaires, to monitor the very early auditory development in children with CIs.

Concluding, technological advances, early age at diagnosis and implantation, and hearing preservation surgical techniques permit the implantation of CIs in children with PD. One of the most gratifying outcomes of PDCI is to restore a child's ability to understand speech even in difficult listening conditions like noise.

Chapter 13

Understanding the partial deafness – different perspectives: subjective, auditory perception and communication, psychological, and social

Joanna Kobosko
Institute of Physiology and Pathology of Hearing

CONTENTS

INTRODUCTION

Partial deafness (PD) is a hearing loss where a patient cannot hear any high-frequency sounds but in lower frequencies has good hearing or hearing loss capable of being compensated with acoustic stimulation (Skarżyński et al. 2003). From the psychological, linguistic, and hearing-and-speech-rehabilitation standpoint, the essential factor is the onset of hearing impairment – whether it is prelingual or postlingual.

When dealing with prelingual PD, that is, the hearing impairment that started before the period of speech and language acquisition, that person has been living with the experience from the earliest childhood. Postlingual PD means that the patient has experienced sudden or gradually progressing hearing loss and the related deterioration of health, already after they mastered the language system, about 6 years of age or later (Kobosko et al. 2017). Postlingual hearing loss cases are a substantial majority among PD patients.

The best results in the treatment of PD are brought about by cochlear implantation to stimulate the high-frequency range electrically, while low frequencies are stimulated in a natural, acoustic way. If the impairment is also present in a lower-frequency range, hybrid devices can be used, combining a cochlear implant (CI) (electric stimulation of high frequencies) and a hearing aid (acoustic stimulation of low frequencies) (Skarżyński & Lorens 2010b).

DOI: 10.1201/9781003164876-13

For persons with PD, the decision about cochlear implantation is a crucial one, and most of them retrospectively judge it as beneficial. *Anna*, an over-thirty-year-old woman with postlingual PD, says: "I believe it has been one of the best decisions in my life. I am satisfied. I have had help, and I can say today that, although I do not have 100% hearing norm, I still have gained a lot" (in: Obszańska 2014, p. 43).

A look at the PD from different perspectives will let us know: (1) what is PD in the experience of patients with that kind of hearing impairment (subjective standpoint), (2) what is the nature of hearing and speech-understanding difficulties in people with PD (perspective related to the auditory perception of speech and communication), (3) how people with PD function psychologically and how do they cope with their impairment (psychological perspective), and (4) what social relationships and social context they have (social perspective). It should be highlighted that auditory capabilities obtained through a CI usually promote many positive changes in these spheres/perspectives of the CI experience. According to the published studies, CI satisfaction in people with PD with a mean CI experience of 4 years was, on average, 79% (Kobosko et al. 2018; Kobosko et al. 2020). It is a similar rate as in other CI users, such as those with profound deafness of postlingual onset (Kobosko et al. 2015). CI users with PD report the largest, in their subjective assessment, benefits in the psychosocial functioning areas: "self-esteem," "activity limitations," and "social interactions" measured with the NCIQ – *Nijmegen Cochlear Implant Questionnaire* (Hinderink et al. 2000, Kobosko et al. 2020).

PARTIAL DEAFNESS FROM THE SUBJECTIVE PERSPECTIVE

To form an idea, what is the PD for a person experiencing it in different areas of life, what difficulties, limitations, experiences, and challenges it entails, is to establish the subjective perspective of that impairment. That idea has been created based on many years of clinical observation of patients with PD and qualitative studies conducted in the form of individual case studies, also on CI users with PD (Obszańska 2014). The subjective perspective on the PD is illustrated here with a testimony of the over-30-year-old woman (in this text, we call her *Anna*, to preserve her anonymity). She had been diagnosed with PD at the age of 14 years; she decided to have the first CI when she was 24 and then the second implant after nine years of using a unilateral CI. *Anna's* statements quoted here represent the CI users with PD, especially with the postlingual onset, who have benefited from this treatment.

PARTIAL DEAFNESS FROM THE PERSPECTIVE OF AUDITORY PERCEPTION OF SPEECH AND COMMUNICATION

PD in the sphere of auditory perception of the environmental sounds and speech may lead to a situation that a person with PD can hear but, in many daily situations, cannot understand verbal communications – they have a feeling of "lack of speech understanding" (Pankowska et al. 2012; Kobosko et al. 2017, 2020). *Anna* points out this important aspect of the problem, saying:

> For many, it is difficult to understand that it is possible to hear and not understand. We are speaking here about a mother tongue, not a foreign language. But yes, it is possible if you have a hearing impairment
>
> (Obszańska 2014 p. 43).

Difficulties manifesting as "lack of speech understanding" in persons with PD involve several aspects: (1) limited ability to receive, differentiate, and recognize the surrounding sounds both in quiet and in the presence of interfering sounds; (2) reception of speech supported by visual channel (observing interlocutor's face, lip reading); (3) limitations in following and recognizing the content of spoken communications in different acoustic conditions; (4) significant limitations in differentiating and recognizing similar-sounding words; (5) disordered prosody and articulation with correct verbal communication using multiword, grammatically correct sentences (Pankowska et al. 2012, Solnica et al. 2012, Solnica & Pankowska 2013). Another fragment of *Anna's* testimony points to that problem:

> I experienced it often, for example, during the lectures. There were moments that I could hear and understand whole sentences, providing the teacher was facing the class. When they turned to the board, continuing the explanations and writing out some formulas or words, I would stop understanding what they said. The voice was audible, same volume, same distance, but the sense of the communication disappeared
>
> Obszańska (2014 p. 43).

It is common for all people with PD that hearing amplification with conventional hearing aids generally produces unsatisfactory or no benefits. This is why they search for ways to improve their hearing, for example, cochlear implantation. *Anna* relates:

> I have tried wearing hearing aids, but they did not help; I could not hear the lost sounds. (…) Each time, hearing aids would amplify what I could already hear well – making it unnaturally loud. They did not help with what I could not hear. It felt awful
>
> Obszańska (2014 p. 42).

After cochlear implantation, PD patients gain the capability of receiving sounds from the whole-frequency range. Well-designed auditory training is necessary to integrate the acoustic sensation obtained through a natural hearing with the sensation delivered through a CI (Pankowska et al. 2012, Solnica et al. 2012, Kobosko et al. 2017).

We should keep in mind that there is a difference between the auditory adaptation process to a CI in the group of patients with PD and the "traditional" group with profound hearing loss in all frequencies, as has been shown on the graph (Figure 13.1). It consists mostly of feelings and assessments of patients after the activation of a speech processor.

In the first period of about 1–2 months from speech processor activation, people with PD feel that their hearing did not improve (subjective "speech understanding"). Most often, they describe it as discomfort in listening to "high" sounds, they "feel overburdened by the excess of sounds, their sharpness," "listening requires even more attention than before," which means "increased hearing effort," they are "tired from listening." Sometimes, these negative sensations are connected to the quality of sounds, which feel "irritating, unnatural, metallic-sounding." *Anna* describes her first experience with a CI with these words:

> I was surprised that it felt different than in a hearing aid, that, although I cannot yet hear well, I accept whatever gets through to me. I accept that silence is so

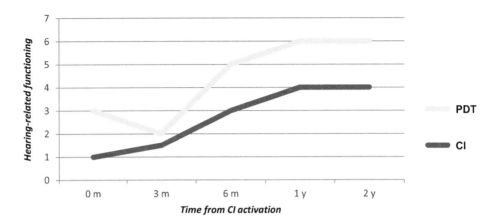

Figure 13.1 Hearing-related functioning of patients with PD and "traditional" patients with postlingual deafness after cochlear implantation – in the period from cochlear implant activation to 2 years after (based on Lorens et al. 2008).

distinct, even loud, and that there are sounds that I had no idea existed because I could never hear them, but now I can. I was born hearing, and I had auditory memory, but I have never heard, for example, a mobile phone. I knew only the ringing of a traditional telephone. I have seen new technologies, but I have never heard how they sound

Obszańska (2014 p. 43).

Further, *Anna* reports: "When I had been using a cochlear implant a little longer, I noticed that I pay less attention to a person's mouth, that I rely more on my 'electric hearing" (Obszańska 2014 p. 44).

There were moments that I felt confused, surprised, embarrassed, irritated, but I tried not to focus on what's difficult but on the overall experience; I surrounded myself with sounds and gave in to their stimulation. Even when it was difficult, I kept the processor on to habituate myself to sounds

Obszańska (2014 p. 45).

Speech and language therapists working with PD patients after cochlear implantation observe that after a short period of such "difficult" adaptation, patients' hearing-related functioning improves fast, including improved speech understanding. For comparison, "traditional" CI users experience gradual hearing improvement from the moment of speech processor activation, but the process is slower and gradual, as shown in Figure 13.1.

From the perspective of years, *Anna*, a woman with the postlingual PD introduced in this chapter, says that the greatest surprise she had after cochlear implantation was related to music: "I was delighted with music and sensations it entailed" (Obszańska 2014 p. 43).

Despite her many years of CI experience and significant benefits from using one, and later two implants, *Anna* still experiences some difficulties in hearing and understanding speech, similarly to other partially deaf CI users:

Sometimes I miss a part of a sentence in a heated discussion. I cannot freely understand when I'm talking on a phone. I miss dialogue in comedy, dubbing, or being a back seat passenger in a car. But there are only some fragments in the whole picture of a sound event

Obszańska (2014 p. 43).

We should keep in mind that a CI will not make a deaf or partially deaf person into a hearing person. It will not "by itself" improve their quality of life, self-esteem, or relations with people. It is a tool that can be optimally used to better hear and understand in the first place speech. *Anna's* testimony quoted here confirms it. Implanted persons with PD benefit from a CI in different degrees, for many reasons, both objective (medical factors) and psychological (such as low self-esteem, depression, insufficient social support, and others). The success of rehabilitation of hearing and speech after cochlear implantation is also significantly dependent on a deaf and hard-of-hearing person's preimplantation psychosocial functioning, even a person with PD.

PARTIAL DEAFNESS FROM THE PSYCHOLOGICAL PERSPECTIVE

Coping with hearing loss and psychosocial adaptation

From a psychological standpoint, postlingually acquired deafness or PD involves a *loss* of hearing and, consequently, a loss of ability and health. This is usually a very stressful experience, often related to an emotional/life crisis. The loss starts the process of grief and mourning, which means coping with the ability loss (Kübler-Ross 2007, Wolski 2010). We can say that it is a foundation of the psychosocial adaptation to a chronic illness or disability (Livneh & Antonak 2005). The process of adaptation to the ability loss, such as deafness or PD, according to Elizabeth Kübler-Ross, has five stages: "shock and denial," "anger," "bargaining," "depression," and "acceptance."

Each of the above-mentioned stages of coping with loss (of hearing) involves a different perception of oneself and own situation, another way of handling the tasks, also those related to the rehabilitation of hearing and speech, such as adapting to a CI. For example, a person who denies being partially (or profoundly) deaf will spend time and energy on searching for a cause of hearing loss and possibilities of "recovering hearing" through miraculous methods and treatments (healers, quacks), and on proving to oneself and others that the problem does not exist or is not yet serious (Rawool 2018). They will have excessive hopes and unrealistic expectations, also those related to the cochlear implantation. We should remember that denial, as a defense mechanism, is a natural reaction to intense stress or trauma, and it is helpful in emotional, gradual coping with a difficult situation. However, denial is not conducive to effective rehabilitation or health in the long term (Livneh 2016).

When the partial or total deafness is prelingual, we are dealing with the task of coping with being a deaf person and the consequences of that fact, "being different" related to deafness and communication as well as socialization experiences. A prelingually, totally, or partially deaf person has been living with hearing loss from birth or early childhood and does not know the hearing norm. Then, we can speak of hearing loss only in the context of its further deterioration. In that group of patients, the denial of deafness or PD is possible when they experience difficulties accepting themselves as a deaf person (Zalewska 2009, Kobosko et al. 2019a). A case study of a 49-year-old man with prelingual PD using a CI (Kobosko et al. 2017) shows the symptoms of denial in his declaration that he can "hear more and better than it is possible," which entails high psychological cost.

Persons with PD often feel that they are living "on the border" of two worlds: "hearing" and "deaf" (Stephens 2009, Kobosko et al. 2017). It may be related to experiencing problems with their own identity as a deaf or "partially" deaf person, as mentioned before. They suffer the reactions of other people who are confused by their behavior ("sometimes she/he can hear, sometimes not?", "is she/he pretending?", "what's wrong with her/him?"). They have to put effort into daily life (strain, stress, anxiety, tiredness) (Carlsson et al. 2015, Williams et al. 2015). *Anna*, quoted earlier in this chapter, describes her progressing PD thus:

> I didn't think I had a problem with hearing, only with other things. I thought I was less efficient, slow, awkward, absent-minded. When I connected what was going on with me with a hearing loss, I had to define myself anew – what kind of person I was
>
> Obszańska (2014 p. 42).

Difficulties and setbacks experienced by people with PD often endanger their self-esteem (Kobosko et al. 2018). *Anna* describes it with these words: "I was unsure, tense, I could not find my place in a group. All the time, I was checking something, making notes, reading more to be on the same level of information as my peers" (Obszańska 2014 p. 42). In the situation of a lasting loss of ability, such as PD, a vital dimension of experiencing self is the feeling of being disabled, which is stronger in persons with acquired impairment and younger, also in postlingual CI users (Kobosko 2015).

For many partially deaf persons who decide to have a CI, the effects of cochlear implantation and hearing and speech rehabilitation are positive and lead to many good changes in life. It finds confirmation in the level of global self-esteem of CI users with PD, which is at the same level as in the general population (Kobosko et al. 2018). For *Anna*, the positive effects of implantation have brought about the reconstruction of her self-image and acceptance of disability, which she describes as follows: "I have reached peace, freedom, and development. I have lots of reasons to be glad. I can be more engaged in different tasks at home, at work, or traveling" (Obszańska 2014 p. 43).

Psychosocial functioning of patients with partial deafness using cochlear implants – study results

Studies on the psychosocial functioning of patients with PD, especially CI users, are sparse. The published studies on the mental health of the deaf and hard of hearing people, including certainly also those with PD, show that their psychosocial functioning is worse than the general population, regardless of whether they are pre- or postlingually deaf and irrespective of the degree of hearing loss (de Graaf & Bijl 2002, Fellinger et al. 2007, Kvam et al. 2007, Fellinger et al. 2012, du Feu & Chovaz 2014, Carlsson et al. 2015). The results of the increasing number of studies suggest, however, that psychosocial functioning of the deaf and hard of hearing persons in the mental health sphere improves after cochlear implantation. The majority of CI users are on a similar level as the general population (Rembar et al. 2012, Kobosko et al. 2015, Bosdriesz et al. 2018, Kobosko et al. 2018).

Results of a pilot study on persons with PD who are not CI users (Cieśla et al. 2016) show that they experience more intense depression (measured with the *Beck Depression Inventory*) and anxiety – considered both as a state and as a trait (measured with the STAI – *State-Trait-Anxiety-Inventory*) than persons with hearing norm. These results suggest also that people with PD have a reduced quality of life (assessed with the questionnaire WHOQOL-BREF – *World Health Organization Quality of Life-BREF*) compared to the reference group comprising people without mental health problems. Decreased quality of life (WHOQOL-BREF) has been noted in two areas under assessment: mental health and physical health. In the area of social and environmental relations, the quality of life of people with PD was similar to that of the general population. Decreased quality of life and significantly higher intensity of depression and anxiety symptoms have been found to be not dependent on sex or the prelingual vs. postlingual onset of deafness.

In another study, the RSES – *Rosenberg Self-Esteem Scale* (Dzwonkowska et al. 2008) – was used to measure the overall self-esteem level in a group of adults with pre- or postlingual and total or partial deafness, implanted after 18 years of age (Kobosko et al. 2018). It has been confirmed empirically that global self-esteem is one of the mental health predictors in the general population (Orth et al. 2012). The results of the discussed study show that persons from the study group had a lower overall self-esteem level than the general population. CI users with PD, however, regardless of the pre- or postlingual onset of impairment, have similar overall self-esteem levels as the general population. Study results show that global self-esteem (RSES) plays an essential role in the perception of CI benefit (NCIQ) by persons with PD with pre- or postlingual onset (Kobosko 2018). The higher the overall self-esteem, the higher the CI benefit obtained in all NCIQ areas in the subjective assessment of implant users with PD. Among the mid-strength relationships, the weakest was observed between the evaluation of benefits in the area of "basic sound perception" (NCIQ) and the global self-esteem (RSES), and the strongest between the "self-esteem" (NCIQ) and the global self-esteem (RSES). On the other hand, there is no relationship between the level of CI satisfaction (measured with a VAS-type scale) and the overall self-esteem (RSES) in the whole group of partially deaf persons. A significant positive correlation has been observed between the overall self-esteem (RSES) and the CI satisfaction only in men with PD, but not in women (Kobosko 2018).

Psychological distress (measured with the GHQ-28 – *General Health Questionnaire*) (Makowska & Merecz 2001) has been studied in a group of people with PD aged 18–60 years, who have been using one CI for four years on average (range 1–10 years). The study group included both people with prelingual and postlingual deafness (Kobosko et al. 2019b, 2020). The results show that in people with PD using a CI, the overall level of psychological distress and the intensity of components – anxiety and insomnia symptoms (GHQ-28 – scale B), social dysfunction symptoms (GHQ-28 – scale C), depression symptoms (GHQ-28 – scale D) – was significantly higher than the Polish norm for the general (working) population (Makowska & Merecz 2001). The only exception was the level of somatic symptoms (GHQ-28 – scale A) (Kobosko et al. 2020).

Moreover, it came out that CI users with prelingual-onset PD experience a similar intensity of overall psychological distress and the above-mentioned psychopathology symptoms (GHQ-28 scales) as the general population. In contrast, these with the postlingual onset of PD obtain significantly higher scores in all tested GHQ-28 scales and overall psychological distress (GHQ-28 total) than the normative population (Kobosko et al. 2019b). A comparison of two groups of people with PD with different onset (prelingual vs. postlingual) shows no differences regarding the intensity of anxiety and insomnia symptoms (GHQ-28 – scale B) and depression (GHQ-28 – scale D). The overall level of psychological distress (GHQ-28 total), social dysfunction symptoms (GHQ-28 – scale C), and somatic symptoms (GHQ-28 – scale A) is on a significantly higher level in the group with postlingual onset (Kobosko 2018, Kobosko et al. 2019b). If the results are analyzed accounting for sex, then women with PD using CIs show a much higher intensity of psychological distress (GHQ-28), while men are on the same level as the general population. Compared to men, women had higher scores in the anxiety and insomnia symptoms scale (GHQ-28 – scale B) (Kobosko et al. 2020).

The intensity of psychological distress (GHQ-28) is related to the subjective assessment of CI benefit and satisfaction in partially deaf CI users. Studies show that perception of CI benefits in the psychosocial sphere, comprising "self-esteem," "activity limitation," and "social interactions" (NCIQ) is in the group of women with PD related to the psychological distress. In men with PD, there is no such relationship. In CI users with PD, regardless of sex and the prelingual or postlingual onset of impairment, there is no relationship between psychological distress and CI satisfaction (Kobosko et al. 2020).

PARTIAL DEAFNESS FROM THE SOCIAL PERSPECTIVE

Persons with PD, similar to many other deaf and hard-of-hearing people, often experience difficulties in the social sphere, that is, in interpersonal relations with peers, colleagues, family, coworkers, and others (Stephens 2009, du Feu & Chovaz 2014, Williams et al. 2015, Domagała-Zyśk 2015). Sometimes they conceal their hearing problems (Mäki-Torkko et al. 2015). *Anna*, a woman with PD, believes that difficulties related to her progressing hearing loss had no effect on the quality of her relationships at school:

> I had good relationships with peers. But I remember that it was difficult to speak in the local dialect, I did not participate in group discussions at breaks, I did not get classroom jokes. Always, when there was a discussion or somebody spoke during the lesson, I had to turn around to catch what they were saying. I rather had many individual contacts, one-to-one
>
> Obszańska (2014 p. 42).

Deaf and hard-of-hearing persons are not always so successful – interpersonal relations are the most susceptible to difficulties and limitations resulting from hearing problems (Stephens 2009, du Feu & Chovaz 2014, Carlsson et al. 2015, Mäki-Torkko et al. 2015, Williams et al. 2015, Dillon & Pryce 2020) in comparison with other kinds of disabilities (Müller-Siekierska 2019). We can say that difficulties in communicating with others by way of hearing lie in the nature of deafness or PD, as is receiving and sending verbal communications, and thus limitations in verbal exchanges in social interactions, even in the case of hearing-impaired persons with high competences in the phonic language (Krakowiak et al. 2009). We should add that in spite of the social and cultural changes of the last decades, the social context of the deaf and hard of hearing people, also people with PD, is still connected with stigmatization, marginalization, isolation, and exclusion (du Feu & Fergusson 2003, Manchaiah et al. 2015, Mäki-Torkko et al. 2015, Dillon & Pryce 2020).

SUMMARY

PD is a multidimensional phenomenon. Treatment and rehabilitation of hearing and speech in patients with PD, even those provided with CIs, should allow for different perspectives of experiencing the PD described in this chapter: subjective, related to the auditory perception of speech and communication, psychological, and social. In people with PD and those using CIs, rehabilitation's effectiveness is connected with coping with hearing loss and the psychosocial adaptation to the PD.

The method of treatment of PD with CIs has proven to bring about very good results, confirmed by the indicators of its effectiveness: subjective high and very high assessment of satisfaction and benefit from the CI and the psychological indices such as the overall self-esteem of CI users with PD evaluated in the studies in comparison with the general population. Significant subjective benefits from the CI are related in the first place to the psychosocial functioning of the partially deaf CI users. However, the persisting increased levels of psychological distress, even after cochlear implantation, indicate difficulties suffered by that group of patients, particularly concerning people with postlingual PD. For this reason, the latter group requires the particular attention of the therapists and other specialists responsible for their hearing and speech rehabilitation as well as professional psychological support.

Chapter 14

Evaluation of partial deafness patients by means of auditory evoked potentials, otoacoustic emissions, and wideband tympanometry

Krzysztof Kochanek, W. Wiktor Jedrzejczak and Lech Śliwa
Institute of Physiology and Pathology of Hearing

CONTENTS

INTRODUCTION

The application of behavioral methods, such as pure-tone audiometry, is the gold standard for assessing hearing sensitivity and auditory perception. Such methods have been routinely used for CI candidates, and patients provided with auditory implants. However, recently, there is a growing number of patients in whom behavioral methods may be difficult to apply or give inaccurate results (Leigh et al. 2019). These include young children and persons with limited communication abilities. In such cases, objective hearing assessment methods may be a reasonable alternative (Piotrowska et al. 2005a, 2009).

One can use electrophysiological methods of hearing testing based on auditory brainstem responses (ABRs) and/or auditory steady-state responses (ASSR) for CI patients and candidates. Acoustic methods include the application of otoacoustic emissions (OAE) and acoustic immittance-related measures.

APPLICATION OF EVOKED AUDITORY BRAINSTEM RESPONSES (ABR)

ABRs have been used for a long time for objective assessment of hearing threshold (Burkard and Don 2015). Presently, one typically uses responses evoked either by wideband stimuli, such as click or chirp used to assess hearing threshold in the frequency range of 2000–4000 Hz, or by short tone-pips or narrow-band chirps to obtain frequency-specific responses (Hatliński et al. 2008, Kochanek 2000, Kochanek et al.

DOI: 10.1201/9781003164876-14

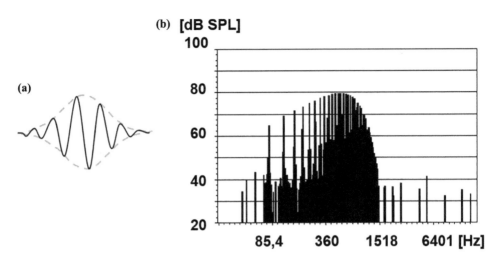

Figure 14.1 (a) Waveform of a typical tone-pip stimulus with nonlinear Gaussian envelope (without plateau) and two-cycle rise time and fall time (contour proportions 2-0-2), (b) the acoustic spectrum of a 500 Hz tone-pip measured in an ear simulator.

2000a, 2000b). Clinical experience indicates that registering ABRs at near-threshold levels (i.e., determining the ABR wave V threshold) is easier when one applies click stimuli or high-frequency tone-pips. It becomes more difficult in low-frequency stimuli, i.e., 500 Hz tone-pips (Kochanek et al. 2000b). This is because the rise time of acoustic pressure produced by a high-frequency stimulus significantly differs from that evoked by a low-frequency tone-pip. If, for example, to elicit ABRs, one uses tone-pips of a nonlinear envelope (Figure 14.1a) at different tone frequencies, i.e., 500 Hz and 4000 Hz, where the rising slope of the envelope contains the same number of tone periods, i.e., two cycles, the stimulus rise time, expressed in time units, is much shorter in the high-frequency stimulus, i.e., equal to 0.5 ms for the 4000 Hz tone-pip compared to 4 ms for the 500 Hz one. The onset of acoustic pressure is then different in the two cases, and so is the degree of synchronization of neural activity in the auditory nerve fibers. Therefore, the two stimuli have radically different efficiency of evoking auditory potentials.

In the case when ABRs are applied to assess hearing threshold in patients with high-frequency hearing loss (such as in the case of PDT patients), one may assume that the activity of the basal turn of the cochlea does not influence the ABRs evoked with short tone-pips of tone frequencies 500 Hz and 1000 Hz. However, the 1000 Hz region's cochlear activity may affect the wave V threshold at 500 Hz. Such an influence can be stronger when one applies a 500 Hz tone-pip of relatively short rise time, i.e., a one-cycle rise time, because the power spectrum of such a short stimulus is relatively wide. It means that the responses originate not only from the 500 Hz region but also from the segment characteristic for 1000 Hz. On the other hand, the increase in the stimulus rise time, i.e., two or four cycles of the 500 Hz tone, will result in a meaningful weakening of synchronization of neural activity and, consequently, a decrease in ABR amplitude. This causes a deterioration of the signal-to-noise ratio (SNR) and increases the wave V detection threshold.

In ABR-based tests for diagnosing hearing in PDT patients used in the Institute of Physiology and Pathology of Hearing, we apply short tone-pip stimuli of 500 Hz and 1000 Hz tone frequency and nonlinear, Gaussian-type envelope (Figure 14.1a). The applied 500 Hz tone-pip has a rise time equal to one cycle, while the 1000 Hz stimulus has a two-cycle rise time. The characteristics of the stimuli have been optimized based on previous research (Hatliński et al. 2008, Kochanek 2000, Kochanek et al. 2000a, 2000b, 2015) that analyzed the correlation between wave V threshold and the audiometric threshold in large populations of normal-hearing persons and hearing-impaired subjects with different hearing loss levels and various shapes of audiograms (flat, low- and high-frequency sloping). The amplifier cutoff frequencies in the acquisition system are set to 200 Hz and 2000 Hz, respectively. Figure 14.1 shows a typical stimulus waveform and an experimentally determined acoustic power spectrum of a 500 Hz tone-pip stimulus.

The following examples illustrate evaluating hearing sensitivity in PDT patients using the ABR method (Piotrowska et al. 2005b). We determined audiometric thresholds in a group of PDT patients and measured ABR thresholds before and after CI surgery. Figure 14.2 shows preoperative and postoperative pure-tone audiograms of five PDT patients. Figure 14.3 presents an example of traces of ABRs, evoked with a 500 Hz tone-pip, registered in a patient before and after the implant operation. One can notice that, in this case, the wave V threshold has insignificantly increased after the implantation (by 10 dB).

Figure 14.4 shows a comparison between wave V thresholds and audiometric thresholds determined in the five previously mentioned PDT patients before and after

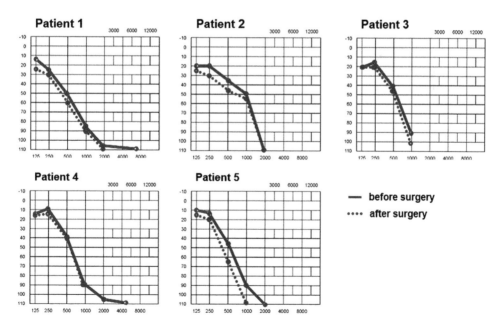

Figure 14.2 Pure-tone audiograms of five selected PDT patients before (continuous lines) and after cochlear implant surgery (dotted lines).

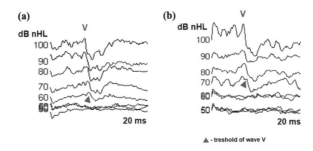

Figure 14.3 Traces of auditory brainstem potentials registered at different stimulus levels in a PDT patient: (a) before, (b) after cochlear implant surgery. The red triangle indicates the level of wave V threshold.

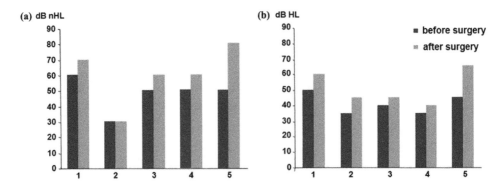

Figure 14.4 (a) Wave V threshold levels in five PDT patients determined before and after cochlear implant surgery, (b) audiometric hearing thresholds determined in the same group of patients. Blue and yellow bars pertain to preoperative and postoperative thresholds, respectively.

CI surgery. As can be seen, the differences between preoperative and postoperative thresholds, both electrophysiological and behavioral, do not exceed 10 dB in four of the patients, #1–4. Only in patient #5, these differences are greater: 20 dB difference between audiometric thresholds and 30 dB difference between wave V thresholds. Nevertheless, the threshold change is similar in both audiometric thresholds and wave V thresholds. Moreover, the comparison of audiometric thresholds and wave V thresholds shows a high consistency between them.

The conformity of preoperative wave V threshold and behavioral threshold to the postoperative ones is also illustrated with graphs in Figure 14.5 that shows the mean values and standard deviations of differences between preoperative and postoperative thresholds. After the operation, the wave V threshold changed slightly more than in the audiometric threshold, and it had an increased variability. Nevertheless, the conformity between the two thresholds was still satisfactory.

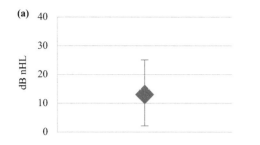
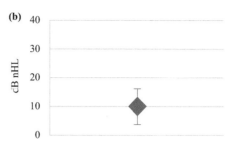

Figure 14.5 (a) Mean value (diamond) and standard deviation (whiskers) of the difference between pre- and postoperative wave V thresholds in the examined group of patients, (b) mean value and standard deviation of the difference between pre- and postoperative audiometric thresholds in the same group.

In summary, the advantages of the ABR method in the assessment of hearing in PDT patients are as follows:

- Good frequency specificity of ABR responses;
- Objective evaluation of hearing threshold in a wide range of hearing loss, from normal hearing up to severe hearing loss;
- Satisfactory precision of hearing threshold evaluation.

Limitations of the method are associated with:

- The limited frequency range in which frequency-specific ABRs can be evoked in typical PDT patients (usually 500 Hz to 1000 Hz),
- Difficulty in diagnosing cases of severe and profound hearing loss (above 90 dB HL) due to the limitations on pulse-type stimuli amplitude.

Then, the ABR method can be considered as the method of choice for objective assessment of hearing in PDT patients belonging to the categories of PDT-AS, PDT-ENS, PDT-EC, and PDT-EAS (Skarżyński et al. 2010).

THE METHOD OF AUDITORY STEADY-STATE RESPONSES (ASSR)

The ASSR method, which has been introduced to clinical audiology more than two decades ago (Picton et al. 2003, Picton 2011, Śliwa et al. 2004, Dimitrijevic and Cone 2015), provides benefits in numerous difficult-to-diagnose cases. In recent years, there is a growing interest in applying the ASSR method in pediatric audiology (Grasel et al. 2015, Kandogan & Dalgic 2012, Yang et al. 2008) and for diagnosing pediatric CI candidates and patients (Ménard et al. 2004, Beck et al. 2015, Kim et al. 2019, Ramos et al. 2015). The main features that differentiate the ASSR method from other electrophysiological methods of hearing testing (like, i.e., the ABR method) are as follows:

- The form of stimuli, which, in the ASSR method, are continuous, modulated tones.
- Method of registration – the potentials of steady-state auditory responses are registered continuously in a long period (tenths of seconds or minutes).
- Method of analysis and evaluation –ASSRs are analyzed in the frequency domain, and the characteristics of the response are evaluated automatically based on statistical criteria.

The typical forms of ASSR stimuli are tones with amplitude (AM) and/or frequency modulation (FM), with sinusoidal or nonlinear envelope. A stimulus example is shown in Figure 14.6. The tone frequency, f_s, is usually one of the typical audiometric frequencies in the range of 250 Hz to 8 kHz. The modulation frequency, f_m, lies in a low-frequency band, from 30 to 100 Hz. Most practical applications use tones with f_m equal to approx. 40 or 80 Hz.

The principle of operation of the acquisition system consists of detecting the presence of an envelope-related component in the registered signal of brain activity. If such an envelope-following component is found, one may assume (at a certain level of significance) that the auditory system has been activated. According to the auditory system's tonotopic organization, the response originates from the region assigned to the tone frequency f_s. As shown in the graph in Figure 14.6b, the presented stimulus is a narrow-band signal, and so are other stimuli used in this method. According to the excitation characteristic, a narrow-band signal activates only the narrow segment of the cochlea assigned to the signal frequency. At the same time, the adjacent segments of the cochlea remain inactivated. Then, the ASSR method provides good frequency specificity allowing for evaluating the actual hearing loss level at a specific frequency. This frequency specificity is comparable to that of pure-tone audiometry.

Evaluation of the hearing threshold in the ASSR method is a two-step procedure (Picton 2003). First, one detects the electrophysiological threshold of the ASSR response. To this end, a series of stimuli at different levels (usually stepping down in 10 dB steps) are presented, similarly as in the ABR method. The ASSR response threshold is assumed the lowest stimulus level at which a statistically significant response appears.

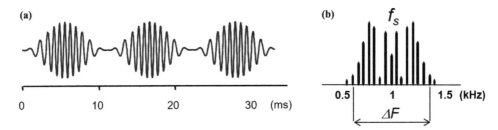

Figure 14.6 (a) Example waveform of ASSR stimulus: AM/FM-modulated tone with tone frequency f_s = 1 kHz and modulation frequency f_m = 80 Hz, (b) the power spectrum of AM/FM-modulated tone stimulus: central frequency f_s = 1 kHz, ½ octave effective power bandwidth ΔF.

Knowing the electrophysiological threshold, one estimates the behavioral hearing threshold (Picton 2011, Hatzopoulos et al. 2010, 2012). The electrophysiological-to-behavioral threshold difference may range from approx. 5 to 30 dB HL or more (Tlumak et al. 2007, Vander Werff et al. 2008). It depends on stimulus frequency, the level of hearing loss, and other factors, including the signal processing method. In most practical-applied instruments, the estimation is performed automatically based on heuristic formulae validated by investigations on a large population of normal-hearing and hearing-impaired subjects.

It must be stressed that the level of registered ASSR potentials is much lower (by order of magnitude) than the level of ABR potentials obtained at the same stimulus level. This leads to a much worse SNR in the registered brain potentials. Consequently, one needs a much longer time of acquisition to effectively distinguish between ASSR signal and the noise originating from spontaneous brain activity and other sources. For the same reason, ASSR potentials exhibit a greater intrasubject and intersubject variability than the ABR potentials and a greater interval of uncertainty when evaluating the behavioral threshold. In the ASSR method, this error interval may range from ±10 dB HL up to ±20 dB HL or more.

The following graphs present an example of application of two electrophysiological methods, ABR and ASSR methods, in a group of PDT patients qualified for CI surgery (Piotrowska et al. 2005b, 2009). In the ABR method, the applied stimuli were tone-pips of Gaussian envelopes with contour proportions 2-0-2 (see Figure 14.1a), presented at tone frequencies of 500 Hz and 1 kHz. The ABR threshold was found by analyzing a series of responses to stimuli at stepping-down levels (see Figure 14.3).

In the ASSR method, one used AM/FM-modulated tones of modulation frequency approx. 40 Hz, and tone frequencies of 250 Hz, 500 Hz, 1 kHz, 2 kHz, and 4 kHz. In the applied measuring system, detection of ASSR envelope-following signal was realized automatically, based on the registered response's spectral analysis, followed by the analysis of phase coherence in the 40 Hz spectrum component (at the modulation frequency) – see Figure 14.7.

Figure 14.8a presents tone audiograms of the investigated group of PDT candidates. As can be seen, the patients belonged to the PDT-EC and PDT-EAS categories. Figure 14.8b presents a juxtaposition of an averaged pure-tone audiogram of the group with averaged electrophysiological ABR and ASSR thresholds. There is also shown an estimated behavioral audiogram derived based on ASSR tests.

Figure 14.9 depicts the mean values and standard deviations of differences between behavioral hearing thresholds and ABR and ASSR electrophysiological thresholds in the examined group of patients. As can be seen, ABR thresholds lie closer to the behavioral ones – the mean threshold difference is about 10–15 dB HL. In the case of ASSRs, the mean threshold difference is higher, up to 30 dB HL.

On the other hand, we can see that the ASSR method made it possible to objectively evaluate hearing sensitivity in a much wider range of frequency than the ABR method (250 Hz to 4 kHz, compared to 500 Hz – 1 kHz in the ABR method). This is because modulated tones at low frequencies (250 Hz or even 125 Hz) are still capable of evoking ASSR potentials. The short-tone stimuli at such low tone frequencies, applied in the ABR method, couldn't effectively synchronize neural activity. It is also

(a)   **(b)**

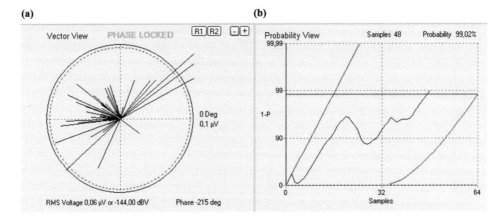

Figure 14.7 A screenshot from an ASSR registering instrument illustrating the method of signal detection: (a) Vector graph of amplitude and phase of the f_m (40 Hz) spectral component in consecutive samples of the registered signal, (b) probability view illustrating the degree of phase coherence; achieving the assumed level of probability (99%) confirms the presence of the ASSR potential.

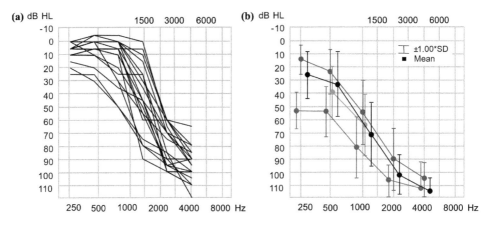

Figure 14.8 (a) Individual tone audiograms of PDT patients in the examined group, (b) average tone audiogram of the examined group (red); average ABR threshold (green); average ASSR threshold (blue); average tone audiogram estimated based on ASSR thresholds (black). Points denote the mean values, while whiskers standard deviations.

worth noticing that modulated tones used as ASSR stimuli have power characteristics similar to pure tones; thus, they can be presented at much higher hearing levels (up to 120 dB HL).

In summary, the advantages of the ASSR method in application to PDT patients are:

• Excellent frequency specificity, which allows for a reliable evaluation of hearing loss at a given frequency, even in patients with steeply sloping audiograms.

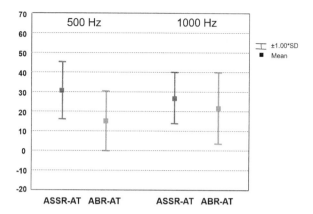

Figure 14.9 Electrophysiological (ASSR, ABR) to behavioral (AT) threshold difference in the examined group of PDT patients. Dots denote the mean values, while whiskers standard deviations.

- Possibility of objective hearing testing at very low audiometric frequencies, even up to 125 Hz; this property is beneficial in PD cases when only low-frequency hearing is preserved.
- Extended range of stimulus hearing level, even up to 120 dB HL, which makes it possible to evaluate hearing in patients with severe and profound hearing loss.

The ASSR method can also be applied to perform objective audiometric tests in free-field conditions in patients with CIs or hearing aids. This is because modulated tone stimuli are easily transmitted through an implant's signal processor (or a hearing aid), contrary to short pulses or tone-pips used in the ABR method. ASSR method then allows for objective evaluation of functioning and the effective gain of the hearing prosthesis.

The drawbacks of the ASSR method consist of:

- The limited accuracy of hearing threshold evaluation, lower than that provided by the ABR method.
- Increased variability of test results, both intra- and intersubjective.
- The relatively long time needed for performing tests.

Despite the mentioned disadvantages, the ASSR method is a valuable tool for objective assessment of hearing in PDT patients, giving satisfactory results when other objective methods fail. It can be applied to all categories of PD, including the PDT-ES type.

APPLICATION OF OTOACOUSTIC EMISSIONS (OAES)

OAEs are sounds that can be recorded in the ear canal and originate from the cochlea (Kemp 1978). They are relatively easy to measure and do not need cooperation from the subject. OAEs are widely used for hearing screening in newborns and young children (e.g., Norton et al. 2000, Ciorba et al. 2008, Śliwa et al. 2011, Trzaskowski et al. 2015). However, their usefulness can be extended (reviewed in Kemp (2002)). One such application is in the diagnosis of PD.

Clinically, two types of OAEs are commonly used: transiently evoked OAEs (TEOAEs) and distortion product OAEs (DPOAEs). TEOAEs are evoked by clicks, and DPOAEs are evoked by two tones. The presence of OAEs means that the hearing threshold is not higher than about 30–40 dB HL. TEOAEs are quite good indicators of hearing in the 1–4 kHz range, and DPOAEs are good at the slightly higher range of 2–6 kHz (Gorga et al. 1993). However, when examining PD patients, we are mainly interested in residual hearing at low frequencies, usually below 1 kHz. Unfortunately, both TEOAEs and DPOAEs perform poorly in this range (Gorga et al. 1993).

To gauge hearing at low frequencies, we can use another type of OAE, namely, tone burst evoked OAEs (TBOAEs). They are evoked by a tone burst – a short-tone stimulus modulated by a nonlinear envelope, usually Gaussian. Tone bursts of low frequency evoke responses that originate from low-frequency regions of the cochlea and can indicate the presence of hearing in this region. Lichtenstein and Stapells (1996) showed that the identification of hearing loss at 0.5 kHz is best obtained by a 0.5 kHz TBOAE, and this extends below the operating range of TEOAEs.

Indeed, 0.5 kHz TBOAEs have proven to be very effective in the case of PD patients (Jedrzejczak et al. 2012). Figure 14.10 shows the frequency ranges covered by 0.5 kHz TBOAEs in comparison with TEOAEs and DPOAEs. There are reports on evoking 0.5 kHz TBOAEs by tone bursts of either 2, 4, or 5 cycles long (Lichtenstein and Stapells 1996, Jedrzejczak et al. 2009, 2013). The recording window can be the standard 20 ms, as for TEOAEs, but it is better to use a 30 ms window, as OAEs of 0.5 kHz have long latency and parts of the response may exceed 20 ms (Jedrzejczak et al. 2009). The response levels of 0.5 kHz TBOAEs are lower than those of TEOAEs in the 1–4 kHz range. The result is that they have smaller SNRs than TEOAEs. The recording time (the number of averages) can be increased to take this effect into account. Also, the criteria for the signal's presence may be lowered, but this needs to be done with caution to avoid recording a signal when there is none. TBOAEs at 0.5 kHz have been shown to be good in separating PD ears from ears with profound hearing loss at

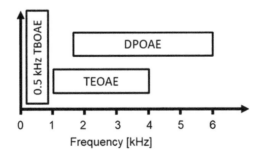

Figure 14.10 Frequency ranges over which different types of OAEs can separate normally hearing ears from ears with hearing loss. TBOAE – tone burst evoked otoacoustic emission; TEOAE – transiently evoked otoacoustic emission; DPOAE – distortion product otoacoustic emission.

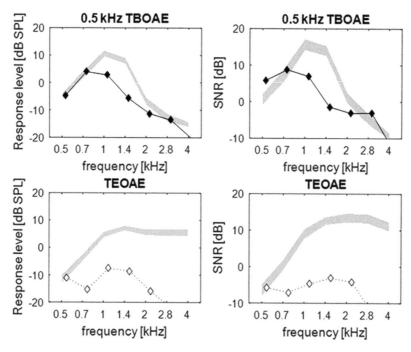

Figure 14.11 OAEs for PD child (data points) superimposed on data from normally hearing children (gray). 0.5 kHz TBOAEs (top row) and TEOAEs (bottom row); average response magnitude (dB SPL, left) and SNR (dB, right).

0.25, 0.5, and 1 kHz (i.e., hearing thresholds better than 25 dB at 0.25, 0.5, and 1 kHz, with steeply falling thresholds beyond) (Jedrzejczak et al. 2012).

TBOAEs at 0.5 kHz may be recorded in all age groups: in newborns (Jedrzejczak et al. 2015a), in children (Jedrzejczak et al. 2013, 2015b), and in adults (Jedrzejczak et al. 2009, 2012). Commercially available systems can be used to measure them (Jedrzejczak et al. 2013).

Figure 14.11 compares otoacoustic emissions – TBOAEs and TEOAEs – in a PD patient with normal-hearing levels up to 1 kHz (10-year-old child) with those of normal-hearing children. The figure shows the standard parameters used in OAE tests: response levels and SNRs for 0.5 kHz. It can be seen that for TEOAEs (bottom row), PD subjects do not show responses – SNRs are below zero, whereas normally hearing subjects present SNRs of around 10 dB in the 1–4 kHz range. The situation is different for 0.5 kHz TBOAEs: here, for PD subjects, SNRs are above zero. The SNRs are lower than for normally hearing subjects, but they are still clearly present.

It can be concluded that 0.5 kHz TBOAEs may be used to distinguish PD subjects from those who have profound hearing loss at all frequencies. The procedure involves making recordings of TEOAEs and 0.5 kHz TBOAEs. Normally hearing subjects will have TEOAEs, while subjects with hearing loss will have absent TEOAEs. Then, when 0.5 kHz TBOAEs are measured, subjects with hearing loss at all frequencies will still not have responses, while PD subjects will show measurable responses.

APPLICATION OF WIDEBAND TYMPANOMETRY

The PD patients achieve benefits of combined electric-acoustic stimulation on the condition that sufficient acoustic hearing is preserved after cochlear implantation. For this reason, one applies minimally invasive surgical techniques (Skarżyński et al. 2006, 2007b, 2010) and special kinds of implant electrodes (Skarżyński et al. 2012a, 2014a). In most cases, natural hearing is well preserved after the operation (Skarżyński et al. 2006); however, a possibility of hearing loss must be taken into consideration.

Although the primary source of postimplantation hearing loss is intercochlear (Adunka & Kiefer 2006, Choi & Oghalai 2005, Eshraghi 2006), there could also be a conductive hearing loss associated with changes in middle-ear immittance properties. Some authors (Greene et al. 2015, Pazen et al. 2017, Saoji et al. 2020) suggest that these factors may be the following: alteration of middle-ear cavity volume (due to the introduction of the facial recess), the presence of the electrode lead, and placement and sealing of the electrode at the round window (that may alter input impedance of the cochlea). In some cases, one also observes postsurgical growth of fibrous tissue that impedes intrascalar fluid movement and consequently raises impedance at the oval window, leading to increased stiffness of the ossicular chain. In consequence, middle-ear impedance may increase, which is connected with the deterioration of sound transmission.

Any degree of conductive hearing loss is of concern because it can affect the low-frequency hearing threshold, thus deteriorating benefits from electric-acoustic stimulation.

Acoustic immittance measures, widely used for assessing middle-ear conditions, allow for detecting different pathologies that affect sound transmission through the middle ear (Margolis & Hunter 1999, Shanks & Shohet 2009, Hunter & Shahnaz 2014). However, classical tympanometry methods are not sufficiently accurate for evaluating subtle changes in middle-ear structure – such that may typically occur after low-invasive CI surgery.

An alternative approach to determining middle-ear function is the application of measures based on acoustic wave energy transmission (Hunter & Shahnaz 2014, Hunter & Stanford 2012, Liu et al. 2008, Rosowski et al. 2013, Rasetshwane & Neely 2012, Rosowski & Wilber 2015). In this method, the measured quantities are wideband energy reflectance (ER) and energy absorbance (EA). EA is the fraction of incident energy absorbed by the middle ear, which depends on its structures' acoustic properties (Allen et al. 2005, Jeng et al. 2008). According to the definition, $ER = 1-EA$. Both quantities can be easily measured over a wide frequency range by applying wideband stimuli (clicks or chirps) as test signals. Compared with traditional admittance tympanometry, measures based on absorbance or reflectance are not sensitive to probe position in the ear canal (assuming there are no energy losses in the ear) and provide a significant amount of information about middle-ear properties at high frequencies, thus making it possible to evaluate middle-ear conditions more comprehensively.

In contemporary devices, wideband EA (or reflectance) can also be measured as a joint function of frequency and ear canal pressure (Liu et al. 2008). In such a mode of operation, air pressure sweeps over a specific range (typically +200 to 300 daPa, similarly as in classic tympanometry), and absorbance-frequency characteristics are measured consecutively at each pressure step. Based on such a data set, one can plot an absorbance-frequency characteristic at a selected ear canal pressure (typically, the ambient pressure or the tympanometric peak pressure, TPP). One can also determine an absorbance-pressure characteristic for a selected frequency band. The graph of absorbance vs. pressure has a single-peak shape, similar to a traditional tympanogram (so, it is sometimes called the wideband absorbance tympanogram). Numerous reports show how to interpret these measures and what diagnostic benefits can be obtained (Keefe et al. 2017, Merchant et al. 2019, Nakajima et al. 2013, Neely et al. 2019, Prieve et al. 2013, Sanford & Brockett 2013, Shahnaz et al. 2009, Śliwa et al. 2020). Application of wideband absorbance measures has proved very useful in diagnosing various middle-ear disorders (Keefe & Simmons 2003, Jeng et al. 2008, Allen et al. 2005, Harris et al. 2005, Merchant et al. 2019, Nakajima et al. 2013, Neely et al. 2019), especially in detecting early forms of otosclerosis (Shahnaz et al. 2009, Keefe et al. 2017, Śliwa et al. 2020).

According to the reasons mentioned above, the application of wideband absorbance can be considered as an effective method for assessing the influence of cochlear implantation on conductive hearing loss. Such an application will be illustrated in the following example.

The study group consisted of 19 PDT patients (11 men, 8 women, aged 52 ± 15 years) admitted to the Oto-Rhino-Laryngosurgery Clinic as candidates for cochlear implantation. All patients underwent comprehensive otologic and audiological examinations dedicated for implant candidates. Additionally, impedance audiometry and wideband absorbance tests were performed pre- and postoperatively. The patients were operated with the low-invasive, six-step Skarzynski method (Skarżyński et al. 2012b), using soft, flexible implant electrodes.

The control group of normal-hearing persons consisted of 126 subjects (38 men, 88 women, aged 30.2 ± 7.2 years), recruited from healthy volunteers. All candidates were comprehensively examined to confirm a lack of hearing impairment. The details on group selection and gender and audiometric characteristics of the control group can be found in another study (Śliwa et al. 2020).

In wideband absorbance measurements, one used the instrument Titan (Interacoustics) with software package IMP440/WBT440. The applied test procedures were as recommended by the manufacturer (Interacoustics 2020). The frequency range for absorbance measurement was 0.226–8 kHz, and the ear canal pressure varied from +200 to –300 daPa (downwards). The stimulus amplitude was about 100 dB peSPL (approx. 65 dB HL), typical for such tests.

The data obtained from the tests were used to determine absorbance-related measures, among them: (1) the characteristics of absorbance vs. frequency, measured at TPP, and (2) middle-ear resonance frequency (FR).

A detailed description of the applied test methods and data analysis can be found in the references (Śliwa & Kochanek 2016, Śliwa et al. 2020).

The following graphs illustrate the results of tests carried out in patients before and after CI surgery.

Figure 14.12 illustrates the differences between absorbance values in the preoperative and postoperative period and between absorbance values in the implanted and contralateral ear. In graph 14.12a, one can see that some changes in absorbance after surgery appear only at high frequencies (above 3,000 Hz). However, all the differences have a random character and are below the level of significance. Similarly, as shown

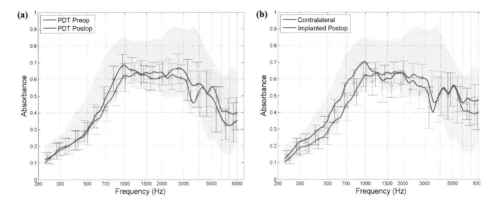

Figure 14.12 (a) Comparison of absorbance-frequency characteristics of implanted ears before surgery (blue line) and after surgery (red line), (b) comparison of absorbance characteristic of the implanted ear after surgery and the characteristic of the contralateral ear. Thick lines are group averages; whiskers denote the confidence intervals of the mean value. Yellow field covers the interval between 10% and 90% percentiles of normal ear absorbance.

in Figure 14.12b, there is some difference between absorbance in implanted and contralateral ear, but it is significant at no frequency. At low frequencies, below 1,000 Hz, nonimplanted ears exhibit a slightly higher absorbance, which might be due to the fact that, generally, in the examined group of patients, the condition of the contralateral ear was closer to normal than that of the ear diagnosed for implantation.

Another quantity that might be sensitive to alterations in middle-ear characteristics arising after cochlear implantation is the middle-ear FR. It depends on the middle-ear vibrating apparatus's mechanical and acoustic properties, primarily on the elements' stiffness and mass. Thus, FR is associated with the middle ear's acoustic impedance, and to some extent, is correlated with EA.

The tests have shown that the differences in FR between all examined groups of ears are small. Average FR is practically identical in implanted ears before and after surgery. It is noticeable that postoperative FRs in PDT patients do not significantly differ from those of normal-hearing ears (Figure 14.13).

The presented results show that the surgery has not significantly altered EA and other immittance-related measures in PDT patients. This conclusion is generally consistent with other authors' findings. Scheperle and Hajicek (2020) suggest that CI surgery may increase middle-ear stiffness, affecting ER (e.g., decreased absorbance). However, their study made on 13 CI recipients has shown that the observed changes in reflectance were within the range of natural variability, so no effect of cochlear implantation could be confirmed. Saoji et al. (2020) found some EA changes after implant surgery in a low-frequency region (500–1,000 Hz). However, their study was performed on only five subjects, so the results' reliability is limited. In another study, Merchant et al. (2020) report on results obtained in a group of 21 CI patients, in whom absorbance characteristics were measured before and after surgery. The authors have found a meaningful decrease in low-frequency absorbance of implanted ears compared to that of a matched group of normal-hearing subjects. The authors attribute this effect

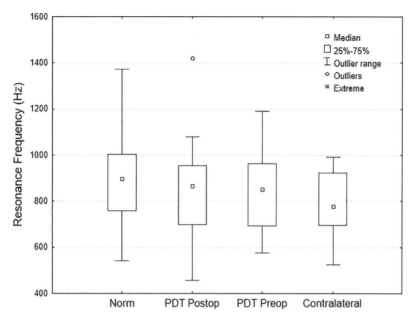

Figure 14.13 Comparison between middle-ear resonance frequency (FR) of implanted ears in PDT patients after surgery (PDT postop) and before surgery (PDT preop), of resonance frequency in a contralateral ear (Contralateral) and normal-hearing ears (Norm). Central point denotes the median, box – 25%–75% range, and whiskers – 5%–95% range.

to the increased cochlear pressure resulting from the presence of an implant electrode. However, in almost all examined patients (except one), one applied a surgical approach through cochleostomy and the electrode's full insertion. This surgical technique significantly differs from that used in patients recruited to the present study. Such a procedure apparently has a much greater effect on the cochlea's impedance, so Merchant's results aren't entirely comparable with the above-presented ones. Greene et al. (2015) present a study done on seven cadaveric ears in fresh-frozen heads. The authors examined middle mechanical and acoustic ear properties, among other things, the effect of CI electrodes on middle-ear absorbance. The results have shown only a minimal effect of implantation, which leads the authors to conclude that middle-ear mechanics remain unchanged after implantation. This conclusion is consistent with the results reported by Pazen et al. (2017). They modeled mechanical properties of the middle and inner ear based on the measurements of acoustic pressure and velocity in cadaveric human temporal bones. Although the tests done on cadaveric preparations were different from the *in vivo* tests, general conclusions are valid.

The above-presented results, as well as findings of other authors who examined absorbance characteristics of the middle ear of PDT patients (Wasson et al. 2018, Chole et al. 2014, Donnelly et al. 2009), clearly indicate that implantation has a minimal effect on middle-ear absorbance, and consequently on energy transmission through the middle ear. One can then expect that the influence of implant electrodes on conductive hearing loss would be negligible. It should be stressed that such results were obtained in the present study in the group of patients implanted with the use of a minimally invasive surgical technique (Skarżyński et al. 2012b). We may conclude that by using this method, one avoids inflicting trauma to the middle-ear conductive structures. The volume of the middle-ear cavity and the cochlea impedance is minimally changed, and there are no harmful host reactions to the electrode. Good preservation of middle-ear absorbance and other immittance-related characteristics is indirect evidence of the advantages of the mentioned implantation method.

SUMMARY

The above-mentioned objective methods – ABRs, ASSRs, OAEs, and wideband tympanometry may be successfully used in PDT patients. Their purpose can be to evaluate the hearing of PDT patients who cannot cooperate (newborns or young children) and provide additional and more precise insights on hearing status than audiometry.

Chapter 15

Auditory cortex, partial hearing loss, and cochlear implants: selected observations and comments

Frank E. Musiek, Jillian N. Bushor, Carrie M. Clancy and Madelyn Schefer
University of Arizona

CONTENTS

INTRODUCTION

High-frequency sensorineural hearing loss (HFSNHL) is one of the most common types and configurations of hearing loss. There are a number of etiologies that are associated with this kind of hearing loss, with presbycusis likely the most common. Symptoms associated with HFSNHL are difficulty understanding speech signals,

DOI: 10.1201/9781003164876-15

hearing in noisy situations, localizing sound sources, and, much of the time, tinnitus. These symptoms for many years were strictly linked to damage to the high-frequency (basal) end of the cochlea. Most commonly, HFSNHL was managed with the application of hearing aids with a high-frequency emphasis. However, the success rate for amplification in HFSNHL has been rather underwhelming.

In approximately the 1980s, some rather important research findings became available, with one of the main contributors being Kent Morest, a well-known auditory neuroanatomist. Morest's research at that time revealed what would become known as trans-synaptic degeneration in the auditory system (Morest 1983). That is, if the hair cells in the cochlea were lost or damaged, this would result in a corresponding loss of cells in the brainstem auditory nuclei via trans-synaptic degeneration. This and other studies, such as those by Webster and Webster (1979) at this time, opened the door to an entirely new way of thinking about HFSNHL and its implications. Evidence was accumulating to indicate that if the cochlear hair cells were damaged, then the ascending neurons connected to those cells would become nonfunctional and would not supply appropriate input to auditory structures in the brainstem. This supported the concept that peripheral hearing loss affected not only the peripheral but also the central auditory system.

Given the findings of cochlear lesions on brainstem auditory nuclei, the next obvious question was what would happen in the auditory cortex in this condition? One of the first papers to address this question about the cortex was one by Robertson and Irvine (1989). This paper and others on this theme will be detailed later, but in an overview, Robertson and Irvine showed an important and interesting finding. They showed in animals that the tonotopic map in the auditory cortex was altered when HFSNHL was induced in the cochlea. The cortex neurons remained functional, but the neural substrate receptive to the high frequencies shifted to become responsive to the last lower frequencies that were intact in the cochlea (see also Schwaber, Garraghty, and Kaas (1993)). Cortical auditory fibers, however, were not responsive to the high-frequency damaged areas in the cochlea. This finding was highly notable and would have a far-reaching impact on both basic science and clinical domains – as will be discussed later. This research serves as the basis for a major portion of this chapter. The Robertson and Irvine study (or at least its key findings) has been replicated and expanded upon; however, another main question arose: could this shift or change in the frequency map be reversed? That is if the input to the auditory cortex could be reestablished, would the neural substrate become responsive to the previous unresponsive frequencies? This key question will also be addressed later in this chapter.

EARLY ANIMAL STUDIES

A historical perspective on cortical reorganization is of value, starting with the Robertson and Irvine classic research. Specifically, the goal of the seminal Robertson and Irvine's (1989) experiment was to investigate changes in the tonotopic organization of the auditory cortex as a consequence of partial unilateral HFSNHL. Similar studies of other sensory systems have revealed that there is plasticity within corresponding regions of the cortex; when input from a specific region of the body is impaired, the area of the cortex that would normally respond to the sensation is deprived (Franck

1980, Kaas et al. 1983, Jenkins & Merzenich 1987). As a result, that portion of the somatosensory cortex will rearrange to become responsive to sensory input from regions of the body that neighbor the site of the lesion. Because cochlear hearing loss results in a similar loss of sensory input to the auditory cortex, Robertson and Irvine (1989) investigated whether or not the auditory cortex demonstrates the same plasticity observed in other sensory systems.

Robertson and Irvine (1989) executed this study by creating cochlear lesions in guinea pigs and utilizing compound action potential (CAP) audiograms to measure the subsequent neural responses related to that region of the cochlea, both before and after the lesion. One group was assessed immediately after the lesion was created, while another group was afforded approximately a 1- to 3-month recovery period. The guinea pigs that were assessed immediately after the lesion were found to have a loss of sensitivity across the high frequencies. The other group of guinea pigs was found to have significantly regained neural sensitivity in the high frequencies following the recovery period, even though there was not a substantial recovery of the damaged cochlea itself. The frequency organizations of the auditory cortices in these animals were comparable to those of normal adult guinea pigs.

Post-lesion, the researchers also dissected and examined the remaining hair cells in the cochlea, recording the locations of the missing or damaged cells with reference to the distance from the basal end of the cochlea. They discovered that both inner and outer hair cells were damaged in cochlear frequency regions that were in agreement with the new frequency maps established in the auditory cortex. In some animals, the damage was not limited to the hair cells; rather, the primary afferent nerve fibers within the osseous spiral lamina have also deteriorated.

Due to the paucity of input in the auditory cortex following the HFSNHL, the neural substrate that correlated to the damaged frequency range was repurposed. For the animals given a recovery period, the region that previously responded to higher frequencies adapted to expanded representations in the cortex that corresponded to the intact regions of the cochlea bordering the lesioned frequency range. These are referred to as edge frequencies and will be discussed further in this chapter. In the animals assessed immediately post-lesion, there was no proof of expanded sensitivity in regard to the edge frequencies. The characteristic frequencies (CFs) of neurons neighboring the lesion were measurable, but with greatly elevated CAP thresholds and broader tuning compared to the original CF.

Robertson and Irvine (1989) concluded that, over time, the plasticity of the cortex allows the neural substrate to adapt to respond to the edge frequencies, a finding supported by the Harrison et al.'s (1991) study examining cortical reorganization in cats following neonatal high-frequency cochlear hearing loss. This finding is comparable to the reorganization demonstrated by the somatosensory system in adult primates as a response to peripheral nerve damage (Merzenich et al. 1983a, 1983b). Thus, the authors suggest that the guinea pigs' cortical capability for the reorganization may be innate to all sensory systems, and it is likely that similar processes occur after partial deafness in humans. Though the study examined reorganization following cochlear lesions, the authors posit that the auditory cortex may not be the primary locus for adaptation. In fact, they suggest that the plasticity of the cortex may reflect changes taking place in structures that are lower in the ascending pathway. Previous studies of somatosensory plasticity in animals found changes in the brainstem and spinal cord, and Robertson cited his unpublished observations that provide early evidence of changes in the inferior colliculus as evaluated in guinea pigs.

Other animal studies

Though the findings of Robertson and Irvine (1989) were foundational in our understanding of auditory plasticity, they were certainly not the last to investigate this phenomenon; many researchers since have attempted to replicate or expand upon the study. In contrast to the cochlear lesions created by Robertson and Irvine (1989), Recanzone et al. (1991) investigated the effects of auditory training on plasticity. They trained adult owl monkeys on frequency discrimination and demonstrated that the trained frequency induced plasticity. The result of the discrimination training was a region of cortical representation for the trained frequency that was two to eight times larger than that of the control animals. The authors conclude that auditory plasticity is a phenomenon that is not only impacted by cases of cochlear hearing loss but that can also be manipulated via auditory training.

In 1993, Schwaber et al. examined neuroplasticity of the auditory cortex in adult primates. Like Robertson and Irvine (1989), they chose to induce cochlear lesions. They employed the chemicals kanamycin and furosemide to deafen macaque monkeys in the high frequencies, mapping the tonotopic organization of the primary auditory cortex after a three-month period allowed for reorganization to take place. That same year, Rajan et al. (1993) confirmed the results of Robertson and Irvine's (1989) study, finding that the tonotopic organization of the primary auditory cortex in cats was altered following a cochlear lesion demonstrating the same expansion of edge frequency representation. They expected a high level of agreement in the tonotopic maps of primary auditory areas for both ipsilateral and contralateral cochlear representations. Interestingly, the authors note that lesioned animals demonstrated differences between ipsilateral and contralateral maps for the regions of the cortex that underwent reorganization, while areas outside the area of contralateral reorganization were found to be congruent and comparable to normal animals. In other words, the region of the cortex that reorganized as a consequence of a contralateral lesion did not display the same changes in sensitivity of its representation of the ipsilateral, unlesioned ear. This is a significant finding with respect to the binaural interactivity of the auditory system. By the time the signal has reached the auditory thalamus, most neurons are receiving bilateral input, which is continued into the cortex. With this evidence, the authors echo Robertson and Irvine's (1989) proposal that the observed cortical reorganization is a reflection of changes occurring subcortically.

A more recent Rajan and Irvine's (2010) study found that, in partially deafened cats who underwent extensive cortical reorganization, the reorganized region was separated into two portions that showed differences in both neuronal sensitivity and responsiveness. In the reorganized cortex that directly bordered the unaffected cortex, neuronal sensitivity and responsiveness to specific frequency inputs were found to be essentially normal. However, the researchers found that neurons further into the deprived cortex demonstrated poorer sensitivity and less responsiveness to the same input.

In an effort to further expand upon the classic studies, Eggermont (2017) dove deeper into the physiological processes underlying brain plasticity by comparing hearing loss in neonates and adult cats. While hearing loss in adults only resulted in tonotopic map reorganization in the thalamus and the cortex, neonates with hearing loss demonstrate changes spanning the entire auditory pathway, including the inferior colliculus. These tonotopic changes are reported to manifest after a recovery period of approximately 3 weeks. Following the acquired hearing loss, there was no longer balance in the cochlear output across frequency, and that imbalance drives an imbalance in excitatory and inhibitory processes. Eggermont (2017) found that in the few days following trauma, excitatory activity had diminished, but there were no significant changes in either inhibitory activity. Interestingly, after a period of 2 months, excitatory activity was still diminished, while inhibitory activity showed substantial growth. This finding suggests that the decrease in inhibition, rather than an increase in excitation, underlies increased spontaneous firing rates, which is a well-documented effect of cochlear hearing loss. This also spotlights the balance between inhibition and excitation in the auditory cortex as a likely key factor in overall function.

Other auditory structures

As Robertson and Irvine (1989) determined, the cortex is not the only area to undergo reorganization following hearing loss. Many researchers since have investigated the involvement of other auditory structures earlier in the pathway. In 1997, Meleca et al. ruled out involvement of the dorsal cochlear nucleus (DCN) in hamsters, concluding that although similar to changes observed in higher-order structures, the changes observed in the tonotopic map of the DCN were not evidence of plasticity. Rather, they found that the changes were simply consequences of the peripheral lesions. In agreement, Rajan and Irvine (1998) concluded that tonotopic changes in the DCN were not driving the changes that have been observed in the cortex. Following these studies, Ma and Young (2006) found changes in excitation and inhibition in the DCN but also failed to find evidence of plasticity.

In an attempt to identify other plastic auditory structures, Wang et al. (2002) found that half of the neurons in the inferior colliculus demonstrated increased spontaneous firing rates following acoustic trauma, a phenomenon the authors explain as an effect of reduced inhibition. To confirm this, the authors applied antagonists specific to inhibitory neurotransmitters and found that the results were comparable to those observed following acoustic trauma. Further, similar results were found by Barsz et al. (2007) in the inferior colliculi of mice and Izquierdo et al. (2008) in rats, providing evidence that tonotopic changes observed following cochlear hearing loss were not a result of plastic changes in the midbrain. Izquierdo et al. (2008) found that the inferior colliculus reorganized in response to the lesion, but the neurons did not return to normal or even near-normal sensitivity or responsiveness. Eggermont (2017) established that excitatory and inhibitory neuronal circuits play a role in the plasticity of the auditory cortex. At the time, Izquiredo et al. (2008) commented on the potential influence but did not specifically investigate these circuits within the inferior colliculus. However, Sturm et al. (2017) did investigate this circuitry. They demonstrated that following damage to the cochlea, excitatory and inhibitory pathways of the inferior colliculus undergo a significant reorganization, functionally resulting in a gap detection deficit. To prevent the development of such central auditory processing deficits,

Sturm et al. (2017) also showed that it is possible to use acoustic enrichment to block changes in the excitatory-inhibitory circuit balance in the inferior colliculus prior to circuit reorganization, which has positive implications for the use of acoustic enrichment following hearing loss.

In contrast to these DCN findings, there is evidence to suggest that the ventral portion of the medial geniculate body (MGBv) has plasticity similar to the cortex. Zhang and Yan (2008) used tones to induce changes in the MGBv. They demonstrated that through corticofugal projections, the auditory cortex played a significant role in the plasticity observed in the MGBv. The results suggest that "thalamocortical circuitry possesses an intrinsic mechanism for input-specific cortical plasticity induced by auditory learning or experience." While they were looking at different structures, Rajan and Irvine (2010) also discussed the influence of the thalamocortical pathway. Recall that they found neuronal sensitivity and responsiveness to be different when measured in areas bordering the lesion compared to those measured further into the deprived cortex. The authors noted that analogous response patterns could be seen following ocular lesions and the resulting reorganization of large deprived areas of the visual cortex. Therefore, noted differences in response properties following a lesion might be generalized to all receptor lesions that result in large areas of cortical deprivation. Thus, the authors suggest it may originate subcortically and "speculate that the two areas of A1 reorganization may reflect differences in the transcortical spatial distribution of thalamo-cortical and horizontal intracortical connections."

Top-down vs. bottom-up influences

The uncertainty regarding where plasticity begins prompted Polley et al. (2006) to investigate the influence of both bottom-up sensory input and top-down inputs on auditory cortical map reorganization. The researchers took a perceptual learning approach to their investigation, training rats to respond to frequency or intensity cues. The animals trained in frequency displayed an expanded representation of the intended frequency range but did not differ in intensity coding, whereas the opposite was true for the group responding to intensity changes. The researchers propose that top-down, task-specific input may interact with bottom-up sensory input to shape auditory plasticity. However, as noted by Kral and Eggermont (2007), bottom-up influences are more significant during sensory system development, and top-down influences drive reorganization in adult systems. This comes with the implication that top-down higher-order influences, which are established with experience, cannot simply be increased to account for deprivation of bottom-up sensory influences. This could mean that the auditory cortex may not have the same capacity for adaptation in those that are congenitally deaf.

Cross-modal adaptation

As we consider auditory cortical plasticity in adult humans, we must consider the potential for cross-modal adaptation and the effects it may have on cochlear implantation. In long-term deafness, the auditory cortex that is not being stimulated will be reassigned to other sensory modalities. To address this, Allman et al. (2009) examined cross-modal reorganization in ferrets. We know that this kind of adaptation occurs in the congenitally deaf, but these researchers aimed to contribute to the lack of research regarding changes in the adult cortex following acquired hearing loss. They found that cross-modal reorganization can indeed occur even after the maturation of the affected sensory systems.

More recently, Land et al. (2016) conducted a study on cross-modal plasticity in congenitally deaf cats, which demonstrated that cross-modal reorganization did not reduce the auditory responsiveness of the area that was adapted. These results suggest that cross-modal reorganization is not likely as destructive to the restoration of auditory input as previously thought and should not deter us from pursuing cochlear implants (CI) for a user with long-term deafness. This is an important finding to explore given that cross-modal reorganization related to the poor residual hearing has been viewed as a contraindication to cochlear implantation and a threat to successful communication outcomes.

On the contrary, Bavelier and Neville (2002) suggest that the nature of the sensory change, when it occurs, and which systems are modified will all influence plastic changes in the system. Thus, while cross-modal reorganization may not be entirely detrimental, understanding the loci and timeline of adaptation within the auditory system can help us to determine the best time for cochlear implantation. The mechanisms underlying plasticity are not all present as we age; for example, adults are less likely to demonstrate subcortical connectivity than a child with cochlear hearing loss. There may be a sensitive period for plasticity, implying that we must pay close attention to the reorganization of the cortex to predict successful reorganization following implantation. The nature of different experiences for different patients can result in different plastic changes. Changes in the visual cortex in postlingually deaf individuals may not be a result of reorganization driven by the changes in auditory perception, but rather it "seems to reflect the greater reliance of cochlear implant users on visual cues during the processing of oral language" (p. 444). In the last two decades, researchers have attempted to assess cortical reorganization using imaging and evoked potentials studies, which will be expanded upon later in this chapter.

Implications for cochlear implant users

Since the advent of auditory plasticity studies in animals, researchers have been trying to predict how their results could extrapolate to humans, especially those who undergo cochlear implantation. Temporal cortical reorganization after partial cochlear hearing loss is a normal process that may be impacted by age or residual hearing. In 1993, Schwaber et al. postulated that residual low-frequency hearing loss in CI patients may lead to potentially cortical reorganization during deprivation such that the whole auditory cortex may become responsive to the low frequencies, requiring the cortex to reorganize once more with the reintroduction of cochlear nerve stimulation. However, they also go on to suggest that fitting hearing aids for a severe to profound high-frequency hearing loss may be pointless if the cortex has already reorganized to respond to lower frequencies. This notion has important clinical implications for those who are dissatisfied with their hearing aids and often refuse to wear them.

In 2017, Eggermont completed a study where he created a noise-induced hearing loss in cats. He found that the cats lost their ability to detect gaps in noise following the hearing loss. Eggermont (2017) states that the resulting deficits in temporal processing acuity and tonotopic reorganization may be detrimental to speech understanding in individuals with hearing loss. He found evidence that if acoustic stimulation is presented directly after the injury, excitatory and inhibitory circuits do not have time to reorganize. Izquierdo (2008) has also reported that "maintaining the stability of the neuronal circuitry for frequency coding in the inferior colliculus may be important for the treatment of noise-induced hearing loss (p. 355)." Ultimately, these findings suggest that exposure to sound therapy may be a viable option for individuals with cochlear hearing loss to halt the development of central auditory processing deficits, but this view awaits further investigation.

Looking back and looking forward: how research has evolved

Back in 1989, Robertson and Irvine performed a study that provoked countless other investigations into reorganization and cortical plasticity following cochlear hearing loss. From the beginning, researchers have been looking for ways to predict how reorganization occurs in humans. Exploring tonotopic maps of the cortex in relation to cochlear lesions evolved into probing cortico-fugal and cortico-cortical pathways, as well as inhibitory and excitatory pathways. From rats to chinchillas to primates, researchers moved ever closer to uncover the underlying mechanisms. Even back in 1989, Robertson and Irvine were searching for ways to project their findings onto humans to understand how changes in plasticity of auditory structures may affect the success of cochlear implantation. They began with animal cortical auditory evoked potentials (CAEPs), examining changes in the tonotopic arrangement of different structures in response to peripheral changes.

As the years progressed and more researchers developed an interest in the phenomenon, it became clear that they needed to determine how they could evaluate human subjects. Researchers made the transition from animal studies to human studies by way of imaging studies. However, imaging has not been the only tool explored. With the evolution of human event-related potentials as a measurement tool, researchers continue to deepen their understanding of the plasticity of various auditory structures. Specifically, they aim to study the reorganization that occurs as a result of hearing loss, following the reorganization that occurs after reintroduction of auditory exposure. These studies have implications for CI users for both pre- and postoperative physiological and behavioral outcomes.

IMAGING

In an effort to expand animal models and investigate cortical reorganization in humans, imaging studies have been a hallmark research approach for evaluating both structural and functional activation in response to sensory stimulation. Major imaging techniques, including functional magnetic resonance imaging (fMRI), positron emission tomography (PET), and functional near-infrared spectroscopy (fNIRS), have been used to measure cortical gray matter activity, while methods such as diffusion tensor imaging (DTI) have been employed to analyze subcortical white matter tracts. This section will discuss the most widely used imaging techniques used in auditory reorganization research while discussing the benefits and limitations of each method.

Foundational animal research has allowed researchers to more accurately predict human anatomical and physiological correlates while steering human research. Neuroimaging studies in both animals and humans have clearly established that primary auditory areas of the cortex include Heschl's gyrus (HG) and planum temporale (PT), both located on the superior plane of the temporal lobe. Primate studies have generated terms of core, belt, and parabelt areas on the superior temporal plane for key auditory regions (Kaas and Hackett 2000). Regardless of terminology, these areas have afferent and efferent projections to peripheral auditory structures. During a period of sensory deprivation, i.e., hearing loss, these projections are deprived of input coming from the peripheral auditory system; consequently, there is less cortical activity in more rostral temporal structures. As a result of neural plasticity, auditory deprivation provides the opportunity for neighboring frequencies that remain, or edge frequencies, to functionally reorganize and to occupy the unstimulated cortical region.

In reviewing activation patterns, one must consider the anatomy of the auditory cortex to understand where expected activation should occur. Along the superior temporal plane, HG, which is found approximately two-thirds anterior to posterior from the temporal pole, houses the primary activation site for auditory reception (Whiteley et al. 2019). Immediately posterior to HG lies PT. Together these two structures comprise the tonotopically organized core, belt, and parabelt areas, with high frequencies mostly concentrated in the anterior fringe and medial aspect of HG and lower frequencies regions in the middle and lateral aspects of HG (Langers et al. 2014, Musiek and Baran 2020).

Imaging methods

fMRI

The use of fMRI in CI research was scarce in the 1990s due to the risk of imaging machinery moving the internal magnet of the CI. With the rapid progression in CI technology through the 21st century, offering MRI compatibility of up to 3.0 Tesla for some devices, fMRI has now been widely used for advancing the understanding of tonotopic mapping in the auditory cortex in regard to auditory rehabilitation with CI. However, it is not the best method as even lower-level MRI machines (1.5 T) can cause discomfort among CI patients (Kim et al. 2015). Neural activity can be tracked in the brain by monitoring changes in blood oxygen levels in response to an auditory stimulus. Greater blood oxygen level dependence (BOLD) correlates with greater cell activity. While this is an efficient method for evaluating functional neural activity, physiologic noise can result in precise quantitative measurements being obscured. Langers et al. (2014) found that while fMRI can be used to map tonotopic fields, individual variability along with scanner noise significantly reduces the chance of exact frequency mapping. fMRI causes large artifacts due to the high magnetic field of the device (artifacts are stronger ipsilaterally), making the temporal cortex difficult to see. The artifact could be improved if the magnet were removed, though this is generally not done for the benefit of the patient, but this would not allow for auditory information to go through the system, and the experimental research would be unsuccessful (Anderson et al. 2017). Regardless, fMRI studies have at least provided enough evidence to determine that there is a tonotopic representation of frequency in the primary auditory cortex with frequencies organized from low to high moving medially from the lateral edge of the plane (Langers & van Dijk 2012).

In an effort to better understand the nature of cortical auditory responses in normal listeners, researchers performing these studies employ varying stimuli, including block tonal stimuli (Norman-Haignere et al. 2013, Seifritz et al. 2006, Upadhyay et al. 2007), broadband natural sounds (De Martino et al. 2013), or continuous or stepwise sweeping tones or other narrowband stimuli (Da Costa et al. 2011, Dick et al. 2012, Hertz and Amedi 2010, as cited by Langers et al. 2014). Utilizing a more complex tone is thought to evoke greater recruitment of cortical activation. For instance, studies utilizing aural speech stimuli with speech reading tasks show not only greater sensory activation but specifically demonstrate multimodal activation of auditory, speech, and visual cortical regions. It is important to consider the complexity and characteristics of the stimulus in any anatomical research. More complex stimuli will correlate with larger recruitment and activation of neural substrates. However, when tasks require other sensory modalities, such as reading speech, activation patterns will naturally incorporate larger networks of activity from other sensory regions as well.

PET

PET evaluates the levels of glucose metabolism in the body by following a chemical tracer in the bloodstream. This method is advantageous for evaluating cortex and small brainstem nuclei for more detailed information in contrast with gross fMRI. However, one limitation of PET evaluation is that because the chemical tracer used to observe metabolism is generally radioactive, the use of PET scans should be limited to about once a year, making longitudinal research a challenge (Anderson et al. 2017, Giraud et al. 2001b).

Recent PET studies have found that following the reorganization of the auditory cortex subsequent to auditory deprivation (i.e., hearing loss), the auditory cortex continues to adapt with the reintroduction of sensory input. When using PET to assess cortical activity following aural rehabilitation (i.e., hearing aids and CI), the evidence suggests that while there is reorganization in the brain as a result of a cross-modal takeover, the changes are thought to occur at a downstream cortical level rather than an upstream brainstem nuclei pathway (Speck et al. 2019).

It should be no surprise to find that there is greater functional reorganization in the cortex contralateral to the more impaired ear as the contralateral pathways are the dominant pathway in the auditory system (Musiek and Baran 2020). In contrast to the connections of the primary auditory cortex and inferior colliculus nuclei to the ipsilateral (more impaired) ear, PET has shown that the contralateral connections from the same structures to the poorer ear display a relative decrease in metabolism. Changes in metabolism were also correlated with the duration of deafness, the effects of which will be discussed in more depth later (Speck et al. 2019).

Some researchers suggest that the reorganization of the auditory cortex, which follows the initial anatomic changes in response to auditory deprivation, partly relies on the introduction of cross-modal information from visual cues (Strelnikov 2015). The brain's ability to integrate audiovisual information is known to improve speech recognition ability in CI populations. Evidence of this interaction can be seen using both PET imaging and behavioral measures of speech recognition ability, where results indicate that deaf individuals have better audiovisual integration capabilities than normal listeners (Strelnikov 2015). Specifically, greater activation of the occipital, superior temporal, and frontal lobes has been observed during speech discrimination tasks, with a gradient of superior temporal lobe activity correlating with greater CI experience (Rouger 2012). Before CI users pursue speech therapy intervention, there is greater activation documented in right hemisphere superior temporal sulcus (STS) in contrast to users with more substantial CI experience, whose levels of right hemisphere STS activation are reduced.

Han et al. (2019) found that in deafened individuals compared to normal-hearing individuals, there is a hypometabolic activity in the inferior colliculus and superior temporal gyri. The decreased metabolic activity in the deafened patients recovered to more normal levels as the duration of their deafness increased. Why does this happen? Interestingly, visual hyperactivity in occipital areas was noted immediately following cochlear injury – perhaps this activity influenced auditory cortex activity.

The auditory cortex appears to be resistant to cross-modal adaptation in postlingually deafened adults, whereas congenital deafness is much more likely to demonstrate neural plasticity throughout the development. This highlights the need for early intervention to take advantage of greater neural plasticity in an unmatured brain. In agreement with Strelnikov et al. (2013), Han and colleagues (2019) propose that speech and language comprehension for CI users is more impacted by the presence of visual cues than in a normal-hearing listener, which is supported by the association between greater visual cortex activity and better post-implant speech perception performance. To echo the suggestions of Land et al. (2016), the heavy influences of audiovisual connections are not maladaptive. They reflect a positive change in neural plasticity as a result of sensory reintroduction following CI use.

These findings suggest that CI users experience reversed neuroplasticity causing greater reactivation of frontal areas and reduced cross-modal activation over time (Rouger 2012). After cochlear implantation, deaf patients experience greater activation of auditory and audiovisual speech processing networks, but also visual speech processing networks to provide efficient word matching by facilitating audio-visuo-motor loop activation along with articulatory-to-phonological information matching (Rouger 2012). Based on these findings, the implications for CI rehabilitation are to provide visual cues during auditory training to encourage auditory recovery and cortical representation. Ultimately, it is not only the level of input that can be provided by the CI itself but the auditory rigor and hierarchical auditory training approach in combination with visual support that will allow CI users to be most successful.

fNIRS

fNIRS has emerged as a new approach for imaging as it is more compatible with CI, which was an early concern for researchers using other methods of imaging. Compatibility is less of a concern in recent years with improvements in implant design and imaging safe procedures that reduce the risk of complications from a CI magnet moving during imaging. There is less electric artifact compared to other imaging methods. Typical imaging devices such as MRI machines generate a lot of ambient noise, which can interfere with the stimulus that the patient is hearing and thus influence cortical activation. fNIRS is virtually silent, and unlike BOLD techniques for fMRI, which measure short-term changes, fNIRS looks at both the oxygenated and deoxygenated hemoglobin and quantifies differences in response to infrared light in order to track changes in the blood for a more accurate assessment of neural activity over time. Increased activation of a region is characterized by greater metabolic demands and, therefore, an influx of oxygenated blood. Unfortunately, a major limitation of this method is that measurements can only be recorded at a maximum depth of about 3 cm, while portions of the auditory cortex can lie deeper than this.

Due to fNIRS being a virtually silent imaging technique, imaging can occur continuously throughout the experiment without acoustic artifacts. One benefit of fNIRS is that it has improved temporal resolution relative to fMRI, meaning greater measurement of activity on and offsets due to the high sampling rate (10 Hz and above). This is also ideal for pediatric imaging research as the interstimulus interval (ISI) is rather short, making the experiment easier on children with short attention spans. This research is typically done using a block or event-related designs. Where data sets can often be limited due to availability or inconsistencies with involved participants, block design fNIRS studies can measure the localized metabolic activity during steady-state processes using different auditory tasks. Additionally, event-related designs using fNIRS can be very informative in oddball acoustic or phonetic experiments with short target stimuli (approximately 200 ms with a 1000 ms ISI). The advantage of event-related fNIRS designs has great promise for future CI research (Basura et al. 2018).

Performance on block tasks using fNIRS, such as recording speech-specific responses during perception tasks, was largely dependent on the CI users' language proficiency rather than their auditory capabilities (Olds et al. 2016). When listening to speech, CI users do not perceive the complete signal. For normal listeners without hearing impairment, understanding a degraded signal is easier because they have the top-down lexical processing to fill in the gaps. For postlingually deafened adults, this same effect is observed; individuals who had typical language development as children and had sufficient language restoration with a CI showed reactivation of the auditory cortex without changes in compensatory processing or neurological reorganization (Bisconti et al. 2016). Some postlingually deafened CI users demonstrate the activation in the auditory cortex during visual stimulation tasks as a consequence of visual processing regions expanding into the deprived auditory regions. The inverse findings have demonstrated that, compared to normal listeners, CI users show greater activation in occipital regions during auditory tasks. This evidence strongly supports the argument of cortical reorganization as a result of neural plasticity. Collectively, this evidence continues to provide a rationale for incorporating visual reinforcements into aural rehabilitation programs to optimize language perception post-implantation (Chen et al. 2016).

DTI/DKI

DTI or diffusion kurtosis imaging (DKI) is a method of evaluating the microstructure within the cortex. This technique measures the distribution of water molecules within cell membranes and fibers in the brain to assess white (myelinated axonal) tracts. There has been some DTI research regarding hearing loss among pre- and postlingually deaf individuals, but more research is needed regarding white matter changes after aural rehabilitation with CI. For individuals with SNHL, DTI is sensitive enough to assess microstructural processes and the following functional changes of the central auditory nervous system (CANS), where traditional MRI or CT scans are unable to demonstrate the same level of detail. Another tool, auditory evoked potentials (AEPs) are used to estimate hearing thresholds and identify the potential site(s) of a lesion; if the pathway traveled by the AEP is disrupted, the stimulus will struggle to reach distal structures. Where AEP may lose the advantage in that sense, DTI can be used to "assess the neuronal deficit regardless of the disrupted locations in the central auditory pathway" (Chang et al. 2004).

The research describing the potential changes in white matter tracts as a component of the reorganization of other auditory structures following hearing loss is ongoing. Some evidence suggests there is a reduction of white matter following SNHL (Hribar et al. 2014); others argue that this does not occur (Li et al. 2012). Though there is some debate as to white matter volume changes, for gray matter changes, Qi et al. (2019) posit that volume may be reduced the longer an individual experiences deafness. DTI has been used in other tangential studies, and there is ample research focusing on evaluating cortical changes in both aging and largely congenitally deaf populations. However, there is a paucity of research evaluating cerebral changes following postlingual HFSNHL hearing loss and subsequent reintroduction of sound (via CI). Future research could have noteworthy implications for how hearing professionals approach aural rehabilitation by considering not only typical aging effects but also the interaction with the duration of deafness and their collective influences on the microstructure of the brain.

Duration of deafness impacting reorganization

Early plasticity research used imaging techniques to study functional activity and neural pathways in animals. Researchers have learned from animal studies that a large factor contributing to neural plasticity and adaptation is the timing of sensory deprivation. Animal studies have indicated that, compared to late-deafened adult animals, congenitally deaf animals experience greater cross-modal interaction as a result of either territorial expansion (Rauschecker 1995) or another method of immature systems redistribute the weight of sensory input to strengthen existing underlying connections (Meredith et al. 2017).

In human studies, prelingual deafness will result in a greater reorganization that spans the auditory system as children's brains are highly plastic. In prelingually deaf individuals, we see primary auditory areas are redistributed to other systems, including the visual cortex (Qi et al. 2019). Research has shown that congenital deafness and cross-modal adaptation does not result in a decreased sensory activation of the adapted region in response to auditory stimuli. However, in postlingually deafened adults, there is a greater chance that the auditory system will not be impacted as much by deprivation due to their auditory systems fully developing during the critical period versus prelingually deaf individuals (Peterson et al. 2013).

These findings could have promising implications for humans and auditory rehabilitation methods, including cochlear implantation, and even predicting outcomes
with intervention, as they suggest that the deprived auditory cortex may still be uti-
lized in both congenitally and late-deafened humans (Anderson et al. 2019). If there
is a better understanding of how sensory systems are interacting prior to implantation, there might be a more patient-specific opportunity to target auditory training
approaches during rehabilitation with a hearing device.

Cross-modal reorganization

There is some debate as to whether cross-modal reorganization is adaptive or maladaptive for the central auditory system following hearing loss. Researchers have
demonstrated using imaging techniques that plasticity in the mature adult brain yields
briefly reduced neuronal activity in the primary auditory cortex and related areas in
response to auditory deprivation (Anderson et al. 2009, Lee et al. 2003). Thus, there is
speculation that this leads to functional reorganization as well. Furthermore, findings
from Lee and colleagues (2003) suggest that preimplantation, stronger cross-modal
activation in auditory areas in response to the visual speech was predictive of poorer
auditory speech understanding post-implantation.

As established by early anatomical studies, there is a stronger audiological representation in the left superior temporal lobe compared to the right (Geschwind and
Levitsky 1968). Considering this laterality construct, it is important to understand the
variance in cortical activation and, therefore, functional reorganization in response
to different monaural deprivation conditions. Zhang et al. (2016) provided evidence of
this cross-modal plasticity. In cases of unilateral sensorineural hearing loss (USNHL),
those who had hearing loss in the left ear demonstrated functional cross-modal reorganization such that the non-auditory-deprived left primary auditory cortex became responsive to visual and sensory stimuli, which was not seen in those with right
UNSHL. This must be taken into account because significant cross-modal reorganization has been documented in the deprived primary auditory cortex and functional
networks, but the current study provides evidence that the non-deprived cortex can
also undergo reorganization following a hearing loss (Zhang et al. 2016). The cross-
modal reorganization is not inherently detrimental to the auditory system. Humans
can adapt to auditory deprivation by engaging in audiovisual interactions. This is referred to as "cooperative advantage," whereby the deprivation of one sense leads to an
enhanced perception of another sense (Merabet et al. 2009).

Reorganization following intervention

Initially, it was thought that sensory cortices were primarily unimodal, only responding to one type of sensory stimuli. With the increase of available research analyzing
sensory deprivation, we now know that in the case of sensory deprivation, specialized brain regions can be recruited and specialized for other sensory modalities (Voss
et al. 2012). Progressive deprivation of auditory stimuli causes deterioration of phonological memory and impedes the dorsal stream (parieto-frontal) in postlingually
deafened adults. They argue the greater the duration of deafness, the more likely the

auditory system relies on the ventral semantic route (i.e., occipito-temporal pathways, including inferior longitudinal fasciculus and uncinate fasciculus) to improve speech understanding (Lazard et al. 2012). Researchers have found that following hearing loss intervention, specifically cochlear implantation, cross-modal reorganization may be interrupted (Strelnikov et al. 2013). In fact, some researchers suggest that following the CI and the reintroduction of sound to the system, the auditory and visual systems can both occupy substrate in the superior temporal plane and end up working together more efficiently (Anderson et al. 2019).

EVOKED POTENTIALS

Evoked potential studies in patients with hearing loss have allowed us to obtain objective assessments of neural response to auditory stimulation in these patients, both before and after intervention with devices like hearing aids or CI. Electrophysiologic assessment in CI recipients can be difficult due to electrical artifacts created by the implant itself. However, Sandmann and colleagues found that AEP evaluation, especially using independent component analysis, in CI recipients held promise for "indicating the maturation (or) reorganization of the auditory system after implantation," the latter of which is most relevant to this chapter (Sandmann et al. 2009 p. 1967).

This avenue of research allows some insight into the anatomic and physiologic correlates of hearing loss and restored auditory function via amplification in the auditory cortex, as well as potentially providing a cross-check to behavioral assessments such as speech perception testing. Evoked potential testing in patients with hearing loss is often used in combination with imaging techniques, including fMRI, fNIRS, and standardized low-resolution electromagnetic tomography (sLORETA), in order to visualize the areas of the brain providing the evoked potential response. This combination of techniques involves recording CAEP latencies and amplitudes, usually for the individual waves comprising the P1-N1-P2 complex. These responses are then mapped to electrical current source reconstructions and dipole moments, which measure the strength of cortical activation.

In cases of partial or high-frequency cochlear hearing loss, the so-called lesion-edge studies have shown that cortical neurons previously responding to frequencies within the range of the hearing loss reallocate themselves to respond to adjacent frequencies, where hearing is better, thereby increasing the cortical area responding to these "edge frequencies." Further evoked potential studies in adult patients have shown additional evidence of cortical resource reallocation, including cross-modal recruitment, in both prelingual and postlingual hearing loss. Evoked potential studies in pediatric patients have shown evidence of neural reorganization induced by auditory deprivation in children with hearing loss, as well as showing evidence of reversed cortical reorganization after early cochlear implantation. These findings are a testament to the neural plasticity of the central auditory system.

Lesion-edge studies

In the early part of the 21st century, attention shifted from animal studies to human studies of cortical reorganization resulting from peripheral hearing loss. Dietrich and colleagues (2001) bridged this gap with a magnetoencephalography (MEG) study of adult patients with acquired HFSNHL and tinnitus. Their results showed that these patients had significantly stronger cortical activation in response to auditory stimuli near the frequency cutoff point between frequencies with normal-hearing sensitivity and frequencies with hearing loss, and relatively weaker cortical activation in response to auditory stimuli at frequencies unaffected by the hearing loss. This response pattern was not seen in normal-hearing control subjects, whose responses were more consistent across all investigated frequencies. The authors theorized that the reorganized response pattern reflected an expanded representation of the "lesion-edge" frequencies in the auditory cortex, caused by re-afferentation, or reassignment, of cortical neurons in frequencies affected by the hearing loss (Dietrich et al. 2001). This study was an early indication that cortical reorganization occurs in humans as a result of peripheral hearing loss or after deprivation of auditory sensory input.

Though CI are not always prescribed for patients with partial hearing loss, evoked potential studies in these patients are potentially useful for understanding cortical changes that might be applicable to all hearing loss configurations. Because the entire auditory system is tonotopically organized, cochlear hearing losses that affect only certain frequencies create changes in the auditory nerve and throughout the CANS in areas that respond to affected frequencies. Lesion-edge studies in patients with HFSNHL have allowed us to directly compare neural responses in cortical areas affected by the cochlear lesion to cortical responses in adjacent, unaffected areas.

In patients with HFSNHL, there is a shift in frequency response at the auditory cortex showing high-volume plasticity. In this situation, more neural substrate becomes responsive to what is often termed the "cutoff frequency" (fc), or the last best hearing frequency before the slope of the hearing loss. As mentioned earlier, neural substrate that was once devoted to the damaged frequencies now shifts to become responsive to the fc. This means more cortical area is available to the fc for the processing of various acoustic stimuli. If more auditory cortex is available to the restricted frequency range near the fc, functional hearing might be expected to be better in that range. Interestingly, Bekesy's experiments on the somatosensory system laid some groundwork for this thinking (von Bekesy and Wever 1960).

There has been evidence to indicate that absolute hearing thresholds may be most sensitive at the fc in situations where sloping hearing loss follows (Thai-Van et al. 2010). In this case, would other auditory function also be improved at or near the fc – for instance, frequency discrimination? McDermott and colleagues answered this question, showing that difference limens (DLs) for frequency were improved at the fc in individuals with HFSNHL (McDermott et al. 1998). Thai-Van and colleagues followed this work with a larger study showing essentially the same results (Thai-Van et al. 2002). In this study, it also appeared that as the slope of the loss became sharper, the DLs for frequency became better (smaller), and this action was noted for low frequencies as well (Thai-Van et al. 2002).

At this stage of "edge frequency" research, it seemed appropriate to realize that the shift in tonotopicity in the auditory cortex to the fc provided more neural substrate at or near the fc and that this translated into better DLs for frequency (and likely other auditory functions) at the fc. This led to the next main question: if hearing was restored at the frequencies with hearing loss, would the changes in auditory cortex substrate be reversed? In other words, if the cortex shifted back to a more normal tonotopic arrangement, would the DLs for frequency at fc become worse, indicating this change?

The answer to these key queries would need to include rehabilitative approaches and devices such as hearing aids and CI.

As Thai-Van et al. reported, patients with HFSNHL were tested for frequency discrimination before receiving amplification and again one month after receiving amplification. As hypothesized, these patients showed alterations in DLs at the fc after amplification, but the post-amplification changes did not occur at other frequencies, which was seen as an indication of possible cortical reorganization after amplification (Thai-Van et al. 2002 and 2010).

Further research into altered DLs at the fc is needed. Specifically, research on DLs at the fc in partial hearing loss before and after cochlear implantation was difficult for these authors to find. However, this measure appears to hold much promise as a clinical index for measuring auditory cortex reorganization as a result of partial hearing loss, as well as examining the reversal of this reorganization after amplification or cochlear implantation. Also, from a methodological perspective, measuring thresholds using Bekesy-like tracking procedures can provide more accuracy than traditional (discrete) approaches for defining edge frequencies and should be employed in future research (see Figure 15.1).

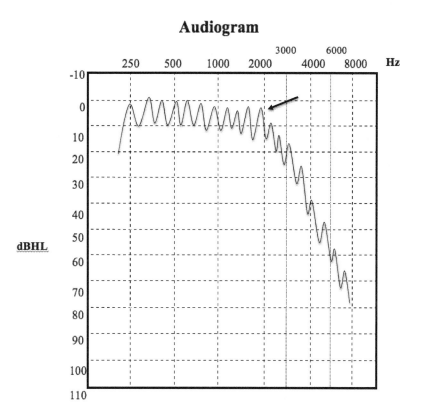

Figure 15.1 Bekesy-like audiometric tracking, with the arrow pointing to the lesion-edge frequency.

Further findings in adult patients

It is well established that cochlear implantation is the highest standard of treatment for adults with severe to profound hearing loss, but individual outcomes following cochlear implantation can vary widely (Wolfe 2020, Boisvert et al. 2020). Despite ample evidence of functional improvement in audibility and speech perception with cochlear implantation, anatomic and physiologic changes corresponding to these functional improvements have not been clarified in the research literature. Further, anatomic and physiologic differences in patients with differing degrees and configurations of hearing loss or differing degrees of success with cochlear implantation also have not been fully explored.

With this knowledge gap in mind, Purdy and Kelly (2016) attempted to find electrophysiologic correlates for longitudinal improvements in behavioral speech perception measures in adult CI users. To this end, they examined middle latency response (MLR), mismatch negativity (MMN), and obligatory CAEP responses to tonal stimuli in postlingually deaf CI users over the first nine months following implantation. They found that the clearest indicator of auditory system plasticity might be the P2 area or amplitude times width of the P2 component. Specifically, P2 latency did not change significantly over time, but amplitude and width both became progressively larger. This change was consistent with steadily improving behavioral speech perception scores over the same time period. However, in a related study, Barlow et al. (2016) found that intensive post-implantation auditory training produced only small gains in behavioral speech perception and no correlating changes in CAEP measurements. Taken together, these studies suggest that further longitudinal research is needed to assess short-term and long-term changes in neural response to sound and that further studies may guide clinical audiologists in mapping these changes onto observed functional outcomes in adult CI recipients. For adult patients with HFSNHL, further CAEP studies using tonal stimuli in addition to speech sounds could be conducted to address the lesion-edge neuroplasticity explored above.

Liebscher and colleagues (2018) examined CAEP responses to single-electrode bursts and monosyllabic word scores in adult CI users to assess how evoked potentials and speech perception are related to a place of stimulation along the implanted electrode. They found that CAEP responses varied significantly by stimulation site and rate, with component amplitudes declining significantly from apical to basal sites and the most robust responses recorded at slow rates of stimulation. They concluded that N1 and N1-P2 amplitudes at medial sites positively correlated with monosyllabic word performance and that P2 latency at apical sites negatively correlated with speech recognition performance. Most interestingly for the purposes of this chapter, this group of researchers also found that "deafness-related neural degeneration" persists after auditory access is restored via cochlear implantation and that this effect is more pronounced for electrical stimulation at the base of the cochlea than for stimulation at the apical end (Liebscher et al. 2018 p. 939). They hypothesized that the reduced CAEP responses to basal stimulation might be attributed to sequential changes in parts of the tonotopically organized CANS responding to high frequencies, which would logically result from longer periods of auditory deprivation in the high frequencies due to cochlear hearing loss (Liebscher et al. 2018).

Cross-modal reallocation

Evoked potential studies have also provided further insight into the nature of cortical reorganization after a peripheral hearing loss in adults. Campbell and Sharma (2013 and 2014) conducted a pair of studies specifically regarding cortical reorganization resulting from postlingual hearing loss. In their first study, Campbell and Sharma (2013) measured speech-evoked CAEPs in eight normal-hearing subjects and nine patients with bilateral mild-moderate HFSNHL. These CAEP measurements were combined with sLORETA imaging, and a behavioral measure of speech-in-noise perception was obtained for each subject or patient. As compared to normal-hearing subjects, patients with hearing loss showed increased P2 latencies, which correlated with increased (worse) behavioral speech-in-noise scores. (The study also revealed increased P2 amplitudes, which the authors attributed to greater perceptual and auditory memory demands, but this explanation related to higher-level processing seems questionable for a response as early as 200 ms.) Along this line, patients with hearing loss also showed a decreased activation in the auditory cortex and an increased activation in the frontal cortex compared to normal-hearing subjects. On this basis, the authors concluded that postlingual mild-moderate HFSNHL might be associated with demonstrable cortical reorganization (Campbell and Sharma 2013).

In their second study, Campbell and Sharma (2014) compared visual evoked potentials (VEPs) to auditory behavioral speech-in-noise measures, specifically QuickSIN scores. In their eight normal-hearing subjects and nine adult patients with postlingual HFSNHL, they found a negative correlation between QuickSIN score and VEP N1 latency, meaning that a shorter latency VEP N1 was associated with worse speech-in-noise performance. In the nine patients with HFSNHL, they found larger VEP component amplitudes, suggesting greater perceptual and memory demands, and decreased component latencies. They further observed that the activation related to these VEPs, visualized via sLORETA, occurred in areas of the cortex typically associated with auditory processing, including all three temporal gyri. Their evidence suggests that cross-modal reorganization of cortical resources begins after even short periods of auditory deprivation and that this cortical reorganization may have implications for functional outcomes in patients with acquired hearing loss (Campbell and Sharma 2014).

In two related studies, Cardon and Sharma (2018) and Glick and Sharma (2020) used VEPs and somatosensory evoked potentials (SEPs) to examine cortical reallocation in adults with mild-moderate age-related hearing loss. These patients showed evidence of cortical recruitment of auditory areas for processing both somatosensory (vibrotactile) and visual stimuli. The latter study also found that in these patients, cross-modal visual recruitment was reversed after intervention with amplification and that this reversal correlated with gains in speech perception and cognition (Glick and Sharma 2020).

There has also been research specifically focused on patients with hearing loss severe enough to indicate cochlear implantation. In these patients, further evidence has been found for cortical resource reallocation after auditory deprivation. A 2006 evoked potential study by Doucet et al. included both prelingually and postlingually deafened CI recipients. Rather than grouping patients by onset or duration of deafness, these patients were split into groups of "good" or "poor" performance on behavioral measures of speech perception. Their VEP results were interpreted to suggest more extensive cross-modal reorganization in patients with poor speech perception and more intramodal reorganization in patients with good speech perception. Additionally, the authors suggested that some patients' lack of success with speech perception after cochlear implantation might be related to the limited availability of cortical areas normally reserved for auditory processing (Doucet et al. 2006).

Chen and colleagues (2017) used combined AEPs, VEPs, and fNIRS to show that, compared to normal-hearing control subjects, CI users displayed a reduced stimulus-specific activation in both auditory and visual processing areas and enhanced adaptation for visual stimuli, but reduced adaptation for auditory stimuli. One interpretation of this data is that CI users process visual information more efficiently than normal-hearing listeners, but that they may process auditory information less efficiently.

Sandmann and colleagues (2012) posited that these cortical resource reallocations to other sensory modalities could be maladaptive for spoken language, making auditory information more difficult to process. But Stropahl et al. (2017) later argued that cortical reallocation to the visual system could be adaptive to the development of visual language modalities such as sign language and to visual aspects of spoken language such as facial expression and speechreading. Again, further longitudinal studies, including data collection before and after cochlear implantation, are needed to elucidate the nature and extent of cross-modal plasticity during and after auditory deprivation.

These cross-modal cortical reallocations make some sense if taken in the context of the dorsal-ventral stream theory of speech processing described by Hickok and Poeppel (2007). According to this theory, the dorsal and ventral streams of the speech processing system anatomically parallel the dorsal and ventral streams of the visual processing system (Hickok and Poeppel 2007, Hebart and Hesselmann 2012). The auditory portion of the ventral speech processing stream runs through the superior and middle temporal lobes bilaterally and is thought to be involved in processing spoken language for comprehension of meaning. The auditory portion of the dorsal stream is less precisely defined but involves auditory structures in the posterior temporal lobe as well as somatosensory areas of the parietal lobe. This stream is thought to incorporate prior sensorimotor knowledge to facilitate and enhance comprehension of oral motor speech productions (Hickok and Poeppel 2007). The close proximity and associations among auditory, visual, and somatosensory areas in both streams provide a logical basis for the findings in the evoked potential studies described above.

Figure 15.2 illustrates the visual and dorsal speech pathways on a theoretical basis, along with the intrahemispheric connective pathways that are likely involved. These might include the superior longitudinal fasciculus, which courses from posteriorly located visual areas along with the arcuate fasciculus towards the frontal lobe, as well as possibly the inferior longitudinal fasciculus, which courses anteriorly from the visual association areas across the auditory areas in the temporal lobe and then to the frontal lobe. Though not pictured in the diagram, connections to the hippocampus, which involves working memory, are also likely and important elements of these pathways.

Relevant findings in pediatric patients

Evoked potential studies in pediatric patients can inform clinical candidacy criteria and prognoses for child and adult CI recipients, as well as providing direction for

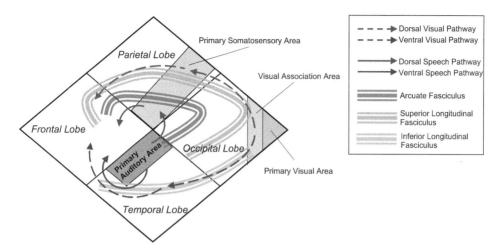

Figure 15.2 Schematic representation of dorsal-ventral visual and speech processing pathways in the brain.

future research in both populations. In congenitally deaf children receiving CI, evoked potential studies have been used to examine the nature of the effects of hearing loss on the auditory cortex and the overall neurodevelopmental effects of auditory deprivation. The following studies of congenital or early childhood auditory deprivation can shed some light on the main question addressed in this chapter: if parts of the auditory cortex are reallocated to respond to other stimulus modalities following auditory deprivation, will that cortical area still be available to auditory stimulation after cochlear implantation restores auditory access?

Research on auditory nervous system plasticity in children using CI dates back at least to the mid-1990s. Ponton and colleagues reported in 1996 that CAEPs in children with CI revealed changes in P1 latency related to age and duration of auditory deprivation. They also found that with the reversal of auditory deprivation via cochlear implantation, P1 latencies resumed a grossly normal maturation pattern (Ponton et al. 1996). Importantly, this study underscored the need for early implantation to reverse auditory deprivation in young children with severe to profound hearing loss who are learning spoken language. However, later evoked potential studies in combination with imaging techniques have revealed major differences in cortical responses to auditory stimuli in children with CI.

Gilley and colleagues (2008) measured synthetic speech-evoked CAEPs in congenitally deaf children, one group who received unilateral CI early (before 4 years of age) and one group who received unilateral CIs later (after 7 years of age). These were compared with CAEP measurements in a control group of normal-hearing children, and CAEP measurements were combined with sLORETA current source reconstructions and dipole source analyses. While normal-hearing children revealed bilateral neural activation in auditory temporal areas in response to speech sounds, children with CI revealed only unilateral activation in the brain hemisphere contralateral to the implant. Further, in the late-implanted children, this neural activation shifted from the expected auditory response areas, specifically HG, to the contralateral parietotemporal cortex, which is associated with both the dorsal visual stream and the dorsal speech processing stream (Gilley et al. 2008, Hickok and Poeppel 2007).

The authors hypothesized that the contralateral-only activation in implanted children might be "evidence of a cortical de-coupling of auditory pathways" resulting from different degrees of auditory deprivation early in life (Gilley et al. 2008 p. 60). They note that this effect was not observed in previous studies of postlingually deafened adult patients, possibly because in these patients, the ipsilateral and contralateral auditory pathways, including the interhemispheric pathway through the corpus callosum, had developed and matured before auditory deprivation took place. More important to our discussion of adult CI recipients is the finding that for late-implanted children, neural activity in response to auditory stimulation occurred in areas of the brain typically reserved for visual motion processing. Like the cross-modal studies presented above, this finding suggests a reorganization of the dorsal-ventral stream, where visual information is rerouted through cortical areas previously associated with auditory language processing, including the temporal gyri and arcuate fasciculus. In addition, it appears that auditory information is subsequently rerouted to alternate proximate cortical areas, including the parietotemporal cortex (Gilley et al. 2008, Axer et al. 2013). Further study of this cortical reorganization pattern should be considered for adult CI candidates after prolonged auditory deprivation and for adult CI patients experiencing limited open-set speech perception outcomes.

In their review of developmental and cross-modal plasticity in children with CI, Sharma et al. (2015) discuss new data using the cortical N1 potential to validate sensitive periods, or periods of increased neural plasticity, for auditory input and auditory nervous system maturation. Earlier research, including the studies cited above, has established the P1 latency as an important marker of auditory nervous system development in young children. In line with the Gilley et al.'s study cited above, Sharma and colleagues suggest here that after 7 years of age, cortical plasticity is reduced, marking the end of a critical sensitive period for auditory input. Specifically, N1 component detectability was interpreted to reflect decreasing auditory nervous system plasticity, as the N1 component was significantly less detectable in children implanted after 7 years of age than in children implanted earlier (Sharma et al. 2015).

Finally, in a review of cross-modal plasticity and hearing loss, Sharma and Glick (2016) describe the reversal of cross-modal plasticity in a case study of a child using a CI for single-sided deafness (SSD). The child considered here was identified at the age of 5 years with a unilateral moderate hearing loss that eventually progressed to severe profound levels, and the child received a CI just before the age of 10 years. Cortical evoked potentials for visual, somatosensory, and auditory synthetic speech stimuli were recorded before and after implantation, along with current density source localizations and behavioral measures of speech perception and sound localization (Sharma et al. 2015). Preimplantation evoked potential sources were consistent with cross-modal recruitment following auditory deprivation, while post-implantation measures revealed activation localized to expected sensory-specific areas (i.e., temporal regions for auditory stimuli). This child also demonstrated excellent speech perception and sound localization with the implant, suggesting that cross-modal plasticity in the reverse direction may have contributed to the degree of benefit from implantation (Sharma and Glick 2016). This case study suggests several avenues for further research, including the examination of differing degrees of plasticity to and from each sensory modality, comparison of plasticity in unilateral and bilateral hearing loss, and age-related effects on plasticity in each of the aforementioned conditions.

Continuing research directions and clinical applications

Unilateral hearing loss and SSD are the main focus of ongoing research and clinical exploration in cochlear implantation. Three recent evoked potential studies highlight the directions and expanding clinical implications of this ongoing research, including the comparison of cortical responses to electrical and acoustic listening in the same subject, the configuration of cortical reorganization in SSD, and cortical reorganization following different interventions for unilateral hearing loss.

Bönitz and colleagues (2018) recorded CAEPs from eight unilaterally deaf CI users who performed a three-stimulus oddball task, both with their normal-hearing ear and separately with their implanted ear. Comparisons were made for the auditory N1 component as well as the later Novelty P3 and Target P3. Electric (CI) listening was associated with reduced amplitudes for the N1 component and the early part of the Novelty P3 component, as compared to acoustic (normal-hearing ear) listening. The authors claim that these results reflect a distinctive CAEP pattern for CI-aided listening, as well as contributing data to the idea of distinct subcomponents for the auditory Novelty P3 response (Bönitz et al. 2018).

Legris and colleagues (2018) undertook a longitudinal study comparing CAEPs in nine adult CI users with SSD and a normal-hearing control group. In the CI patients, speech-evoked CAEPs were measured prior to implantation and again at intervals of 6 and 12 months post-implantation. Behavioral speech-in-noise measures were also taken at each interval. Results revealed increased CAEP amplitudes at electrodes contralateral to the implanted ear after implantation for all CI users, while peak latencies at temporal and mastoid sites remained significantly longer than in normal-hearing controls. Patients with left-side CI showed consistent but statistically insignificant increases in N1 amplitude at 12 months post-implantation compared to baseline, and scalp potential topography in these patients revealed bilateral activation at N1 latencies at 6 and 12 months post-implantation. Patients with right-side CI did not show increased N1 amplitude over time, but scalp topography revealed increased positivity at contralateral temporal electrodes at 12 months post-activation. All patients showed increased speech recognition in spatially separated noise at 12 months post-implantation. The authors hypothesized that these asymmetric activation patterns, along with improved speech perception, may reflect adaptive cortical reorganization following the restoration of binaural function with cochlear implantation (Legris et al. 2018).

Finally, another study by Legris et al. (2019) examined cortical auditory responses in patients with unilateral hearing loss using three different amplification devices: contralateral routing of signal (CROS) hearing aids, bone-anchored hearing aids (BAHA), and CI. Speech-evoked CAEPs were recorded with and without amplification for each patient and compared to normal-hearing controls, and behavioral speech-in-noise measures were taken for each patient. Results showed that cochlear implantation was associated with the largest effects on CAEPs, specifically N1 peak amplitude, as well as improved speech-in-noise understanding. The authors suggested that further longitudinal studies in adult CI patients with SSD could elucidate the progression of cortical reorganization after implantation (Legris et al. 2019).

These studies highlight the expanded use of cochlear implantation as a rehabilitation strategy for degrees and configurations of hearing impairment beyond the typical candidacy criteria of bilateral severe-profound SNHL and reduced speech perception ability. Adult patients with HFSNHL, unilateral hearing loss, or SSD can experience degraded functional speech perception in many environments, as well as altered central auditory processing of sound and speech. Cochlear implantation can mitigate these changes, even if the mechanisms behind them are not yet fully understood. In terms of auditory nervous system research, these patients provide a unique opportunity to examine how changes in functional hearing might correlate with changes in the auditory cortex resulting from varying degrees and configurations of hearing loss. In cases of HFSNHL, these studies allow us the opportunity to examine specific alterations to the tonotopic organization of the CANS. Studies of patients with SSD can help us to separate and analyze changes to the inter- and intrahemispheric auditory pathways in the brain induced by unilateral auditory deprivation. For patients with both SSD and HFSNHL, cochlear implantation is quickly becoming a viable option for restoration of auditory access, as well as potential restoration of corresponding physiologic activity in the auditory cortex. This potential restoration of neural activity has implications not only for speech and language processing but for other conditions associated with hearing loss, including dementia and age-related changes in auditory processing.

SUMMARY

In this chapter, we have overviewed some key research on the effect of HFSNHL and hearing loss in general on the auditory cortex and related cortices in the brain. Pioneering studies on cortical reorganization as a result of hearing loss have been carefully profiled. These studies served as a springboard for subsequent studies on the concepts of cortical restructuring and "lesion-edge frequencies," using evoked potentials and imaging methodology. This research has also produced interesting interactions when CI are applied to adult patients with partial hearing loss as well as severe to profound hearing loss, and in pediatric populations. Cochlear implantation has been shown to influence the plastic reorganization of the brain to perhaps allow a more natural cortical organization and related functional hearing ability. Cortical reorganization within and across sensory modalities have been explored as promising research avenues that deserve further investigation.

Though this chapter captures many of the research advances in brain reorganization related to hearing loss and subsequent rehabilitation of hearing loss, much remains unknown. Studies focusing on auditory cortex dynamics related to partial and complete hearing loss as well as cross-modal plasticity appear to hold great promise for marked advancement in cochlear implantation.

Bibliography

Abdala, C. and Y.S. Sininger. 1996. The development of cochlear frequency resolution in the human auditory system. *Ear Hearing* 17, no. 5: 374–85.

Abramides, P.A., R.S.M. Bittar, R.K. Tsuji, R.F. Bento. 2015. Caloric test as a predictor tool of postural control in CI users. *Acta Oto-Laryngol* 135, no. 7: 685–91.

Adunka, O. and J. Kiefer. 2006. Impact of electrode insertion depth on intracochlear trauma. *Otolaryng Head Neck* 135: 374–82.

Adunka, O., J. Kiefer, M. Unkelbach, A. Radeloff, W. Gstoettner. 2005. Evaluating cochlear implant trauma to the scala vestibule. *Clin Otolaryngol* 30: 121–27.

Allen, J.B., P.S. Jeng, H. Levitt. 2005. Evaluation of human middle ear function via an acoustic power assessment. *J Rehabil Res Dev* 42 (4 Suppl. 2): 63–78.

Alles, M. J. R. C., M. A. der Gaag and R. J. Stokroos. 2006. Intratympanic steroid therapy for inner ear diseases, a review of the literature. *Eur Arch Oto-Rhino-L* 263, no. 9: 791–97.

Allman, B.L., L.P. Keniston, M.A. Meredith. 2009. Adult deafness induces somatosensory conversion of ferret auditory cortex. *Proc Natl Acad Sci – Biol* 106, no. 14: 5295–930.

American Educational Research Association, American Psychological Association, National Council on Measurement in Education, Joint Committee on Standards for Educational and Psychological Testing (U.S.). 2014. *Standards for Educational and Psychological Testing*. Washington, DC: American Educational Research Association.

Anderson, C.A., D.S. Lazard., D.E. Hartley. 2017. Plasticity in bilateral superior temporal cortex: Effects of deafness and cochlear implantation on auditory and visual speech processing. *Hearing Res* 343: 138–49.

Anderson, C.A., I.M. Wiggins, P.T. Kitterick, D.E. Hartley. 2019. Pre-operative brain imaging using functional near-infrared spectroscopy helps predict cochlear implant outcome in deaf adults. *JARO-J Assoc Res Oto* 20: 511–28.

Andresen, E. 2000. Criteria for assessing the tools of disability outcomes research. *Arch Phys Med Rehab* 81 (Suppl. 2): S15–S20.

Aschendorff, A., J. Kromeier, T. Klenzner, R. Laszig. 2007. Quality control after insertion of the nucleus contour and contour advance electrode in adults. *Ear Hearing* 28 (2 Suppl. l): 75S–79S.

Avci, E., T. Nauwelaers, T. Lenarz et al. 2014. Variations in microanatomy of the human cochlea. *J Comp Neurol* 522: 3245–61.

Axer, H., C.M. Klingner, A. Prescher. 2013. Fiber anatomy of dorsal and ventral language streams. *Brain Lang* 127, no. 2: 192–204.

Bagatto, M., C. Brown, S. Moodie, S. Scollie. 2011. External validation of the LittlEARS® Auditory Questionnaire with English-speaking families of Canadian children with normal hearing. *Int J Pediatr Otorhi* 75: 815–17.

Barbara, M., P. Mancini, A. Nattioni, S. Monini, D. Ballantyne, R. Filipo. 2000. Residual hearing after cochlear implantation. *Adv Oto-Rhino-Laryng* 57: 385–88.

Barlow, N., S.C. Purdy, M. Sharma, E. Giles, V. Narne. 2016. The effect of short-term auditory training on speech in noise perception and cortical auditory evoked potentials in adults with cochlear implants. *Semin Hear* 37, no. 1: 84–98.

Barsz, K., W.W. Wilson, J.P. Walton. 2007. Reorganization of receptive fields following hearing loss in inferior colliculus neurons. *Neuroscience* 147, no. 2: 532–45.

Basura, G.J., X.-S. Hu, J. San Juan, A.-M. Tessier. 2018. Human central auditory plasticity: a review of functional near-infrared spectroscopy (fNIRS) to measure performance and tinnitus perception. *Laryngoscope Investig Otolaryngol* 3, no. 6: 463–72.

Baumann, S., M. Meyer, L. Jäncke. 2008. Enhancement of auditory-evoked potentials in musicians reflects an influence of expertise but not selective attention. *J Cogn Neurosci* 20, no. 12: 2238–49.

Bavelier, D. and H.J. Neville. 2002. Cross-modal plasticity: where and how? *Nat Rev Neurosci* 3: 443–52.

Beck, R. M., S.S. Grasel, H.F. Ramos et al. 2015. Are auditory steady-state responses a good tool prior to pediatric cochlear implantation? *Int J Pediatr Otorhi* 79, no. 8: 1257–62.

Bekinschtein, P., C.A. Oomen, L.M. Saksida, T.J. Bussey. 2011. Effects of environmental enrichment and voluntary exercise on neurogenesis, learning and memory, and pattern separation: BDNF as a critical variable? *Semin Cell Dev Biol* 22, no. 5: 536–42.

Bell, L.S., F. Barker, H. Heselton, E. MacKenzie, D. Dewhurst, A. Sanderson. 2015. A study of the relationship between the video head impulse test and air calorics. *Eur Arch Oto-Rhino-L* 272, no. 5: 1287–94.

Beroun, A., S. Mitra, P. Michaluk, B. Pijet, M. Stefaniuk, L. Kaczmarek. 2019. MMPs in learning and memory and neuropsychiatric disorders. *Cell Mol Life Sci* 76, no. 16: 3207–28.

Biedron, S., A. Prescher, J. Ilgner, M. Westhofen. 2010. The internal dimensions of the cochlear scalae with special reference to cochlear electrode insertion trauma. *Otol Neurotol* 31: 731–37.

Bisconti S., M. Shulkin, X.-S. Hu, G. Basura, P. Kileny, I. Kovelman. 2016. Functional near-infrared spectroscopy brain imaging investigation of phonological awareness and passage comprehension abilities in adult recipients of cochlear implants. *J Speech Lang Hear R* 59: 239–53.

Blamey, P., F. Artieres, D. Başkent et al. 2012. Factors affecting auditory performance of postlinguistically deaf adults using cochlear implants: an update with 2251 patients. *Audiol Neuro-Otol* 18, no. 1: 36–47.

Boggess, W.J., J.E. Baker, T.J. Balkany. 1989. Loss of residual hearing after cochlear implantation. *Laryngoscope* 99: 1002–5.

Boisvert, I., M. Reis, A. Au, R. Cowan, R.C. Dowell. 2020. Cochlear implantation outcomes in adults: A scoping review. *PLOS ONE* 15, no. 5: e0232421.

Bönitz, H., B. Kopp, A. Buechner, T. Lunner, B. Lyxell, M. Finke. 2018. Event-related neuronal responses to acoustic novelty in single-sided deaf cochlear implant users: initial findings. *Clin Neurophysiol* 129, no. 1: 133–42.

Boothroyd, A. 2007. Adult aural rehabilitation: what is it and does it work? *Trends Amplif* 11, no. 2: 63–71.

Bosdriesz, J.R., M. Stam, C. Smits et al. 2018. Psychosocial health of cochlear implant users compared to that of adults with and without hearing aids: results of a nationwide cohort study. *Clin Otolaryngol* 43, no. 3: 828–34.

Bozdagi O., V. Nagy, K.T. Kwei, G.W. Huntley. 2007. In vivo roles for matrix metalloproteinase-9 in mature hippocampal synaptic physiology and plasticity. *J Neurophysiol* 98: 334–44.

Brandt, E. and A. Pope (ed). 1997. *Enabling America: Assessing the role of rehabilitation science and engineering*. Washington, DC: National Academy.

Brown, R.F., T.E. Hullar, J.H. Cadieux, R.A. Chole. 2010. Residual hearing preservation after pediatric cochlear implantation. *Otol Neurotol* 31: 1221–6.

Brunton L., B. Knollman and R. Hilal-Dandan. 2017. *Goodman and Gilman's: The Pharmacological Basis of Therapeutics*, 13th Edition. New York: McGraw-Hill Education.

Buchman, C.A., J. Joy, A. Hodges, F.F. Telischi, T.J. Balkany. 2004. Vestibular effects of cochlear implantation. *Laryngoscope* 114, no. 103: 1–22.

Burkard, R. F. and M. Don. 2015. Introduction to auditory evoked potentials. In *Handbook of clinical audiology*, ed. J. Katz, 187–206. Philadelphia, PA: Wolters Kluwer.

Burton, H., A. Wineland, M. Bhattacharya, J. Nicklaus, K.S. Garcia, J.F. Piccirillo. 2012. Altered networks in bothersome tinnitus: a functional connectivity study. *BMC Neurosci* 13, no. 3: 1–15.

Campbell, J. and A. Sharma. 2013 Compensatory changes in cortical resource allocation in adults with hearing loss. *Front Syst Neurosci* 7: 71.

Campbell, J. and A. Sharma. 2014. Cross-modal re-organization in adults with early stage hearing loss. *PLOS ONE* 9, no. 2: e90594.

Cardon, G. and A. Sharma. 2018. Somatosensory cross-modal reorganization in adults with age-related, early-stage hearing loss. *Front Hum Neurosci* 12: 172.

Carlsson, P.I., J. Hjaldahl., A. Magnuson et al. 2015. Severe to profound hearing impairment: quality of life, psychosocial consequences and audiological rehabilitation. *Disabil Rehabil* 37, no. 20: 1849–56.

Chang, Y.M., S.H. Lee, Y.J. Lee et al. 2004. Auditory neural pathway evaluation on sensorineural hearing loss using diffusion tensor imaging. *Neuroreport* 15, no. 11: 1699–703.

Cheeran, B., P. Talelli, F. Mori et al. 2008. A common polymorphism in the brain-derived neurotrophic factor gene (BDNF) modulates human cortical plasticity and the response to rTMS. *J Physiol* 586, no. 23: 5717–25.

Chen L.C., P. Sandmann, J. Thorne, M. Bleichner, S. Debener. 2016. Cross-modal functional reorganization of visual and auditory cortex in adult cochlear implant users identified with fNIRS. *Neural Plast* 2016:4382656.

Chen, L.C., M. Stropahl, M. Schönwiesner, S. Debener. 2017. Enhanced visual adaptation in cochlear implant users revealed by concurrent EEG-fNIRS. *Neuroimage* 146: 600–8.

Ching, T.Y.C., H. Dillon, D. Byrne. 1998. Speech recognition of hearing-impaired listeners: Prediction from audibility and the limited role of high-frequency amplification. *J Acoust Soc Am* 103: 1128–40.

Ching, T. and M. Hill. 2007. The Parents' Evaluation of Aural/Oral Performance of Children (PEACH) scale: normative data. *J Am Acad Audiol* 18: 220–35.

Chisolm, T.H., C.E. Johnson, J.L. Danhauer et al. 2007. A systematic review of health-related quality of life and hearing aids: final report of the American Academy of Audiology Task Force on the Health-Related Quality of Life Benefits of Amplification in Adults. *J Am Acad Audiol* 18: 151–83.

Cho, H. S., K.-Y. Lee, H. Choi, J. H. Jang, and S. H. Lee. 2016. Dexamethasone is one of the factors minimizing the inner ear damage from electrode insertion in cochlear implantation. *Audiol Neuro-Otol* 21, no. 3: 178–86.

Choi, C.H. and J.S. Oghalai. 2005. Predicting the effect of post-implant cochlear fibrosis on residual hearing. *Hearing Res* 205: 193–200.

Chole, R.A., T.E. Hullar, L.G. Potts. 2014. Conductive component after cochlear implantation in patients with residual hearing conservation. *Am J Audiol* 23: 359–64.

Chrousos, G. P. 2015. Adrenocorticosteroids & adrenocortical antagonists. In *Basic & clinical pharmacology*, ed. B.G. Katzung and A.J. Trevor, 680–95. New York: McGraw-Hill Companies, Inc.

Cieśla, K., M. Lewandowska, H. Skarżyński. 2016. Health-related quality of life and mental distress in patients with partial deafness: preliminary findings. *Eur Arch Oto-Rhino-L* 273, no. 3: 767–76.

Ciorba, A., S. Hatzopoulos, M. Busi, P. Guerrini, J. Petruccelli, A. Martini. 2008. The universal newborn hearing screening program at the University Hospital of Ferrara: focus on costs and software solutions. *Int J Pediatr Otorhi* 72, no. 6: 807–16.

Colebatch, J.G. and G.M. Halmagyi. 1992. Vestibular evoked potentials in human neck muscles before and after unilateral vestibular deafferention. *Neurology* 42: 1635–6.

Colletti, V., S.D. Soli, M. Carner, L. Colletti. 2006. Treatment of mixed hearing losses via implantation of a vibratory transducer on the round window. *Int J Audiol* 45, no. 10: 600–8.

Coninx, F., V. Weichbold, L. Tsiakpini et al. 2009. Validation of the LittlEARS® Auditory Questionnaire in children with normal hearing. *Int J Pediatr Otorhi* 73: 1761–8.

Coordes, A., D. Basta, R. Götze et al. 2012. Sound-induced vertigo after cochlear implantation. *Otol Neurotol* 33: 335–42.

Cullen, R.D., C. Higgins, E. Buss et al. 2004. Cochlear implantation in patients with substantial residual hearing. *Laryngoscope* 114: 2218–23.

Da Costa, S., W. van der Zwaag, J.P. Marques, R.S.J. Frackowiak, S. Clarke, M. Saenz. 2011. Human primary auditory cortex follows the shape of Heschl's gyrus. *J Neurosci* 31: 14067–75.

Davis, J.M., J. Elfenbein, R. Schum, R.A. Bentler. 1986. Effects of mild and moderate hearing impairments on language, educational, and psychosocial behavior of children. *J Speech Hear Disord* 51: 53–62.

de Graaf, R. and R.V. Bijl. 2002. Determinants of mental distress in adults with a severe auditory impairment: differences between prelingual and postlingual deafness. *Psychosom Med* 64: 61–70.

De Martino, F., M. Moerel, P.F. van de Moortele et al. 2013. Spatial organization of frequency preference and selectivity in the human inferior colliculus. *Nat Commun* 4: 1386.

Della Santina, Ch., A. Migliaccio, R. Hayden et al. 2010. Current and future management of bilateral loss of vestibular sensation: an update on the Johns Hopkins Multichannel Vestibular Prosthesis Project. *Cochlear Implants Int* 11 (Suppl. 2): 2–11.

Dettman, S.J., W.A. D'Costa, R.C. Dowell, E.J. Winton, K.L. Hill, S.S. Williams. 2004. Cochlear implants for children with significant residual hearing. *Arch Otolaryngol* 130: 612– 18.

Dettman, S.J., D. Pinder, R.J.S. Briggs, R.C. Dowell, J.R. Leigh. 2007. Communication development in children who receive the cochlear implant younger than 12 months: risks versus benefits. *Ear Hearing* 28 (2 Suppl.): 11S–18S.

Dick, F., T. Tierney, A. Lutti, O. Josephs, M.I. Sereno, N. Weiskopf. 2012. In vivo functional and myeloarchitectonic mapping of human primary auditory areas. *J Neurosci* 32: 16095–105.

Dietrich, V., M. Nieschalk, W. Stoll, R. Rajan, C. Pantev. 2001. Cortical reorganization in patients with high frequency cochlear hearing loss. *Hearing Res* 158, no. 1–2: 95–101.

Dillon H. 2001. *Hearing Aids*. Stuttgart: Thieme Publishers.

Dillon, B. and H. Pryce. 2020. What makes someone choose cochlear implantation? An exploration of factors that inform patient decision making. *Int J Audiol* 59: 1, 24–32.

Dimitrijevic A. and B. Cone. 2015. Auditory Steady-State Response. In *Handbook of clinical audiology*, ed. J. Katz, 267–95. Philadelphia, PA: Wolters Kluwer.

Domagała-Zyśk, E. 2015. [Social relations of deaf and hard-of-hearing persons in work environment] Relacje społeczne osób niesłyszących i słabosłyszących w środowisku pracy. *Człowiek – Niepełnosprawność – Społeczeństwo* 1, no. 27: 61–72 [Polish].

Donnelly, N., A. Bibas, D. Jiang et al. 2009. Effect of cochlear implant electrode insertion on middle-ear function as measured by intra-operative laser Doppler vibrometry. *J Laryngol Otol* 123: 723–9.

Dorman, M.F., R.H. Gifford. 2010. Combining acoustic and electric stimulation in the service of speech recognition. *Int J Audiol* 49, no. 12: 912–19.

Doucet, M.E., F. Bergeron, M. Lassonde, P. Ferron, F. Lepore. 2006. Cross-modal reorganization and speech perception in cochlear implant users. *Brain* 129, no. 12: 3376–83.

Douchement, D., A. Terranti, J. Lamblin, et al. 2015. Dexamethasone eluting electrodes for cochlear implantation: effect on residual hearing. *Cochlear Implants Int* 16, no. 4: 195–200.

Dowell, R.C., S.J. Dettman, P.J. Blamey, E.J. Barker, G.M. Clark. 2002. Speech perception outcomes in children using cochlear implants: prediction of long term outcomes. *Cochlear Implants Int* 3: 1–18.

du Feu, M. and C. Chovaz. 2014 *Mental Health and Deafness*. Oxford: Oxford University Press.

du Feu, M. and K. Fergusson. 2003. Sensory impairment and mental health. *Adv Psychiatr Treat* 9, no. 2: 95–103.

Dziembowska, M., J. Milek, A. Janusz et al. 2012. Activity-dependent local translation of matrix metalloproteinase-9. *J Neuroscience* 32: 14538–47.

Dzwonkowska, I., K. Łachowicz-Tabaczek, M. Łaguna. 2008. [*Self-Esteem and Its Measurement. Polish Adaptation of the M. Rosenberg SES Scale*] *Samoocena i jej pomiar. Polska adaptacja skali SES M. Rosenberga*. Warsaw: Pracownia Testów Psychologicznych.

Eggermont, J.J. 1991. Frequency dependent maturation of the cochlea and brainstem evoked potentials. *Acta Oto-Laryngol* 111: 220–4.

Eggermont, J.J. 2017. Acquired hearing loss and brain plasticity. *Hearing Res* 343: 176–90.

Eggermont, J. J., D. K. Brown, C.W. Ponton, B.P. Kimberley. 1996. Comparison of distortion product otoacoustic emission (DPOAE) and auditory brainstem response (ABR) traveling wave delay measurements suggests frequency-specific synapse maturation. *Ear Hearing* 17: 386–94.

Eggermont, J.J. and J.K. Moore. 2012. Morphological and Functional Development of the Auditory Nervous System. In *Human auditory development*, ed. L. Werner, R.R. Fay, A.N. Popper, 61–106. New York: Springer.

Eisenberg, L. S., K.I. Kirk, A.S. Martinez et al. 2004. Communication abilities of children with aided residual hearing. Comparison with cochlear implant users. *Arch Otolaryngol* 130: 563–9.

Eisenberg, L., A. Schaefer-Martinez, G. Sennarouglu. 1998. Establishing new criteria in selecting children for a cochlear implant: performance of platinum hearing aid users. *Paper Presented at the 7th Symposium on Cochlear Implants in Children*, Iowa City.

Elfenbein, J.L., M.A. Hardin-Jones, J.M. Davis. 1994. Oral communication skills of children who are hard of hearing. *J Speech Hear Res* 37: 216–26.

Eshraghi, A.A. Prevention of cochlear implant electrode damage. 2006. *Curr Opin Otolaryngo* 14: 323–8.

Eshragi, A.A., D.M. Lang, J. Roell et al. 2015. Mechanisms of programmed cell death signaling in hair cells and support cells post-electrode insertion trauma. *Acta Oto-Laryngol* 135: 328–34.

Estabrooks, W., H.M. Morrison, K. MacIver-Lux. 2020. *Auditory-Verbal Therapy: An Overview. Auditory-Verbal Therapy: Science, Research, and Practice*. San Diego: Plural Publishing, Inc.

Ethel, I.M. and D.W. Ethel. 2007. Matrix metalloproteinases in brain development and remodeling: synaptic functions and targets. *J Neurosci Res* 85, no. 13: 2913–23.

Fellinger, J., D. Holzinger, J. Gerich et al. 2007. Mental distress and quality of life in the hard of hearing. *Acta Psychiat Scand* 115: 243–5.

Fellinger, J., D. Holzinger, R. Pollard. 2012. Mental health of deaf people. *Lancet* 379: 1037–44.

Ferrer-Ferrer M. and A. Ditaytev. 2018. Shaping synapses by the neural extracellular matrix. *Front Neuroanat* 12: 40.

Fina, M., M. Skinner, J.A. Goebel et al. 2003. Vestibular dysfunction after cochlear implantation. *Otol Neurotol* 24: 234–42.

Finley, C.C., T.A. Holden, L.K. Holden et al. 2008. Role of electrode placement as a contributor to variability in cochlear implant outcomes. *Otol Neurotol* 29, no. 7: 920–8.

Fitzpatrick E., R. McCrae, D. Schramm. 2006. A retrospective study of cochlear implant outcomes in children with residual hearing. *BMC Ear Nose Throat Disord* 6, no. 1: 7.

Fowler, E.P. 1950. Sudden deafness. *Ann Oto Rhinol Laryn* 59, no. 4: 980–7.

Franck, J.J. 1980. Functional reorganization of cat somatic sensory-motor cortex (SmI) after selective dorsal root rhizotomies. *Brain Res* 186: 923–44.

Fraysse, B., A. Ramos Macias, O. Sterkers et al. 2006. Residual hearing conservation and electroacoustic stimulation with the nucleus 24 contour advance cochlear implant. *Otol Neurotol* 27: 624–33.

Friedmann. D.R., R. Peng, Y. Fang, S.O. McMenomey, J.T. Roland, S.B. Waltzman S.B. 2015. Effects of loss of residual hearing on speech performance with the CI422 and the Hybrid-L electrode. *Cochlear Implants Int* 16, no. 5: 277–84.

Gantz, B.J. and L.S. Davidson. 2006. Effects of stimulus level on the speech perceptionabilities of children using cochlear implants or digital hearing aids. *Ear Hearing* 27: 493–507.

Gantz, B.J., J.T. Rubinstein, R.S. Tyler et al. 2000. Long-term results of cochlear implants in children with residual hearing. *Ann Oto Rhinol Laryn Suppl.* 185: 33–36.

Gantz, B.J. and C.W. Turner. 2003. Combining acoustic and electric hearing. *Laryngoscope* 113: 1726–30.

Gantz, B.J. and C.W. Turner. 2004. Combining acoustic and electrical speech processing: Iowa/Nucleus hybrid implant. *Acta Oto-Laryngol* 124: 344–47.

Gantz, B.J., C. Turner, K. Gfeller. 2004. Expanding cochlear implant technology: combined electrical and acoustical speech processing. *Cochlear Implants Int* 5 (Suppl. 1): 8–14.

Gantz, B.J., C. Turner, K.E. Gfeller, M.W. Lowder. 2005. Preservation of hearing in cochlear implant surgery: advantages of combined electrical and acoustical speech processing. *Laryngoscope* 115: 796–802.

García Negro, A.S., J.L. Padilla Garcia, M. Sainz Quevedo. 2016. Production and evaluation of a Spanish version of the LittlEARS Auditory Questionnaire for the assessment of auditory development in children. *Int J Pediatr Otorhi* 83: 99–103.

Geal-Dor, M., R. Jbarah, S. Meilijson, C. Adelman, H. Levi. 2011. The Hebrew and the Arabic version of the LittlEARS® Auditory Questionnaire for the assessment of auditory development: results in normal hearing children and children with cochlear implants. *Int J Pediatr Otorhi* 75: 1327–32.

Gifford, R.H., M.F. Dorman, H. Skarżyński et al. 2013. Cochlear implantation with hearing preservation yields significant benefit for speech recognition in complex listening environments. *Ear Hearing* 34, no. 4: 413–25.

Gifford, R.H., M.F. Dorman, A.J. Spahr, S.P. Bacon, H. Skarżyński, A. Lorens. 2008. Hearing preservation surgery: psychophysical estimates of cochlear damage in recipients of a short electrode array. *J Acoust Soc Am* 124, no. 4: 2164–73.

Gillespie, M.B. and L.B. Minor. 1999. Prognosis in bilateral vestibular hypofunction. *Laryngoscope* 109: 35–41.

Gilley, P.M., A. Sharma, M.F. Dorman. 2008. Cortical reorganization in children with cochlear implants. *Brain Res* 1239: 56–65.

Giordano, P., S. Hatzopoulos, N. Giarbini et al. 2014. A soft-surgery approach to minimize hearing damage caused by the insertion of a cochlear implant electrode: a guinea pig animal model. *Otol Neurotol* 35: 1440–5.

Giraud, A.L, C.J. Price, J.M. Graham, R.S. Frackowiak. 2001a. Functional plasticity of language-related brain areas after cochlear implantation. *Brain* 124(7): 1307–16.

Giraud, A.L., E. Truy, R.S.J. Frackowiak. 2001b. Imaging plasticity in cochlear implant patients. *Audiol Neuro-Otol* 6: 381–93.

Glasser, M.F. and D.C. Van Essen. 2011. Mapping human cortical areas in vivo based on myelin content as revealed by T1- and T2-weighted MRI. *J Neurosci* 31, no. 32: 11597–616.

Glick, H.A. and A. Sharma. 2020. Cortical neuroplasticity and cognitive function in early-stage, mild-moderate hearing loss: Evidence of neurocognitive benefit from hearing aid use. *Front Neurosci* 14: 93.

Gordon, K.A., B.C. Papsin, R.V. Harrison. 2006. An evoked potential study of the developmental time course of the auditory nerve and brain stem in children using cochlear implants. *Audiol Neuro-Otol* 11: 7–23.

Gorga, M.P., S.T. Neely, B.M. Bergman et al. 1993. A comparison of transient-evoked and distortion product otoacoustic emissions in normal-hearing and hearing-impaired subjects. *J Acoust Soc Am* 94, no. 5: 2639–48.

Grasel, S.S., E.R. de Almeida, R.M. Beck et al. 2015. Are auditory steady-state responses useful to evaluate severe-to-profound hearing loss in children? *Biomed Res Int* 2015: 579206.

Gratacap, M., B. Thierry, I. Rouillon, S. Marlin, N. Garabedian, N. Loundon. 2015. Pediatric cochlear implantation in residual hearing candidates. *Ann Oto Rhinol Laryn* 124, no. 6: 443–51.

Greene, N.T., J.K. Mattingly, H.A. Jenkins, D.J. Tollin, J.R. Easter, S.P. Cass. 2015. Cochlear implant electrode effect on sound energy transfer within the cochlea during acoustic stimulation. *Otol Neurotol* 36: 1554–61.

Greenwood, D.D. 1997. The Mel Scale's disqualifying bias and a consistency of pitch-difference equisections in 1956 with equal cochlear distances and equal frequency ratios. *Hearing Res* 103, no. 1–2: 199–224.

Gstoettner, W.K., J. Kiefer, W. Baumgartner, S. Pok, S. Peters, O. Adunka. 2004. Hearing preservation in cochlear implantation for electric acoustic stimulation. *Acta Oto-Laryngol* 124: 348–52.

Gstoettner, W.K., P. Van de Heyning, A.F. O'Connor et al. 2008. Electric acoustic stimulation of the auditory system: Results of a multi-centre investigation. *Acta Oto-Laryngol* 128, no. 9: 968–75.

Guiraud J., J. Besle, L. Arnold et al. 2007. Evidence of a tonotopic organisation of the auditory cortex in cochlear implant users. *J Neurosci* 27, no. 29: 7838–46.

Hall, D.A. 2014. Editorial. Special issue in Hearing Research: human auditory neuroimaging, *Hearing Res* 307: 1–3.

Hall, D.A., C.P. Lanting, D.E.H. Hartley. 2014. Using fMRI to Examine Central Auditory Plasticity. In *Advanced brain neuroimaging topics in health and disease – methods and application*, ed. D. Papageorgiou, G.I. Christopoilos, S.M. Smirnakis, London: IntechOpen.

Halpin, S. and S.D. Rauch. 2009. Clinical implications of a damaged cochlea: pure tone thresholds vs. information-carrying capacity. *Otolaryng Head Neck* 140, no. 4: 473–6.

Hamid, M. and D. Trune. 2008. Issues, indications, and controversies regarding intratympanic steroid perfusion. *Curr Opin Otolaryngo* 16, no. 5: 434–40.

Hamzavi, J., W.D. Baumgartner, S.M. Pok, P. Franz, W. Gstöttner W.K. 2003. Variables affecting speech perception in postlingually deaf adults following cochlear implantation. *Acta Oto-Laryngol* 123: 493–98.

Han, J.H., H.J. Lee, H.J. Kang, S.H. Oh, D.S. Lee. 2019. Brain plasticity can predict the cochlear implant outcome in adult-onset deafness. *Front Hum Neurosci* 13: 38.

Hariri, A.R., T.E. Goldberg, V.S. Mattay et al. 2003. Brain-derived neurotrophic factor val 66 met polymorphism affects human memory-related hippocampal activity and predicts memory performance. *J Neurosci* 23, no. 17: 6690–94.

Harris, P.K., K.M. Hutchinson, J. Moravec. 2005. The use of tympanometry and pneumatic otoscopy for predicting middle ear disease. *Am J Audiol* 14: 3–13.

Harrison, R.V., A. Nagasawa, D.W. Smith, S.G. Stanton, R.J. Mount. 1991. Reorganization of auditory cortex after neonatal high frequency cochlear hearing loss. *Hearing Res* 54: 11–19.

Hatliński, G.J., K. Kochanek, A. Piłka, W. Bochenek. 2008. Application of tone-pip stimuli of different rise-times for wave V identification in auditory brainstem responses (ABR) procedures. *Biocybern Biomed Eng* 28, no. 4: 51–7.

Hatzopoulos, S., J. Petruccelli, L. Śliwa, W.W. Jędrzejczak, K. Kochanek, H. Skarżyński. 2012. Hearing threshold prediction with Auditory Steady State Responses and estimation of correction functions to compensate for differences with behavioral data, in adult subjects. Part 1: Audera and Chartr EP devices. *Med Sci Monitor* 18, no. 7: 47–53.

Hatzopoulos, S., S. Prosser, A. Ciorba et al. 2010. Threshold estimation in adult normal- and impaired hearing subjects using auditory steady-state responses. *Med Sci Monitor* 16, no. 1: 21–7.

Hebart, M.N. and G. Hesselmann. 2012. What visual information is processed in the human dorsal stream? *J Neurosci* 32, no. 24: 8107–9.

Herdener M., F. Esposito, K. Scheffler et al. 2013. Spatial representations of temporal and spectral sound cues in human auditory cortex. *Cortex* 49, no. 10: 2822–33.

Herholz, S.C. and R.J. Zatorre. 2012. Musical training as a framework for brain plasticity: behavior, function, and structure. *Neuron* 76, no. 3: 486–502.

Hertz, U. and A. Amedi, 2010. Disentangling unisensory and multisensory components in audiovisual integration using a novel multifrequency fMRI spectral analysis. *Neuroimage* 52: 617–32.

Hickok, G. and D. Poeppel. 2007. The cortical organization of speech processing. *Nat Rev Neurosci* 8, no. 5: 393–402.

Hinderink, J.B., P.F. Krabbe, P. Van Den Broek. 2000. Development and application of a health-related quality-of-life instrument for adults with cochlear implants: the Nijmegen cochlear implant questionnaire. *Otolaryng Head Neck* 123, no. 6: 756–65.

Holt, R.F. and M.A. Svirsky. 2008. An exploratory look at pediatric cochlear implantation: is earliest always best? *Ear Hearing* 29, no. 4: 492–511.

Holtmaat, A. and P. Caroni. 2016. Functional and structural underpinnings of neuronal assembly formation in learning. *Nat Neurosci* 19, no. 12: 1553–62.

Honeder, C., C. Zhu, H. Schöpper, et al. 2016. Effects of sustained release dexamethasone hydrogels in hearing preservation cochlear implantation. *Hearing Res* 341: 43–9.

Hribar, M., D. Suput, A.A Carvalho, S. Battelino, A. Vovk. 2014. Structural alterations of brain grey and white matter in early deaf adults. *Hearing Res* 318: 1–10.

Humphries, C., E. Liebenthal, J.R. Binder. 2010. Tonotopic organization of human auditory cortex. *Neuroimage* 50, no. 3: 1202–11.

Hunter, L.L. and C.A. Sanford. 2012. Tympanometry and Wideband Acoustic Immittance. In *Handbook of clinical audiology*, ed. J. Katz, 137–65. Philadelphia, PA: Wolters Kluwer.

Hunter, L.L. and N. Shahnaz. 2014. *Acoustic Immittance Measures. Basic and Advanced Practice*. San Diego, CA: Plural Publishing.

Huttenlocher, P.R. and A.S. Dabholkar. 1997. Regional differences in synaptogenesis in human cerebral cortex. *J Comp Neurol* 387, no. 2: 167–78.

Ilberg C. von, J. Kiefer, J. Tillein et al. 1999. Electric-acoustic stimulation of the auditory system. New technology for severe hearing loss. *ORL J Oto-Rhino-Lary* 61, no. 6: 334–40.

Illing, R.B. and N. Rosskothen-Kuhl. 2008. The Cochlear Implant in Action: molecular changes induced in the rat central auditory system. Cochlear implant research updates. In *Cochlear implant research updates*, ed. C. Umat and R.A. Tange. London: IntechOpen.

Incerti, P.V., T.Y.C. Ching, R. Cowan. 2013. A systematic review of electric-acoustic stimulation: device fitting ranges, outcomes, and clinical fitting practices. *Trends Amplif* 17, no. 1: 3–26.

Interacoustics. 2020. Titan v.3.3. Instructions for use. http://www.interacoustics. com/download/titan/titan-manuals/260-instructions-for-use-titan-en/file.

International Test Commission. 2000. International Guidelines for Test Use. http://www. intestcom.org.

Ito, J. 1998. Influence of the multichannel cochlear implant on vestibular function. *Otolaryng Head Neck* 118, no. 6: 900–2.

Izquierdo, M.A., P.M. Gutierrez-Conde, M.A. Merchan, M.S. Malmierca. 2008. Non-plastic reorganization of frequency coding in the inferior colliculus of the rat following noise-induced hearing loss. *Neuroscience* 154, no. 1: 355–69.

Jacobson, G., D. McCaslin, E. Piker, J. Gruenwald, S. Grantham, L. Tegel. 2011. Patterns of abnormality in cVEMP, oVEMP, and Caloric Teste may provide topological information about vestibular impairment. *J Am Acad Audiol* 22: 601–11.

James, C.J., K. Albegger, R. Battmer et al. 2005. Preservation of residual hearing with cochlear implantation: how and why. *Acta Oto-Laryngol* 125: 481–91.

James, C.J., B. Fraysse, O. Deguine. 2006. Combined electroacoustic stimulation in conventional candidates for cochlear implantation. *Audiol Neuro-Otol* 11 (Suppl. 1): 57–62.

Jedrzejczak, W.W., K. Kochanek, B. Trzaskowski, E. Piłka, P.H. Skarżyński, H. Skarżyński. 2012. Tone-burst and click-evoked otoacoustic emissions in subjects with hearing loss above 0.25, 0.5, and 1 kHz. *Ear Hearing* 33, no. 6: 757–67.

Jedrzejczak, W.W., W. Konopka, K. Kochanek, H. Skarżyński. 2015a. Otoacoustic emissions in newborns evoked by 0.5 kHz tone bursts. *Int J Pediatr Otorhi* 79, no. 9: 1522–6.

Jedrzejczak, W.W., A. Lorens, A. Piotrowska, K. Kochanek, H. Skarżyński. 2009. Otoacoustic emissions evoked by 0.5 kHz tone bursts. *J Acoust Soc Am* 125, no. 5: 3158–65.

Jedrzejczak, W.W., E. Piłka, P.H. Skarżyński, L. Olszewski, H. Skarżyński. 2015b. Tone burst evoked otoacoustic emissions in different age-groups of schoolchildren. *Int J Pediatr Otorhi* 79, no. 8: 1310–5.

Jedrzejczak, W.W., A. Piotrowska, K. Kochanek, L. Śliwa, H. Skarżyński. 2013. Low-frequency otoacoustic emissions in schoolchildren measured by two commercial devices. *Int J Pediatr Otorhi* 77, no. 10: 1724–8.

Jeng, P.S., J.B. Allen, J.A. Lapsley Miller, H. Levitt. 2008. Wideband power reflectance and power transmittance as tools for assessing middle-ear function. *ASHA Perspect Hear Hear Disord Childhood* 18, no. 2: 44–57.

Kaas, J.H. and T.A. Hackett. 2000. Subdivision of auditory cortex and processing streams in primates. *P Natl Acad Sci USA* 90, no. 22: 11793–9.

Kaas, J.H., M.M. Merzenich, H.P. Killackey. 1983. The reorganization of somatosensory cortex following peripheral nerve damage in adult and developing mammals. *Annu Rev Neurosci* 6: 325–56.

Kandogan, T. and A. Dalgic. 2012. Reliability of Auditory Steady-State Response (ASSR): Comparing Thresholds of Auditory Steady-State Response (ASSR) with Auditory Brainstem Response (ABR) in Children with Severe Hearing Loss. *Indian J Otolaryngol* 65 (Suppl. 3): 604–7.

Keefe, D.H., K.L. Archer, K.K. Schmid, D.F. Fitzpatrick, M.P. Feeney, L.L. Hunter. 2017. Identifying otosclerosis with aural acoustical tests of absorbance, group delay, acoustic reflex threshold, and otoacoustic emissions. *J Am Acad Audiol* 28: 838–60.

Keefe, D.H. and J.L. Simmons. 2003. Energy transmittance predicts conductive hearing loss in older children and adults. *J Acoust Soc Am* 114, no. 6, Pt. 1: 3217–38.

Kemp, D.T. 1978. Stimulated acoustic emissions from within the human auditory system. *J Acoust Soc Am* 64, no. 5: 1386–91.

Kemp, D.T. 2002. Otoacoustic emissions, their origin in cochlear function, and use. *Brit Med Bull* 63: 223–41.

Kennedy, D.W. 1987. Multichannel intracochlear electrodes: mechanism of insertion trauma. *Laryngoscope* 97, no. 1: 42–9.

Kiefer, J., W. Gstöttner, W. Baumgartner, S.M. Pok, J. Tillein, Q. Ye, C. von Ilberg. 2004. Conservation of low frequency hearing in cochlear implantation. *Acta Oto-Laryngol* 4, no. 124: 272–80.

Kiefer, J., Ch. von Ilberg, B. Reimer et al. 1998. Results of cochlear implantation in patients with severe to profound hearing loss – Implications for patients selection. *Audiology* 37: 382–95.

Kim, B.G., J.W. Kim, J.J. Park, S.H. Kim, H.N. Kim, J.Y. Choi. 2015. Adverse events and discomfort during magnetic resonance imaging in cochlear implant recipients. *JAMA Otolaryngol* 141, no. 1: 45–52.

Kim, Y.S., S.A. Han, H. Woo, et al. 2019. Effects of residual hearing on the auditory steady state response for cochlear implantation in children. *J Audiol Otol* 23, no. 3: 153–9.

King, A.J., S. Teki, B.D.B. Willmore. 2018. Recent advances in understanding the auditory cortex. *F1000Research* 7 (F1000 Faculty Rev): 1555.

Kobosko, J. 2015. [The experience of disability vs. self-esteem and depression symptoms in postlingually deaf adults using cochlear implants] Poczucie niepełnosprawności a percepcja siebie i objawy depresji u osób dorosłych z głuchotą postlingwalną korzystających z implantu ślimakowego. *Now Audiofonol* 4, no. 1: 41–54 [Polish].

Kobosko, J. 2018. [Persons with partial deafness using the CI vs. self-esteem and stress-coping strategies] Osoby z częściową głuchotą korzystające z CI a samoocena i strategie radzenia sobie ze stresem. Unpublished study results.

Kobosko, J., A. Geremek-Samsonowicz, B. Kochański, A. Pankowska, H. Skarżyński. 2019a. [Acceptance of self as a deaf person vs. subjective assessment of cochlear implant benefits and satisfaction in adults with prelingual deafness]. Akceptacja siebie jako osoby głuchej a subiektywna ocena korzyści i satysfakcji z implantu ślimakowego u osób dorosłych z głuchotą prelingwalną. *Now Audiofonol* 8, no. 4: 22–31 [Polish].

Kobosko, J., W.W. Jedrzejczak, A. Barej, A. Pankowska, A. Geremek-Samsonowicz, H. Skarżyński. 2020. Cochlear implants in adults with partial deafness: subjective benefits but associated psychological distress. *Eur Arch Oto-Rhino-L.* Online ahead of print.

Kobosko, J., W.W. Jedrzejczak, A. Geremek-Samsonowicz, A. Pankowska, H. Skarżyński. 2019b. [Mental health and deafness – study of the adult cochlear implant users with partial or profound deafness using the GHQ-28 questionnaire] Zdrowie psychiczne a głuchota – badania nad dorosłymi użytkownikami implantu ślimakowego z głuchotą częściową lub głęboką z wykorzystaniem kwestionariusza GHQ-28. *Poster presented at the APS Conference*, Warsaw [Polish].

Kobosko, J., W.W. Jedrzejczak, E. Gos, A. Geremek-Samsonowicz, M. Ludwikowski, H. Skarżyński. 2018. Self-esteem in the deaf who have become cochlear implant users as adults. *PLOS ONE* 13, no. 9: e0203680.

Kobosko, J., W.W. Jedrzejczak, W. Pilka, A. Pankowska, H. Skarżyński. 2015. Satisfaction with cochlear implants in postlingually deaf adults and its nonaudiological predictors: psychological distress, coping strategies, and self-esteem. *Ear Hearing* 36, no. 5: 605–18.

Kobosko, J., A. Pankowska, Ł. Olszewski, A. Geremek-Samsonowicz, H. Skarżyński. 2017. [Subjective and objective assessment of cochlear implant benefits in adults with partial deafness of prelingual onset] Subiektywna i obiektywna ocena korzyści z implantu ślimakowego u osób dorosłych z częściową głuchotą o początku prelingwalnym. *Now Audiofonol* 6, no. 4: 31–42 [Polish].

Kochanek, K. 2000. Evaluation of hearing threshold with application of auditory brainstem potentials in frequency range of 500–4000 Hz. *PhD Diss.*, Medical University of Warsaw.

Kochanek, K., G. Janczewski, H. Skarżyński, A. Grzanka, E. Orkan-Łęcka, A. Piłka. 2000a. [The Relationship Between Hearing Sensitivity and ABR Thresholds in Group of Subjects with Different Configuration of Audiogram] Związek pomiędzy progiem słyszenia i progiem odpowiedzi ABR w różnych konfiguracjach audiogramów osób z ubytkami słuchu typu ślimakowego. *Audiofonologia* 18: 73–88 [Polish].

Kochanek, K., G. Janczewski, H. Skarżyński, A. Grzanka, A. Piłka, W. Orkan-Łęcka. 2000b. [The normative values of wave V latency-intensity functions of auditory brainstem responses elicited by click and 500 and 1000 Hz tone pips] Normy latencji fali V słuchowych potencjałów wywołanych pnia mózgu dla trzasku oraz krótkich tonów o częstotliwościach 500 I 1000 Hz. *Audiofonologia* 18: 167–76 [Polish].

Kochanek, K., A. Piłka, E. Orkan-Łęcka, L. Śliwa, H. Skarżyński. 2015. [The concept of ABR method for detection of retrocochlear hearing impairments based on responses evoked by tone pips] Koncepcja metody słuchowych potencjałów wywołanych pnia mózgu z wykorzystaniem krótkich tonów dla potrzeb wykrywania zaburzeń pozaślimakowych słuchu. *Otorynolaryngologia* 14, no. 3: 127–35 [Polish].

Koka, K., A.A. Saoji, L.M. Litwak. 2017. Electrocochleography in cochlear implant recipients with residual hearing: comparison with audiometric thresholds. *Ear Hearing* 38, no. 3: e161–e167.

Konorski J. 1948. *Conditioned Reflexes and Neuron Organization*. New York: Cambridge University Press.

Korver A.M.H., R.J.H. Smith, G. Van Camp et al. 2017. Congenital hearing loss. *Nat Rev Dis Primers* 3: 16094.

Krakowiak, K., E. Muzyka, P. Wojda. 2009. [How to talk with a hard-of-hearing person? – conditions for effective communication] Jak rozmawiać z osobą niesłyszącą? – warunki skutecznej komunikacji. In [*Deaf and hard-of-hearing young adults in a family and surrounding world – for therapists, teachers, educators and parents*] *Młodzież głucha i słabosłysząca w rodzinie i otaczającym świecie – dla terapeutów, nauczycieli, wychowawców i rodziców*, ed. J. Kobosko, 199–211. Warszawa: Stowarzyszenie Usłyszeć Świat.

Kral, A. and J.J. Eggermont. 2007. What's to lose and what's to learn: Development under auditory deprivation, cochlear implants and limits of cortical plasticity. *Brain Res Rev* 56, no. 1: 259–69.

Kral, A., R. Hartmann, J. Tillein, S. Heid, R. Klinke. 2000. Congenital auditory deprivation reduces synaptic activity within the auditory cortex in a layer-specific manner. *Cereb Cortex* 10: 714–26.

Kral A., W.G. Kronenberger, D.B. Pisoni, G.M. O'Donoghue. 2016. Neurocognitive factors in sensory restoration of early deafness: a connectome model. *Lancet Neurol* 15, no. 6: 610–21.

Kral, A., and G.M. O'Donoghue. 2010. Profound deafness in childhood. *N Engl J Med* 363, no. 15: 1430–50.

Kral, A. and A. Sharma. 2012. Developmental neuroplasticity after cochlear implantation. *Trends Neurosci* 35, no. 2: 111–22.

Kral, A. and J. Tillein. 2006. Brain plasticity under cochlear implant stimulation. In *Cochlear and brainstem implants*, ed. A.R. Møller, 89–108. Basel: Karger.

Kral, A., P. A. Yusuf, R. Land. 2017. Higher-order auditory areas in congenital deafness: Top-down interactions and corticocortical decoupling. *Hearing Res* 343: 50–63.

Krause, E., J.P.R. Louza, J. Wechtenbruch, R. Gürkov. 2010. Influence of cochlear implantation on peripheral vestibular receptor function. *Otolaryng Head Neck* 142, no. 6: 809–13.

Krause, E., J. Wechtenbruch, T. Rader, R. Gürkov. 2009. Influence of cochlear implantation on sacculus function. *Otolaryng Head Neck* 140, no. 1: 108–13.

Kronenberger, W.G., J. Beer, I. Castellanos et al. 2014. Neurocognitive risk in children with cochlear implants. *JAMA Otolaryngol* 140: 608–15.

Kübler-Ross, E. 2007. [*Conversations about Death and Dying*] *Rozmowy o śmierci i umieraniu*. Poznań: Media Rodzina [Polish].

Kubo, T., K. Yamamoto, T. Iwaki et al. 2001. Different forms of dizziness occurring after cochlear implant. *Eur Arch Oto-Rhino-L* 258: 9–12.

Kusuma, S., S. Liou, D.S. Haynes. 2005. Disequilibrium after cochlear implantation caused by a perilymph fistula. *Laryngoscope* 115, no. 1: 25–6.

Kvam, M.H., M. Loeb, K. Tambs. 2007. Mental health in deaf adults: symptoms of anxiety and depression among hearing and deaf individuals. *J Deaf Stud Deaf Edu* 12: 1–7.

Lamblin, N., C. Bauters, X. Hermant, J.-M. Lablanche, N. Helbecque, P. Amouyel. 2002. Polymorphisms in the promoter regions of MMP-2, MMP-3, MMP-9 and MMP-12 genes as determinants of aneurysmal coronary artery disease. *J Am Coll Cardiol* 40: 43–8.

Land, R., P. Baumhoff, J. Tillein, S.G. Lomber, P. Hubka, A. Kral. 2016. Cross-modal plasticity in higher-order auditory cortex of congenitally deaf cats does not limit auditory responsiveness to cochlear implants. *J Neurosci* 36, no. 23: 6175–85.

Lange, G. 1989. Gentamicin and other ototoxic antibiotics for the transtympanic treatment of Ménière's disease. *Arch Oto-Rhino-Laryn* 246, no. 5: 269–70.

Langers, D.R. and P. van Dijk. 2012. Mapping the tonotopic organization in human auditory cortex with minimally salient acoustic stimulation. *Cereb Cortex* 22: 2024–38 (E-pub 2011).

Langers, D.R., P. van Dijk, E.S. Schoenmaker, W.H. Backes. 2007. fMRI activation in relation to sound intensity and loudness. *Neuroimage* 35, no. 2: 709–18.

Langers, D., E. de Kleine, P. van Dijk. 2012. Tinnitus does not require macroscopic tonotopic map reorganization. *Front Syst Neurosci* 6: 1–15.

Langers, D.R., K. Krumbholz, R.W. Bowtell, D.A. Hall. 2014. Neuroimaging paradigms for tonotopic mapping (I): The influence of sound stimulus. *Neuroimage* 100: 650–62.

Lazard, D.S., A.L. Giraud, D. Gnansia, B. Meyer, O. Sterkers. 2012. Understanding the deafened brain: Implications for cochlear implant rehabilitation. *Eur Ann Otorhinolary* 129, no. 2: 98–103.

Lazard D.S., H.J. Lee, M. Gaebler, C.A. Kell, E. Truy, A.L. Giraud. 2010. Phonological processing in post-lingual deafness and cochlear implant outcome. *Neuroimage*, 49, no. 4: 3443–51.

Lazard D.S., H.J. Lee, E. Truy, A.L. Guiraud. 2013. Bilateral reorganization of posterior temporal cortices in post-lingual deafness and its relation to cochlear implant outcome. *Hum Brain Mapp* 34, no. 5: 1208–19.

Lee, J.S., D.S. Lee, S.H. Oh et al. 2003. PET evidence of neuroplasticity in adult auditory cortex of postlingual deafness. *J Nucl Med* 44: 1435–39.

Legris, E., J. Galvin, S. Roux et al. 2018. Cortical reorganization after cochlear implantation for adults with single-sided deafness. *PLOS ONE* 13, no. 9: e0204402.

Legris, E., S. Roux, J.-M. Aoustin, J. Galvin, D. Bakhos. 2019. Cortical auditory responses according to hearing rehabilitation in unilateral hearing loss. *Eur Ann Otorhinolary* 136, no. 6: 439–45.

Leigh, J., R. Farrell, D. Courtenaym, R. Dowell, R. Briggs. 2019. Relationship between objective and behavioral audiology for young children being assessed for cochlear implantation: implications for CI candidacy assessment. *Otol Neurotol* 40, no. 3: e252–e259.

Li, J.H., W.J. Li, J.F. Xian et al. 2012. Cortical thickness analysis and optimized voxel-based morphometry in children and adolescents with prelingually profound sensorineural hearing loss. *Brain Res* 1430: 35–42.

Liberman, M.C. and L.W. Dodds. 1984. Single-neuron labeling and chronic cochlear pathology. III. Stereocilia damage and alterations of threshold tuning curves. *Hearing Res* 16: 55–74.

Lichtenstein, V. and D.R. Stapells 1996. Frequency-specific identification of hearing loss using transient-evoked otoacoustic emissions to clicks and tones. *Hearing Res* 98, no. 1–2: 125–36.

Liebau, A. and S. K. Plontke. 2015. Lokale Medikamententherapie bei Innenohrschwerhörigkeit. *HNO* 63(6): 396–401.

Liebscher, T., K. Alberter, U. Hoppe. 2018. Cortical auditory evoked potentials in cochlear implant listeners via single electrode stimulation in relation to speech perception. *Int J Audiol* 57, no. 12: 939–46.

Limb, C.J., H.F. Francis, L.R. Lustig, J.K. Niparko, H. Jammal. 2005. Benign positional vertigo after cochlear implantation. *Otolaryng Head Neck* 132, no. 5: 741–45.

Liu, Y., C. Jolly, S. Braun et al. 2016. In vitro and in vivo pharmacokinetic study of a Dexamethasone-releasing silicone for cochlear implants. *Eur Arch Oto-Rhino-L* 273, no. 7: 1745–53.

Liu, Y.W., Ch.A. Sanford, J.C. Ellison, D.F. Fitzpatrick, M.P. Gorga, D.H. Keefe. 2008. Wideband absorbance tympanometry using pressure sweeps: system development and results on adults with normal hearing. *J Acoust Soc Am* 124, no. 6: 3708–19.

Livneh, H. 2016. Denial in medical conditions: a synopsis of its components. *Ann Psychiatry Ment Health* 4, no. 7: 1084.

Livneh, H., and R.F. Antonak. 2005. Psychosocial adaptation to chronic illness and disability: a primer for counselors. *J Couns Dev* 83, no. 1: 12–20.

Lorens, A. 2014. [Model of audiological rehabilitation after cochlar implantation based on the International Classification of Functioning, Disability and Health (ICF)] Model rehabilitacji audiologicznej po wszczepieniu implantu ślimakowego opracowany na podstawie

Międzynarodowej Klasyfikacji Funkcjonowania, Niepełnosprawności i Zdrowia (ICF). *Now Audiofonol* 3, no. 5: 77–90 [Polish].

Lorens, A., A. Geremek, A. Walkowiak, H. Skarżyński. 2000. Residual acoustic hearing before and after cochlear implantation. Paper presented at the 4th European Congress of Oto-Rhino-Laryngology Head and Neck Surgery "Past – Present – Future" EUFOS 2000, Berlin, Germany.

Lorens, A., A. Obrycka, H. Skarżyński. 2020. Assessment of early auditory development in children after cochlear implantation. In *Advances in Audiology and Hearing Science*, ed. S. Hatzopoulos, A. Ciorba, M. Krumm. Vol. 2, 3–24. Palm Bay, Florida: Apple Academic Press.

Lorens, A., A. Piotrowska, H. Skarżyński. 2004. Optimization of electric stimulation parameters in patients with partial deafness. *Proceedings of 8th World Multiconference on Systemics, Cybernetics and Informatics*. Orlando, USA.

Lorens, A., A. Piotrowska, H. Skarżyński, A. Obrycka. 2005. [Application of implantable prostheses in treatment of hearing impairments] Zastosowanie elektronicznych protez wszczepialnych w leczeniu niedosłuchów. *Polski Merkuriusz Lekarski* 19, no. 111: 487–89 [Polish].

Lorens, A., A. Piotrowska, A. Walkowiak, A. Czyżewski, L. Śliwa. 2001. The psychophysical measurements of frequency selectivity from cochlear implanted patients. *Structures – Waves – Biomedical Engineering* 10, no. 2:79–80.

Lorens, A., M. Polak, A. Piotrowska, H. Skarżyński. 2008. Outcomes of treatment of partial deafness with cochlear implantation: A DUET study. *Laryngoscope* 11892: 288–94.

Lorens, A., H. Skarżyński, A. Czyżewski. 1999. Frequency selectivity of the auditory nerve determined by the electric stimulation. Paper presented at the Audio Engineering Society (AES) 106 Convention, Munich, Germany. AES Paper 4875.

Lorens A., M. Zgoda, H. Skarżyński. 2012. A new audio processor for combined electric and acoustic stimulation for the treatment of partial deafness. *Acta Oto-Laryngol* 132, no. 7: 739–50.

Ma, W.D. and E.D. Young. 2006. Dorsal cochlear nucleus response properties following acoustic trauma: Response maps and spontaneous activity. *Hearing Res* 216–217: 176–88.

McCall, A. and B. Yates. 2011. Compensation following bilateral vestibular damage. *Front Neurol* 2: 88.

McDermott, H.J., M. Lech, M.S. Kornblum, and D.R.F. Irvine. 1998. Loudness perception and frequency discrimination in subjects with steeply sloping hearing loss: possible correlates of neural plasticity. *J Acoust Soc Am* 104, no. 4: 2314–25.

MacDougall, H.G., K.P. Weber, L.A. McGarvie, G.M. Halmagyi, I.S. Cuthoys. 2009. The video head impulse test: Diagnostic accuracy in peripheral vestibulopathy. *Neurology* 73: 1134–41.

Mäki-Torkko, E.M., S. Vestergren, H. Harder, B. Lyxell. 2015. From isolation and dependence to autonomy–expectations before and experiences after cochlear implantation in adult cochlear implant users and their significant others. *Disabil Rehabil* 37, no. 6: 541–7.

Makowska, Z. and D. Merecz. 2001. [Polish adaptation of Goldberg's general health questionnaires GHQ-12 and GHQ-28] Adaptacja ogólnego kwestionariusza zdrowia Goldberga GHQ-12 i GHQ-28 na język polski. In [*Mental health assessment using David Goldberg's questionnaires, Part 2*] Ocena zdrowia psychicznego na podstawie badań kwestionariuszami Davida Goldberga, cz. 2, ed. Z. Makowska and D. Merecz. Łódź: Oficyna Wydawnicza Instytutu Medycyny Pracy [Polish].

Manchaiah, V., G. Stein, B. Danermark et al. 2015. Positive, neutral, and negative connotations associated with social representation of 'hearing loss' and 'hearing aids'. *J Audiol Otol* 19, no. 3: 132–7.

Mandalà, M., L. Colletti, G. Tonoli, V. Colletti. 2012. Electrocochleography during cochlear implantation for hearing preservation. *Otolaryng Head Neck* 146, no. 5: 774–81.

Mangham, C.A. 1987. Effect of cochlear prostheses on vestibuloocular reflexes to rotation. *Ann Oto Rhinol Laryn* Suppl 12: 101–4.

Margolis, R.H. and L.L. Hunter. 1999. Tympanometry: basic principles and clinical practice. In *Contemporary Perspectives in Hearing Assessment*, ed. F.E Musiek and W.F. Rintelmann, 89–130. Boston, MA: Allyn and Bacon.

Meinzen-Derr, J., S. Wiley, J. Creighton, D. Choo. 2007. Auditory skills checklist: clinical tool for monitoring functional auditory skill development in young children with cochlear implants. *Ann Oto Rhinol Laryn* 116, no. 11: 812–18.

Meleca, R.J., J.A. Kaltenbach, P.R. Falzarano. 1997. Changes in the tonotopic map of the dorsal cochlear nucleus in hamsters with hair cell loss and radial nerve bundle degeneration. *Brain Res* 750, no. 1–2: 201–13.

Melvin, T.-A.N., C.C. Della Santina, J.P. Carey, A.A. Migliaccio. 2009. The effects of cochlear implantation on vestibular function. *Otol Neurotol* 30, no. 1: 87–94.

Ménard, M., S. Gallego, E. Truy, C. Berger-Vachon, J.D. Durrant, L. Collet. 2004. Auditory steady-state response evaluation of auditory thresholds in cochlear implant patients. *Int J Audiol* 43 (Suppl. 1): S39–43.

Merabet, L.B. and A. Pascual-Leone. 2010. Neural reorganization following sensory loss: the opportunity of change. *Nat Rev Neurosci* 11, no. 1: 44–52.

Merchant, G.R., J.H. Siegel, S.T. Neely, J.J. Rosowski, H.H. Nakajima. 2019. Effect of middle ear pathology on high-frequency ear-canal reflectance measurements in the frequency and time domains. *JARO-J Assoc Res Oto* 20: 529–52.

Merchant, G.R., K.M. Schulz, J.N. Patterson, D. Fitzpatrick, K.I. Janky. 2020. Effect of cochlear implantation on vestibular evoked myogenic potentials and wideband acoustic immittance. *Ear Hearing* 41, no. 5: 1111–24.

Meredith, M.A., H.R. Clemo, S.G. Lomber. 2017. Is territorial expansion a mechanism for crossmodal plasticity? *Eur J Neurosci* 45, no. 9: 1165–76.

Merzenich, M.M., J.H. Kaas, J.T. Wall, M. Sur, R.J. Nelson, D.J. Felleman. 1983a. Progression of change following median nerve section in the cortical representation of the hand in areas 3b and 1 in adult owl and squirrel monkeys. *Neuroscience* 10: 639–65.

Merzenich, M.M., J.H. Kaas, J.T. Wall, R.J. Nelson, M. Sur, D.J. Felleman. 1983b. Topographic reorganization of somatosensory cortical areas 3h and 1 in adult monkeys following restricted deafferentation. *Neuroscience* 8: 33–55.

Migliaccio, A.A., C.C. Della Santina, J.P. Carey, J.K. Niparko, L.B. Minor. 2005. The vestibulo-ocular reflex response to head impulses rarely decreases after cochlear implantation. *Otol Neurotol* 26, no. 4: 655–60.

Miller, G.A. and P.A. Nicely. 1955. An analysis of perceptual confusions among some English consonants. *J Acoust Soc Am* 27: 338–52.

Minichiello, L. 2009. TrkB signaling pathways in LTP and learning. *Nat Rev Neurosci* 10, no. 12: 850–60.

Moerel M., F. De Martino, E. Formisano. 2012. Processing of natural sounds in human auditory cortex: tonotopy, spectral tuning, and relation to voice sensitivity. *J Neurosci* 32, no. 41: 14205–16.

Mondain, M., M. Sillon, A. Vieu et al. 2002. Cochlear implantation in prelingually deafened children with residual hearing. *Int J Pediatr Otorhi* 63: 91– 7.

Moore, B.C.J. 1995. *Perceptual Consequences of Cochlear Damage*, New York: Oxford University Press.

Morest, D.K. and B.A. Bohne. 1983. Noise-induced degeneration in the brain and representation of inner and outer hair cells. *Hearing Res* 9, no. 2: 145–51.

Morosan, P., J. Rademacher, A. Schleicher, K. Amunts, T. Schormann, K. Zilles. 2001. Human primary auditory cortex: cytoarchitectonic subdivisions and mapping into a spatial reference system. *Neuroimage* 13, no. 4: 684–701.

Müller-Siekierska, D. 2019. [*Styles of Functioning of Young People with Hearing Loss in Close Interpersonal Relations*] *Style funkcjonowania młodych osób z uszkodzeniami słuchu w bliskich relacjach interpersonalnych*. Łódź: Wydawnictwo Uniwersytetu Łódzkiego [Polish].

Munck, A., P. M. Guyre and N. J. Holbrook. 1984. Physiological functions of glucocorticoids in stress and their relation to pharmacological actions. *Endocr Rev* 5, no. 1: 25–44.

Musiek, F.E. and J.A. Baran. 2020. *The Auditory System: Anatomy, Physiology, and Clinical Correlates.* 2nd edition. San Diego, CA: Plural Publishing.

Nagi, S.Z. 1991. Disability concepts revised: Implications for prevention. In *Disability in America: toward a national agenda for prevention*, ed. A. Pope A and A. Tarlov, 309–28. Washington, DC: National Academy Press.

Nagy, V., O. Bozdagi, A. Matynia et al. 2006. Matrix-metalloproteinase-9 is required for hippocampal late-phase long-term potentiation and memory. *J Neurosci* 26, no. 7: 1923–34.

Nakajima, H.H., J.J. Rosowski, N. Shanaz, L.L. Hunter. 2013. Assessment of ear disorders using power reflectance. *Ear Hearing* 34 (Suppl. 1): 48S–53S.

Neely, S.T., S.E. Fultz, J.G. Kopun, N.M. Lenzen, D.M. Rasetshwane. 2019. Cochlear reflectance and otoacoustic emission predictions of hearing loss. *Ear Hearing* 40, no. 4: 951–60.

Niparko, J.K., E.A. Tobey, D.J. Thal et al. 2010. Spoken language development in children following cochlear implantation. *JAMA* 303, no. 15: 1498–506.

Norbury, C.F., D.V. Bishop, J. Briscoe. 2001. Production of English finite verb morphology: a comparison of SLI and mild-moderate hearing impairment. *J Speech Lang Hear R* 44: 165–78.

Norman-Haignere, S., N. Kanwisher, J.H. McDermott. 2013. Cortical pitch regions in humans respond primarily to resolved harmonics and are located in specific tonotopic regions of anterior auditory cortex. *J Neurosci* 33: 19451–69.

Norton, S.J., M.P. Gorga, J.E. Widen et al. 2000. Identification of neonatal hearing impairment: summary and recommendations. *Ear Hearing* 21, no. 5: 529–35.

O'Leary, M.J., J. Fayad, W.F. House, F.H. Linthicum. 1991. Electrode insertion trauma in cochlear implantation. *Ann Oto Rhinol Laryn* 100: 695–99.

Obrycka, A., A. Lorens, J.L. Padilla García, A. Piotrowska, H. Skarżyński. 2017. Validation of the LittlEARS Auditory Questionnaire in cochlear implanted infants and toddlers. *Int J Pediatr Otorhi* 93: 107–16.

Obrycka, A., J.L. Padilla Garcia, A. Pankowska, A. Lorens, H. Skarżyński. 2009. Production and evaluation of a Polish version of the LittlEars questionnaire for the assessment of auditory development in infants. *Int J Pediatr Otorhi* 73: 1035–42.

Obrycka, A., J.L. Padilla Garcia, J. Putkiewicz-Aleksandrowicz, A. Lorens, H. Skarżyński. 2012. Partial deafness treatment in children: a preliminary report of the parents' perspective. *J Hear Sci* 2, no. 2: 61–9.

Obszańska, A. 2014. [Life experience of a patient before and after partial deafness treatment (PDT) – case study] Życie osoby z częściową głuchotą przed wszczepieniem i po wszczepieniu implantu ślimakowego – studium przypadku. *Now Audiofonol* 3, no. 3: 39–4.

Ogawa, S., T.M. Lee, A.R. Kay, D.W. Tank. 1990. Brain magnetic resonance imaging with contrast dependent on blood oxygenation. *P Natl Acad Sci USA* 87, no. 24: 9868–72.

Okulski, P., T.M. Jay, J. Jaworski et al. 2007. TIMP-1 abolishes MMP-9 dependent long-lasting long-term potentiaton in the prefrontal cortex. *Biol Psychiat* 62: 359–62.

Olds, C., L. Pollonini, H. Abaya et al. 2016. Cortical activation patterns correlate with speech understanding after cochlear implantation. *Ear Hearing* 37, no. 3: 160–72.

Olsho, L.W., E. G. Koch, E.A. Carter, C.F. Halpin, N.B. Spetner. 1988. Pure-tone sensitivity of human infants. *J Acoust Soc Am* 84, no. 4: 1316–24.

Orth, U., R.W. Robins, K.F. Widaman. 2012. Life-span development of self-esteem and its effects on important life outcomes. *J Pers Soc Psychol* 102, no. 6: 1271–88.

Osberger, M.J., M. Maso, L.I.C Sam. 1993. Speech intelligibility of children with cochlear implants, tactile aids, or hearing aids. *J Speech Hear Res* 36: 186–203.

Oziębło, D., A. Obrycka, A. Lorens, H. Skarżyński, M. Ołdak. 2020. Cochlear implantation outcome in children with DFNB1 locus pathogenic variants. *J Clin Med* 9, no. 1: 228.

Pankowska, A., A. Barej, A. Lutek, M. Zgoda, E. Zielińska. 2013. [Auditory-Verbal Therapy in the speech and language therapy of children with hearing deficiencies – history, principles and practice] Metoda audytywno-werbalna w rehabilitacji słuchu i mowy dzieci z wadą słuchu – historia, zasady i praktyka. *Now Audiofonol* 2, no. 4: 22–27 [Polish].

Pankowska, A., A. Geremek-Samsonowicz, J. Ćwiklińska, H. Skarżyński. 2014. [Partial deafness – group of patients and aspects of hearing rehabilitation] Częściowa głuchota – grupy pacjentów i aspekty rehabilitacji słuchu. In *[A child with hearing impairment and central auditory processing disorder. Selected problems] Dziecko z wadą słuchu oraz Centralnymi Zaburzeniami Przetwarzania Słuchowego (CAPD). Wybrane problemy*, ed. J. Skibska, 97–110. Kraków: LIBRON – Filip Lohner [Polish].

Pankowska, A., J. Solnica, H. Skarżyński. 2012. [Application of the modified profile of hearing abilities in the follow-up of the effects of hearing rehabilitation in adult patients with partial deafness using cochlear implant system – a preliminary report] Wykorzystanie zmodyfikowanego profilu umiejętności słuchowych w obserwacji efektów rehabilitacji słuchu dorosłych pacjentów z częściową głuchotą korzystających z systemu implantu ślimakowego – doniesienie wstępne. *Now Audiofonol* 1, no. 1: 38–45 [Polish].

Pantev, C., H. Okamoto, H. Teismann. 2012. Tinnitus: the dark side of the auditory cortex plasticity. *Ann NY Acad Sci* 1252: 253–8.

Pantev, C., R. Oostenveld, A. Engelien, B. Ross, L.E. Roberts, M. Hoke. 1998. Increased auditory cortical representation in musicians. *Nature* 23: 811–14.

Parietti-Winkler, C., A. Lion, B. Montaut-Verient, R. Grosjean, G.C. Gauchard. 2015. Effects of unilateral cochlear implantation on balance control and sensory organization in adult patients with profound hearing loss. *Biomed Res Int* 2015: 621845.11.

Parkes W.J., J.J. Gnanasegaram, S.L. Cushing, C.L. McKnight, B.C. Papsin, K.A. Gordon KA. 2017. Vestibular-evoked myogenic potential testing as an objective measure of vestibular stimulation with cochlear implants. *Laryngoscope* 127, no. 2: 75–81.

Pazen, D., A. Anagiotos, M. Nünning, A.-O. Gostian, M. Ortmann, D. Beutner. 2017. The impact of a cochlear implant electrode array on the middle ear transfer function. *Ear Hearing* 38, no. 4: e241–e255.

Penhune V.B., R.J. Zatorre, J.D. MacDonald, A.C. Evans. 1996. Interhemispheric anatomical differences in human primary auditory cortex: probabilistic mapping and volume measurement from magnetic resonance scans. *Cereb Cortex* 6, no. 5: 661–72.

Petersen, B., A. Gjedde, M. Wallentin, P. Vuust. 2013. Cortical plasticity after cochlear implantation. *Neural Plast* 2013: 318521.

Phillips, Ch., L. Ling, T. Oxford et al. 2015. Longitudinal performance of an implantable vestibular prosthesis. *Hearing Res* 322: 200–11.

Picton T.W. 2011. Auditory steady state and following responses: dancing to the rhythms. In *Human auditory evoked potentials*, T.W. Picton, 283–331. San Diego, CA: Plural Publishing.

Picton, T.W., M.S. John, A. Dimitrijevic, D. Purcell. 2003. Human auditory steady-state responses. *Int J Audiol* 42: 177–219.

Piker, E.G., R.W. Baloh, D.L. Witsell, D.B. Garrison, W.T. Lee. 2015. Assessment of the clinical utility of cervical and ocular vestibular evoked myogenic potential testing in elderly patients. *Otol Neurotol* 36, no. 7: 1238–44.

Piotrowska, A., K. Kochanek, W.W. Jędrzejczak, A. Lorens, L. Śliwa, H. Skarżyński. 2009. Preservation of low frequency hearing after cochlear implantation in behavioral and objective measurements. *Paper presented at 9th European Symposium on Pediatric Cochlear Implantation*, Warsaw.

Piotrowska, A., K. Kochanek, A. Lorens, H. Skarżyński, L. Śliwa. 2005a. Estimation of auditory sensitivity for partially-deafened cochlear implant candidates using behavioral and objective measurements. *Paper presented at XIX IERASG Biennial Symposium*, Havana.

Piotrowska, A., K. Kochanek, A. Lorens, H. Skarżyński, L. Śliwa. 2005b. Behavioral and objective measurements of low-frequency hearing preservation after cochlear implantation. *Paper presented at XIX IERASG Biennial Symposium*, Havana.

Plontke, S. K., G. Götze, T. Rahne, A. Liebau. 2017. Intracochlear drug delivery in combination with cochlear implants. *HNO* 65, no. 1: 19–28.

Polley, D.B., E.E. Steinberg, M.M. Merzenich. 2006. Perceptual learning directs auditory cortical map reorganization through top-down influences. *J Neurosci* 26, no. 18: 4970–82.

Ponton, C.W., M. Don, J.J. Eggermont, M D. Waring, A. Masuda. 1996. Maturation of human cortical auditory function: differences between normal-hearing children and children with cochlear implants. *Ear Hearing* 17, no. 5: 430–37.

Prentiss, S., K. Sykes, H. Staecker. 2010. Partial deafness cochlear implantation at the University of Kansas: techniques and outcomes. *J Am Acad Audiol* 21, no. 3: 197–203.

Price, C.J. 2012. A review and synthesis of the first 20 years of PET and fMRI studies of heard speech, spoken language and reading. *Neuroimage* 62, no. 2: 816–47.

Prieve, B.A., M.P. Feeney, S. Stenfelt, N. Shahnaz. 2013. Prediction of conductive hearing loss using wideband acoustic immittance. *Ear Hearing* 34 (Suppl. 1): 54S–59S.

Purdy, S.C. and A.S. Kelly. 2016. Change in speech perception and auditory evoked potentials over time after unilateral cochlear implantation in postlingually deaf adults. *Semin Hear* 37, no. 1: 62.

Putkiewicz, J., A. Piotrowska, A. Lorens, A. Pankowska, A. Obrycka, H. Skarżyński. 2011. [A child with partial deafness in school and peer relatioships] *Dziecko z częściową głuchotą w aspekcie relacji szkolnych i rówieśniczych*. In *[Towards the communication community of the deaf and hearing persons] Ku wspólnocie komunikacyjnej niesłyszących i słyszących*, ed. K. Krakowiak and A. Dziurda-Multan, 97–99. Lublin: Wydawnictwo Katolickiego Uniwersytetu Lubelskiego [Polish].

Qi, R., L. Su, L. Zou, J. Yang, S. Zheng. 2019. Altered gray matter volume and white matter integrity in sensorineural hearing loss patients: A VBM and TBSS Study. *Otol Neurotol* 40, no. 6: e569–e574.

Rademacher, J., P. Morosan, T. Schormann et al. 2001. Probabilistic mapping and volume measurement of human primary auditory cortex. *Neuroimage* 13, no. 4: 669–83.

Rah, Y.C., M. Y. Lee, S. H. Kim et al. 2016. Extended use of systemic steroid is beneficial in preserving hearing in guinea pigs after cochlear implant. *Acta Oto-Laryngol* 136, no. 12: 1213–19.

Rajan, R. and D.R. Irvine. 1998. Neuronal responses across cortical field A1 in plasticity induced by peripheral auditory organ damage. *Audiol Neuro-Otol* 3, no. 2: 123–44.

Rajan, R. and D.R. Irvine. 2010. Severe and extensive neonatal hearing loss in cats results in auditory cortex plasticity that differentiates into two regions. *Eur J Neurosci* 31, no. 11): 1999–2013.

Rajan, R., D.R. Irvine., L.Z. Wise, P. Heil. 1993. Effect of unilateral partial cochlear lesions in adult cats on the representation of lesioned and unlesioned cochleas in primary auditory cortex. *J Comput Neurosci* 338: 17–49.

Rajan, G., D. Tavora-Vieira, W.D. Baumgartner et al. 2018. Hearing preservation cochlear implantation in children: The Hearring Group consensus and practice guide. *Cochlear Implants Int* 19, no. 1: 1–13.

Ramos, H.F., S.S. Grasel, R.M. Beck et al. 2015. Evaluation of residual hearing in cochlear implants candidates using auditory steady-state response. *Acta Oto-Laryngol* 135, no. 3: 246–53.

Rasetshwane, D.M. and S.T. Neely. 2012. Measurements of wide-band cochlear reflectance in humans. *JARO-J Assoc Res Oto* 13: 591–607.

Rauschecker, J.P. 1995. Compensatory plasticity and sensory substitution in the cerebral cortex. *Trends Neurosci* 18, no. 1: 36–43.

Ravicz, M.E., J.R. Melcher, N.Y. Kiang. 2000. Acoustic noise during functional magnetic resonance imaging. *J Acoust Soc Am* 108: 1683–96.

Rawool, V. 2018. Denial by patients of hearing loss and their rejection of hearing health care: a review. *J Hear Sci* 8, no. 3: 9–23.

Recanzone, G.H., C.E. Schreiner, M.M. Merzenich. 1993. Plasticity in the frequency representation of primary auditory cortex following discrimination training in adult owl monkeys. *J Neurosci* 13, no. 1: 87–103.

Reinhard, S.M., K. Razak, I. Ethell. 2015. A delicate balance: role of MMP9 in brain development and pathophysiology of neurodevelopmental disorders. *Front Cell Neurosci* 9: 280.

Rembar, S.H., O. Lind, P. Romundstad, A.S. Helvik. 2012. Psychological well-being among cochlear implant users: A comparison with the general population. *Cochlear Implants Int* 13: 41–8.

Rijke, W.J., A.M. Vermeulen, K. Wendrich, E. Mylanus, M.C. Langereis, G.J. van der Wilt. 2019. Capability of deaf children with a cochlear implant. *Disabil Rehabil* 14: 1–6.

Rivera, S., M. Khrestchatisky, L. Kaczmarek, G.A. Rosenberg, D.M. Jaworski. 2010. Metzincin proteases and their inhibitors: foes or friends in nervous system physiology? *Neuroscience* 30, no. 46: 15337–57.

Rizer, F.M., P.N. Arkis, W.H. Lippy, A.G. Schuring. 1988. Postoperative audiometric evaluation of cochlear implant patients. *Otolaryng Head Neck* 98: 203–6.

Roberts, L.E., D.J. Bosnyak, D.C. Thompson. 2012. Neural plasticity expressed in central auditory structures with and without tinnitus. *Front Syst Neurosci* 6: 40.

Robertson, D. and D.R. Irvine. 1989. Plasticity of frequency organization in auditory cortex of guinea pigs with partial unilateral deafness. *J Comput Neurosci* 282, no. 3: 456–71.

Rosowski, J.J., S. Stenfelt, D. Lilly. 2013. An overview of wideband immittance measurements techniques and terminology: you say absorbance, I say reflectance. *Ear Hearing* 34 (Suppl. 1): 9S–16S.

Rosowski, J.J. and L.A. Wilber. 2015. Acoustic immittance, absorbance and reflectance in the human ear canal. *Semin Hear* 36, no. 1: 11–28.

Rouger, J., S. Lagleyre, J.F. Demonet, B. Fraysse, O. Deguine, P. Barone. 2012. Evolution of crossmodal reorganization of the voice area in cochlear-implanted deaf patients. *Hum Brain Mapp* 33: 1929–40.

Rybakowski, J.K., M. Skibińska, P. Kapelski, L. Kaczmarek, J. Hauser. 2009. Functional polymorphism of the matrix metalloproteinase-9 (MMP-9) gene in schizophrenia. *Schizophr Res* 109: 90–93.

Salt, A. N. and S. K. Plontke. 2018. Pharmacokinetic principles in the inner ear: influence of drug properties on intratympanic applications. *Hearing Res* 368: 28–40.

Sandmann, P., N. Dillier, T. Eichele et al. 2012. Visual activation of auditory cortex reflects maladaptive plasticity in cochlear implant users. *Brain* 135, no. 2: 555–68.

Sandmann, P., T. Eichele, M. Buechler et al. 2009. Evaluation of evoked potentials to dyadic tones after cochlear implantation. *Brain* 132, no. 7: 1967–79.

Sanford, Ch.A. and J.E. Brockett. 2014. Characteristics of wideband acoustic immittance in patients with middle-ear dysfunction. *J Am Acad Audiol* 25: 425–440.

Santi, P.A., M.A. Ruggero, D.A. Nelson, C.W. Turner. 1982. Kanamycin and bumetanide ototoxicity; anatomical, physiological, and behavioral correlates. *Hearing Res* 7: 261–79.

Saoji, A.A., S.B. Shapiro, C.C. Finley, K. Koka, A.M. Cassis. 2020. Changes in wide-band tympanometry absorbance following cochlear implantation. *Otol Neurotol* 41, no. 6: e680–e685.

Scheperle, R.A. and J.J. Hajicek. 2020. Wideband acoustic immittance in cochlear implant recipients: reflectance and stapedial reflexes. *Ear Hearing* 41, no. 4: 883–95.

Schuknecht, H.F. 1978. Delayed endolymphatic hydrops. *Ann Oto Rhinol Laryn* 7, no. 6: 743–48.

Schwaber, M.K., P.E. Garraghty, J.H. Kaas. 1993. Neuroplasticity of the adult primate auditory cortex following cochlear hearing loss. *Am J Otolaryng* 14, no. 3: 252–8.

Seghier, M.L., B. Colette, F. Lazeyras, A. Sigrist, M. Pelizzone. 2005. fMRI evidence for activation of multiple cortical regions in the primary auditory cortex of deaf subjects users of multichannel cochlear implant. *Cereb Cortex* 15: 40–8.

Seifritz, E., F. Di Salle, F. Esposito, M. Herdener, J.G. Neuhoff, K. Scheffler. 2006. Enhancing BOLD response in the auditory system by neurophysiologically tuned fMRI sequence. *Neuroimage* 29: 1013–22.

Sellars, S.L. and P. Beighton. 1978. The aetiology of partial deafness in childhood. *S Afr Med J* 54, no. 20: 811–3.

Shahnaz, N., K. Bork, L. Polka, N. Longridge, D. Bell, B.D. Westerberg. 2009. Energy reflectance and tympanometry in normal and otosclerotic ears. *Ear Hearing* 30, no. 2: 219–33.

Shanks, J. and J. Shohet. 2009. Tympanometry in clinical practice. In *Handbook of clinical audiology*, ed. J. Katz, 157–89. Philadelphia, PA: Wolters Kluwer.

Sharma, A., J. Campbell, G. Cardon. 2015. Developmental and cross-modal plasticity in deafness: evidence from the P1 and N1 event-related potentials in cochlear implanted children. *Int J Psychophysiol* 95, no. 2: 135–44.

Sharma, A. and M.F. Dorman. 2006. Central auditory development in children with cochlear implants: clinical implications. *Adv Oto-Rhino-Laryng* 64: 66–88.

Sharma, A., M.F. Dorman, A. Kral. 2005. The influence of a sensitive period on central auditory development in children with unilateral and bilateral cochlear implants. *Hearing Res* 203, no. 1–2: 134–43.

Sharma, A., M.F. Dorman, A.J. Spahr. 2002. Sensitive period for the development of central auditory system in children with cochlear implants: implications for age of implantation. *Ear Hearing* 23, no. 6: 532–39.

Sharma, A., P. Gilley, M.F. Dorman, R. Baldwin. 2007. Deprivation-induced cortical reorganization in children with cochlear implants. *Int J Audiol* 46: 494–99.

Sharma, A. and H. Glick. 2016. Cross-modal re-organization in clinical populations with hearing loss. *Brain Sci* 6, no. 1: 4.

Sharma, A., H. Glick, E. Deeves, E. Duncan. 2015. The P1 biomarker for assessing cortical maturation in pediatric hearing loss: A review. *Otorinolaringologia* 65, no. 4: 103.

Skarżyńska, M.B., P.H. Skarżyński, B. Król et al. 2018. Preservation of hearing following cochlear implantation using different steroid therapy regimens: a prospective clinical study. *Med Sci Monitor* 24: 2437.

Skarżyński, H. 2012. Ten years' experience with a new strategy of partial deafness treatment. *J Hear Sci* 2, no. 2: 11–18.

Skarżyński, H. 2018. Implantable hearing aids. In *Master techniques in otolaryngology – head and neck surgery. Otology, neurotology, and lateral skull base surgery*, ed. J.T. Roland Jr and E.N. Myers, Warsaw: Wolters Kluwer.

Skarżyński, H., A. Geremek, M. Malesińska, O. Klasek, J. Piotrowski. 1994. Indications for cochlear implants in children. *Head and Neck Diseases* 3: 88–92.

Skarżyński, H., A. Geremek, J. Szuchnik, M. Posłuszna-Owcarz, A. Lorens, E. Michałowska. 1997a. Patients selection protocol for cochlear implantation. *Central East Eur J Oto-Rhino-Laryngol Head Neck Surgery* II, no. 3/4: 126–31.

Skarżyński, H. and A. Lorens. 2010a. Electric acoustic stimulation in children. *Adv Oto-Rhino-Laryng* 67: 135–43.

Skarżyński, H. and A. Lorens. 2010b. Partial deafness treatment. *Cochlear Implants Int* 11, no. 1: 29–41.

Skarżyński, H., A. Lorens, P. D'Haese et al. 2002. Preservation of residual hearing in children and post-lingually deafened adults after cochlear implantation: an initial study. *ORL J Oto-Rhino-Lary* 64: 247–53.

Skarżyński, H., A. Lorens, B. Dziendziel, J.J. Rajchel, M. Matusiak, P.H. Skarżyński. 2019a. Electro-natural stimulation in partial deafness treatment of adult cochlear implant users: long-term hearing preservation results. *ORL J Oto-Rhino-Lary* 81, no. 2–3: 63–72.

Skarżyński, H., A. Lorens, B. Dziendziel, P.H. Skarżyński. 2019b. Electro-natural stimulation (ENS) in partial deafness treatment: pediatric case series. *Otol Neurotol* 40, no. 2: 171–76.

Skarżyński, H., A. Lorens, B. Dziendziel, P.H. Skarżyński. 2015. Expanding pediatric cochlear implant candidacy: a case study of electro-natural stimulation (ENS) in partial deafness treatment. *Int J Pediatr Otorhi* 79, no. 11: 1896–900.

Skarżyński, H., A. Lorens, M. Matusiak, M. Porowski, P.H. Skarżyński, C.J. James. 2012a. Partial deafness treatment with the nucleus straight research array cochlear implant. *Audiol Neuro-Otol* 17: 82–91.

Skarżyński, H., A. Lorens, M. Matusiak, M. Porowski, P.H. Skarżyński, C.J. James. 2014a. Cochlear implantation with the Nucleus Slim Straight electrode in subjects with residual low-frequency hearing. *Ear Hearing* 35, no. 2: 33–43.

Skarżyński, H., A. Lorens, A. Piotrowska. 2000. Residual acoustic hearing in the ear before and after cochlear implantation. *Paper presented at the 5th European Symposium on Paediatric Cochlear Implantation*, Antwerp, Belgium.

Skarżyński, H., A. Lorens, A. Piotrowska. 2003. A new method of partial deafness treatment. *Med Sci Monitor* 9, no. 4: CS20–24.

Skarżyński, H., A. Lorens, A. Piotrowska. 2004a. Preservation of low-frequency hearing in partial deafness cochlear implantation. Extended Abstracts from the VIII International Cochlear Implant Conference, Indianapolis, USA. *Int Congress Series* 1273: 239–42.

Skarżyński, H., A. Lorens, A. Piotrowska. 2005. [Cochlear implants] Wszczepy ślimakowe. In *[Clinical audiology] Audiologia kliniczna*, ed. M. Śliwińska-Kowalska. Mediton [Polish].

Skarżyński, H., A. Lorens, A. Piotrowska, I. Anderson. 2006. Partial deafness cochlear implantation provides benefit to a new population of individuals with hearing loss. *Acta Oto-Laryngol* 126, no. 9: 934–40.

Skarżyński, H., A. Lorens, A. Piotrowska, I. Anderson. 2007a. Partial deafness cochlear implantation in children. *Int J Pediatr Otorhi* 71: 1407–13.

Skarżyński, H., A. Lorens, A. Piotrowska, I. Anderson. 2007b. Preservation of low frequency hearing in partial deafness cochlear implantation (PDCI) using the round window surgical approach. *Acta Oto-Laryngol* 127, no. 1: 41–8.

Skarżyński, H., A. Lorens, A. Piotrowska, R. Podskarbi-Fayette. 2009. Results of partial deafness cochlear implantation using various electrode designs. *Audiol Neuro-Otol* 14 (Suppl. 1): 39–45.

Skarżyński, H., A. Lorens, A. Piotrowska, P.H. Skarżyński. 2010. Hearing preservation in partial deafness treatment. *Med Sci Monitor* 16, no. 11: CR555–562.

Skarżyński, H., A. Lorens, P.H. Skarżyński. 2014b. Electro-natural stimulation (ENS) in partial deafness treatment: a case study. *J Hear Sci* 4, no. 4: 67–71.

Skarżyński, H., A. Lorens, M. Zgoda, A. Piotrowska, P.H. Skarżyński, A. Szkiełkowska. 2011. Atraumatic round window deep insertion of cochlear electrodes. *Acta Oto-Laryngol* 131, no. 7: 740–49.

Skarżyński, H., M. Matusiak, A. Lorens, M. Furmanek, A. Piłka, P.H. Skarżyński. 2016. Preservation of cochlear structures and hearing when using the Nucleus Slim Straight Electrode (CI422) in children. *J Laryngol Otol* 130, no. 4: 332–39.

Skarżyński, H., M. Matusiak, A. Piotrowska, P.H. Skarżyński. 2012b. Surgical techniques in partial deafness treatment. *J Hear Sci* 2, no. 3: 9–13.

Skarżyński, H., L. Olszewski, P.H. Skarżyński et al. 2014c. Direct round window stimulation with the Med-El Vibrant Soundbridge: 5 years of experience using a technique without interposed fascia. *Eur Arch Oto-Rhino-L* 271, no. 3: 477–82.

Skarżyński, H. and R. Podskarbi-Fayette. 2010. A new cochlear implant electrode design for preservation of residual hearing: a temporal bone study. *Acta Oto-Laryngol* 130: 435–42.

Skarżyński, H., J. Szuchnik, M. Mueller-Malesińska. 2004b. *Implanty ślimakowe – rehabilitacja*. Warszawa: Stowarzyszenie Przyjaciół Osób Niesłyszących i Niedosłyszących Człowiek – Człowiekowi.

Skarżyński, H., P. Van de Heyning, S. Agrawal et al. 2013. Towards a consensus on a hearing preservation classification system. *Acta Oto-Laryngol* 133 (Suppl. 564): 3–13.

Skarżyński, H., T. Wolak, A. Pluta et al. 2012c. Functional magnetic resonance imaging of auditory cortex in partial deafness treatment. *J Hear Sci* 2, no. 2: 53–60.

Skarżyński, H., R. Zawadzki, J. Szuchnik, A. Geremek, A. Lorens. 1997b. Analysis of the selected surgical aspects in 102 implanted patients at different ages. *Paper presented at the 5th International Cochlear Implant Conference*, New York, USA.

Skarżyński, P.H. 2012. [Study of auditory fatique using the fMRI technique]. Badanie zjawiska zmęczenia słuchowego metodą fMRI. *PhD Diss.*, Warsaw Medical University.

Skarżyński, P.H., H. Skarżyński, B. Dziendziel, J.J. Rajchel, E. Gos, A. Lorens. 2019. Hearing Preservation with the use of Flex20 and Flex24 electrodes in patients with partial deafness. *Otol Neurotol* 40, no. 9: 1153–59.

Skarżyński, P.H., T. Wolak, H. Skarżyński et al. 2013. Application of the functional magnetic resonance imaging fMRI for the assessment of the primary auditory cortex function in partial deafness patients - a preliminary study. *J Int Adv Otol* 9, no. 2: 153–60.

Solnica, J., J. Kobosko, A. Pankowska, M. Zgoda, H. Skarżyński. 2012. [Effectiveness of the auditory training in persons with partial deafness after cochlear implantation in the assessment of patients and speech-and-language therapists] Efektywność treningu słuchowego osób z częściową głuchotą po wszczepieniu implantu ślimakowego w ocenie pacjentów i logopedów. *Now Audiofonol* 1, no. 1: 31–7.

Solnica, J. and A. Pankowska. 2013. [Hearing rehabilitation of patients with partial deafness using cochlear implants – proposal of the language material for training activities. The report from the speech-and-language therapy praxis] Rehabilitacja słuchowa pacjentów z częściową głuchotą korzystających z implantu ślimakowego - propozycja materiału językowego do zajęć. Doniesienie z praktyki logopedycznej. *Now Audiofonol* 2, no. 1: 63–9.

Sosna, M., G. Tacikowska, K. Pietrasik, H. Skarżyński, A. Lorens, P.H. Skarżyński. 2019b. Effect on vestibular function of cochlear implantation by partial deafness treatment-electro acoustic stimulation (PDT-EAS). *Eur Arch Oto-Rhino-L* 276, no. 7: 1951–9.

Sosna, M., G. Tacikowska, K. Pietrasik, H. Skarżyński, P.H. Skarżyński. 2019a. Vestibular status in partial deafness. *Braz J Otorhinolar* S1808-8694(19)30143-0.

Speck, I., S. Arndt, J. Thurow et al. 2020. 18F-FDG PET imaging of the inferior colliculus in asymmetric hearing loss. *J Nucl Med* 61, no. 3: 418–22.

St Jean, P.L., X.C. Zhang, B.K. Hart et al. 1995. Characterisation of a dinucleotide repeat in the 92kDa type collagenase gene (CLG4B), localisation of CLG4B to chromosome 20 and the role of CLG4B in aortic aneurysmal disease. *Ann Hum Genet* 59: 17–24.

Stelmachowicz, P.G., A.L. Pittman, B.M. Hoover et al. 2004. The importance of high-frequency audibility in the speech and language development of children with hearing loss. *Arch Otolaryngol* 130: 556–62.

Stephens, D. 2009. *Living with Hearing Difficulties: The Process of Enablement*. Hoboken, New Jersey: John Wiley & Sons.

Stephens, D. and R. Hétu. 1991. Impairment, disability and handicap in audiology: towards a consensus. *Audiology* 30: 185–200.

Stredler-Brown, A. and D. Johnson. 2001. *Functional auditory performance indicators: an integrated approach to auditory development*. http://www.tsbvi.edu/attachments/FunctionalAud itoryPerformanceIndicators.pdf.

Strelnikov, K., J. Rouger, J.F. Demonet et al. 2013. Visual activity predicts auditory recovery from deafness after adult cochlear implantation. *Brain* 136: 3682–95.

Strelnikov, K., J. Rouger, S. Lagleyre et al. 2015. Increased audiovisual integration in cochlear-implanted deaf patients: independent components analysis of longitudinal positron emission tomography data. *J Neurosci* 41, no. 5: 677–85.

Striem-Amit, E., U. Hertz, A. Amedi. 2011. Extensive cochleotopic mapping of human auditory cortical fields obtained with phase-encoded fMRI. *PLOS ONE* 6: e17832.

Stropahl, M., L.C. Chen, S. Debener. 2017. Cortical reorganization in postlingually deaf cochlear implant users: Intra-modal and cross-modal considerations. *Hearing Res* 343: 128–37.

Sturm, J.J., Y. Zhang-Hooks., H. Roos, T. Nguyen, K. Kandler. 2017. Noise trauma-induced behavioral gap detection deficits correlate with reorganization of excitatory and inhibitory local circuits in the inferior colliculus and are prevented by acoustic enrichment. *J Neurosci* 37, no. 26: 6314–30.

Sweeney, A.D., M. L. Carlson, M. G. Zuniga et al. 2015. Impact of perioperative oral steroid use on low-frequency hearing preservation after cochlear implantation. *Otol Neurotol* 36, no. 9: 1480–85.

Sweetow, R. and C.V. Palmer. 2005. Efficacy of individual auditory training in adults: a systematic review of the evidence. *J Am Acad Audiol* 16: 494–504.

Szklarczyk, A., J. Lapinska, M. Rylski, R.D. McKay, L. Kaczmarek. 2002. Matrix metalloproteinase-9 undergoes expression and activation during dendritic remodeling in adult hippocampus. *J Neurosci* 22: 920–30.

Śliwa, L., S. Hatzopoulos, K. Kochanek, A. Piłka, A. Senderski, P.H. Skarżyński. 2011. Comparison of audiometric and objective methods in hearing screening of school children. A preliminary study. *Int J Pediatr Otorhi* 75, no. 4: 483–8.

Śliwa, L. and K. Kochanek. 2016. New methods in acoustic immittance measurements. Part II. Wideband reflectance tympanometry. *Now Audiofonol* 5, no. 4: 11–23 [Polish].

Śliwa, L., K. Kochanek, W.W. Jędrzejczak, K. Mrugała, H. Skarżyński. 2020. Measurement of wideband absorbance as a test for otosclerosis. *J Clin Med* 9: 1908.

Śliwa, L., K. Kochanek, A. Piotrowska, A. Piłka. 2004. Fundamentals of Auditory Steady State Responses (ASSR) registration and application methods. *Audiofonologia* 26: 21–8 [Polish].

Talairach, J. and P. Tournoux. 1988. *Co-planar Stereotaxic Atlas of the Human Brain*. New York: Thieme.

Talavage, T.M., J. Gonzalez-Castillo, S.K. Scott. 2014. Auditory neuroimaging with fMRI and PET. *Hearing Res* 307: 4–15.

Talavage, T.M., M.I. Sereno, J.R. Melcher, P.J. Ledden, B.R. Rosen, A.M. Sale. 2004. Tonotopic organization in human auditory cortex revealed by progressions of frequency sensitivity. *J Neurophysiol* 91, no. 3: 1282–96.

Thai-Van, H., C. Micheyl, A. Norena, L. Collet. 2002. Local improvement in auditory frequency discrimination is associated with hearing-loss slope in subjects with cochlear damage. *Brain* 125, no. 3: 524–37.

Thai-Van, H., E. Veuillet, A. Norena, J. Guiraud, L. Collet. 2010. Plasticity of tonotopic maps in humans: influence of hearing loss, hearing aids and cochlear implants. *Acta Oto-Laryngol* 130, no. 3: 333–7.

Tharpe, A. M. and D.H. Ashmead. 2001. A longitudinal investigation of infant auditory sensitivity. *Am J Audiol* 10, no. 2: 104–12.

Tien, H.-C. and F.H. Linthicum. 2002. Histopathologic changes in the vestibule after cochlear implantation. *Otolaryng Head Neck* 127: 260–64.

Tlumak, A.I., E. Rubinstein. J.D. Durrant. 2007. Meta-analysis of variables that affect accuracy of threshold estimation via measurement of the auditory steady-state response (ASSR). *Int J Audiol* 46, no. 11: 692–710.

Todd, N.P., S.M. Rosengren, S.T. Aw, J.G. Colebatch. 2007. Ocular vestibular evoked myogenic potentials (OVEMPs) produced by air- and bone-conducted sound. *Clin Neurophysiol* 118: 381–90.

Todt, I., D. Basta, A. Ernst. 2008. Does the surgical approach in cochlear implantation influence the occurrence of postoperative vertigo? *Otolaryng Head Neck* 138, no. 1: 8–12.

Trehub, S.E., B.A. Schneider, B.A. Morrengiello, L.A. Thorpe. 1988. Auditory sensitivity in school-age children. *J Exp Child Psychol* 46: 273–85.

Trzaskowski, B., E. Piłka, W.W. Jedrzejczak, H. Skarżyński. 2015. Criteria for detection of transiently evoked otoacoustic emissions in schoolchildren. *Int J Pediatr Otorhi* 79, no. 9: 1455–61.

Turner, C.W. 2006. Hearing loss and the limits of amplification. *Audiol Neuro-Otol* 11 (Suppl. 1): 2–5.

Upadhyay, J., M. Ducros, T.A. Knaus et al. 2007. Function and connectivity in human primary auditory cortex: a combined fMRI and DTI study at 3 Tesla. *Cereb Cortex* 17: 2420–32.

Vafadari, B., A. Salamian, L. Kaczmarek. 2016. MMP-9 in translation: from molecule to brain physiology, pathology, and therapy. *J Neurochem* 139 (Suppl. 2): 91–114.

Van de Heyning, P., O. Adunka, S.L. Arauz et al. 2013. Standards of practice in the field of hearing implants. *Cochlear Implants Int* 14 (Suppl. 2): 1–5.

van der Marel, K.S., J.J. Briaire, B.M. Verbist, T.J. Muurling, J.H.M. Frijns. 2015. The influence of cochlear implant electrode position on performance. *Audiol Neuro-Otol* 20, no. 3: 202–11.

Vander Werff, K., T. Johnson, C. Brown. 2008. Behavioral threshold estimation for auditory steady-state response testing. In *Auditory steady-state response. Generation, recording, and clinical applications*, ed. G. Rance, 125–49. San Diego, CA: Plural Publishing.

Vandooren, J., P.E. Van den Steen, G. Opdenakker. 2013. Biochemistry and molecular biology of gelatinase B or matrix metalloproteinase-9 (MMP-9): the next decade. *Crit Rev Biochem Mol Biol* 48, no. 3: 222–72.

Vermeire, K., I. Anderson, M. Flynn, P. Van de Heyning. 2008. The influence of different speech processor and hearing aid settings on speech perception outcomes in electric acoustic stimulation patients. *Ear Hearing* 29: 76–86.

Viccaro, M., P. Mancini, R. La Gamma et al. 2007. Positional vertigo and cochlear implantation. *Otol Neurotol* 28: 764–67.

Von Békésy, G. and E.G. Wever. 1960. *Experiments in Hearing*. New York: McGraw-Hill.

Voss, P. and R.J. Zatorre. 2012. Organization and reorganization of sensory-deprived cortex. *Curr Biol* 22, no. 5: R168–R173.

Walkowiak, A., A. Lorens, A. Wąsowski, A. Obrycka, M. Zgoda, A, Piotrowska. 2004. Spread of excitation (SOE) – a new method of assessment of auditory nerve function. *Structures – Waves – Human Health* 13, no. 2: 161–66.

Waltzman, S.B., N.L. Cohen, R.H. Gomolin, W.H. Shapiro, S.R. Ozdamar, R.A. Hoffman. 1994. Long-term results of early cochlear implantation in congenitally and prelingually deafened children. *Am J Otol* 15 (Suppl. 2): 9–13.

Wang, J., H. An, M.W. Mayo et al. 2007. LZAP, a putative tumor suppressor, selectively inhibits NF-kappaB. *Cancer Cell* 12: 239–51.

Wang, J., D. Ding, R.J. Salvi. 2002. Functional reorganization in chinchilla inferior colliculus associated with chronic and acute cochlear damage. *Hearing Res* 186, no. 1–2: 238–49.

Wang, L., X. Sun, W. Liang, J. Chen, W. Zheng. 2013. Validation of the Mandarin version of the LittlEARS Auditory Questionnaire. *Int J Pediatr Otorhi* 77: 1350–54.

Wasson, J.D., L. Campbell, S. Chambers et al. 2018. Effect of cochlear implantation on middle ear function: a three-month prospective study. *Laryngoscope* 128: 1207–12.

Webster, J. C. and J.A. Cidlowski. 1999. Mechanisms of glucocorticoid-receptor-mediated repression of gene expression. *Trends Endocrin Met* 10, no. 10: 396–402.

Webster, D. B., and M. Webster. 1979. Effects of neonatal conductive hearing loss on brain stem auditory nuclei. *Ann Oto Rhinol Laryn* 88, no. 5: 684–88.

Weichbold, V., L. Tsiakpini, F. Coninx, P. D'Haese. 2005. Development of a parent questionnaire for assessment of auditory behaviour of infants up to two years of age. *Laryngo Rhino Otol* 84: 328–34.

Whiteley, A., B. Wong, B. St. George et al. 2019. Establishing a visual guideline for the locus of the auditory cortex in humans. *Poster presented at the American Auditory Society Scientific and Technology Meeting*, Scottsdale, United States.

Whitney, S.L., P.J. Sparto, J.M. Furman. 2020. Vestibular rehabilitation and factors that can affect outcome. *Semin Neurol* 40, no. 1: 165–72.

Williams, K.C., E. Falkum, E.W. Martinsen. 2015. Fear of negative evaluation, avoidance and mental distress among hearing-impaired employees. *Rehabil Psychol* 60, no. 1: 51–8.

Willingham, E. and S. Manolidis. 2004. Preservation of residual hearing in cochlear implantation. *Otolaryng Head Neck* 131: 267–68.

Wilson, B.S. 2012. Treatments for partial deafness using combined electric and acoustic stimulation of the auditory system. *J Hear Sci* 2, no. 2: 19–32.

Wiłkość, M., A. Szałkowska, M. Skibińska, L. Zając-Lamparska, M. Maciukiewicz, A. Araszkiewicz. 2016. BDNF gene polymorphisms and haplotypes in relations to cognitive performance in Polish healthy subjects. *Acta Neurobiol Exp* 76: 43–52.

Wolak, T., K. Cieśla, A. Lorens et al. 2017b. Tonotopic organization of the auditory cortex in sloping sensorineural hearing loss. *Hearing Res* 355: 81–96.

Wolak, T., K. Cieśla, A. Pluta, E. Włodarczyk, B. Biswal, H. Skarżyński. 2019. Altered functional connectivity in patients with sloping sensorineural hearing loss. *Front Hum Neurosci* 13.

Wolak, T., K. Cieśla, M. Rusiniak et al. 2016. Influence of acoustic overstimulation on central auditory system: an functional Magnetic Resonance Imaging (fMRI) study. *Med Sci Monitor* 22: 4623–35.

Wolak, T., K. Cieśla, J. Wójcik, H. Skarżyński. 2017a. Effect of sound intensity on level of activation in auditory cortex as measured by fMRI. *J Hear Sci* 7, no. 4: 20–7.

Wolfe, J. 2020. *Cochlear Implants: Audiologic Management and Considerations for Implantable Hearing Devices.* San Diego, CA: Plural Publishing, Incorporated.

Wolski, P. 2010. [*Loss of ability. Coping with the acquired disability and occupational activation*] *Utrata sprawności. Radzenie sobie z niepełnosprawnością nabytą a aktywizacja zawodowa.* Warszawa: Wydawnictwo Naukowe SCHOLAR.

Wong, P.C.M. 2010. Neuroimaging and the Listening Brain. *The ASHA Leader* 15: 14–17.

Woods, D.L. and C. Alain. 2009. Functional imaging of human auditory cortex. *Curr Opin Otolaryngo* 17: 407–11.

Woods, D.L., G.C. Stecker, T. Rinne et al. 2009. Functional maps of human auditory cortex: Effects of acoustic features and attention. *PLOS ONE* 4, no. 4: e5183.

Yang, C.H., H.C. Chen, C.F. Hwang. 2008. The prediction of hearing thresholds with auditory steady-state responses for cochlear implanted children. *Int J Pediatr Otorhi* 72, no. 5: 609–17.

Zalewska, M. 2009. [Mechanisms of personality disorders in deaf adolescents who have hearing parents – a clinical case study of a deaf boy child] Mechanizmy zaburzeń tożsamości u młodzieży głuchej mającej słyszących rodziców – kliniczne studium głuchego chłopca. In [*Deaf and hard-of-hearing young adults in a family and surrounding world*] *Młodzież głucha i słabosłysząca w rodzinie i otaczającym świecie*, ed. J. Kobosko. 78–83. Warszawa: Stowarzyszenie Usłyszeć Świat.

Zawawi, F., F. Alobaid, T. Leroux, A.G. Zeitouni. 2014. Patients reported outcome post-cochlear implantation: how severe is their dizziness? *Otolaryng Head Neck* 43: 49.

Zeng F.-G. 2004. Trends in cochlear implants. *Trends Amplif* 8, no. 1: 1–34.

Zeng, F.-G., A.N. Popper, R.R. Fay. 2004. *Cochlear Implants: Auditory Prostheses and Electric Hearing.* New York: New Springer-Verlag.

Zhang, Y., and J. Yan. 2008. Corticothalamic feedback for sound-specific plasticity of auditory thalamic neurons elicited by tones paired with basal forebrain stimulation. *Cereb Cortex* 18, no. (7): 1521–1528.

Zimmerman-Phillips, S., M. Osberger, A. Robbins A. 1997. *Infant-Toddler Meaningful Auditory Integration Scale.* Sylmar, CA: Advanced Bionics Corp.

Index

ABR *see* auditory brainstem responses
acoustic immittance 354, 364, 366, 368
acoustic stimuli 5, 24, 32, 33, 309, 325, 326, 329, 332, 384
air-bone gap 38
air conduction threshold 18, 38, 40, 299
antromastoidectomy 6, 48, 49, 50
  limited conservative 5, 49
ASSR *see* auditory steady-state responses
atticotomy 46, 47
audiogram 37, 55, 313, 359, 360
  sloping 314, 333, 355, 360, 384
audiometer range 17, 19, 54, 55
audiometry 4, 11, 17, 26, 32, 39, 285, 289, 326, 353, 358, 365, 368
auditory brainstem responses (ABR) 4, 5, 18, 59, 60–62, 67, 74, 353–361
auditory cortex *see* auditory; cortex
auditory development 35, 325, 331, 332–341
auditory memory *see* auditory; memory
auditory steady-state responses (ASSR) 337, 353, 357–361
auditory training 11, 307, 325–329, 345, 372, 379, 382, 386
auditory-verbal therapy (AVT) 328
auricle (pinna) 37, 38, 40, 41, 42, 46, 47, 48, 49, 86, 93

BAHA *see* bone-anchored hearing aid
balance dysfunction 293, 296
behavioral measures 353, 356, 359, 361, 376, 379, 383, 386, 387, 390, 391
Benign Paroxysmal Positional Vertigo (BPPV) 295, 296
bilateral cochlear implantation *see* bilateral; cochlear implantation
blood-labyrinth barrier (BLB) 282, 284, 285, 286
blood-oxygenation-level-dependent signal *see* BOLD signal
BOLD signal 306, 311, 377, 380

bone-anchored hearing aid (BAHA) 38, 39, 40, 41, 42, 391
bone conduction implant 2, 3, 4, 37, 38, 39, 40, 43, 51
  inclusion criteria 38–39, 51
  surgical technique 40–44
bone conduction threshold 39, 40
bone niche *see* bony bed
bony bed 5, 8, 9, 43, 44, 45, 46, 48, 49
BPPV *see* Benign Paroxysmal Positional Vertigo

CAEP *see* cortical auditory evoked potentials
caloric test 294, 295, 298–301
candidacy criteria *see* cochlear implants; inclusion criteria
central nervous system (CNS) 16, 34, 306, 309, 310, 320, 381, 390
cervical vestibular evoked myogenic potential (cVEMP) 294, 295, 298–301
cochlea 5, 16, 20, 24, 25, 29, 32, 39, 53, 284, 286, 288, 294, 296, 300, 309–312, 317, 321, 336, 339, 341, 358, 361, 362, 364, 367, 368, 370, 371, 373
  basal turn 296, 336, 340, 354, 370, 371, 386
cochlear implant 1, 3, 5, 10, 15, 16, 19, 21–25, 35, 53, 293, 304, 314, 325, 327, 328, 336, 338–340, 343, 346, 348, 377, 379, 381, 384
  benefit 22, 23, 321, 327, 340, 341, 344–347, 349–351, 364, 390
  candidacy 16, 294, 327, 337, 353, 357, 375, 388, 390, 392
  experience 21, 334, 338, 339, 344, 346, 349, 379
  program in Poland 2–13, 16, 38
  satisfaction 344, 345, 349–351
  surgery *see* cochlear implantation
  users 15, 21, 23, 24, 32, 53, 293, 296, 298, 300, 327, 328, 344, 346, 348, 349, 351, 353, 366, 375–377, 379, 380, 383, 386–388, 391